T0257614

Dermatology: Principles and Practice

Dermatology: Principles and Practice

Edited by Heidi Mueller

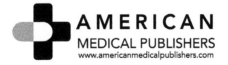

AMERICAN
MEDICAL PUBLISHERS
www.americanmedicalpublishers.com

American Medical Publishers,
41 Flatbush Avenue,
1st Floor, New York,
NY 11217, USA

Visit us on the World Wide Web at:
www.americanmedicalpublishers.com

© American Medical Publishers, 2022

This book contains information obtained from authentic and highly regarded sources. Copyright for all individual chapters remain with the respective authors as indicated. All chapters are published with permission under the Creative Commons Attribution License or equivalent. A wide variety of references are listed. Permission and sources are indicated; for detailed attributions, please refer to the permissions page and list of contributors. Reasonable efforts have been made to publish reliable data and information, but the authors, editors and publisher cannot assume any responsibility for the validity of all materials or the consequences of their use.

ISBN: 978-1-63927-065-1

Trademark Notice: Registered trademark of products or corporate names are used only for explanation and identification without intent to infringe.

Cataloging-in-Publication Data

Dermatology : principles and practice / edited by Heidi Mueller.
    p. cm.
Includes bibliographical references and index.
ISBN 978-1-63927-065-1
1. Dermatology. 2. Skin--Diseases. 3. Skin--Diseases--Treatment. 4. Dermatology--Case studies.
5. Skin--Diseases--Case studies. I. Mueller, Heidi.
RL72 .D47 2022

616.5--dc23

Table of Contents

Preface

The branch of medical science which deals with the functions and structures of skin, nails, and hair, as well as their diseases, is referred to as dermatology. It includes both medications and surgeries. Various fields of dermatology include cosmetic dermatology, dermatopathology, immunodermatology, Mohs surgery, pediatric dermatology and dermatoepidemiology. Major therapies provided under the field of dermatology include excision and treatment of skin cancer, and cryosurgery which treats warts and another dermatosis. Several other therapies include hair removal with laser, hair transplantation, laser therapies for the birthmark or tattoo removal and photodynamic therapy. It also includes procedures like autologous melanocyte transplant known as vitiligo surgery. This book traces the progress of this field and highlights some of its key concepts and applications. It strives to provide a fair idea about this discipline and to help develop a better understanding of the latest advances within dermatology. Those in search of information to further their knowledge will be greatly assisted by this book.

This book is a comprehensive compilation of works of different researchers from varied parts of the world. It includes valuable experiences of the researchers with the sole objective of providing the readers (learners) with a proper knowledge of the concerned field. This book will be beneficial in evoking inspiration and enhancing the knowledge of the interested readers.

In the end, I would like to extend my heartiest thanks to the authors who worked with great determination on their chapters. I also appreciate the publisher's support in the course of the book. I would also like to deeply acknowledge my family who stood by me as a source of inspiration during the project.

Editor

A Case Series of Bowen's Disease Treated with the Combination of Cryosurgery and Ingenol Mebutate and Followed Up with Optical Coherence Tomography

Georgios Gaitanis ⓘ,[1] Theodora Tsironi,[1]
Panagiota Spyridonos,[2] and Ioannis D. Bassukas ⓘ [1]

[1]Department of Skin and Venereal Diseases, Faculty of Medicine, School of Health Sciences, University of Ioannina, Ioannina, Greece
[2]Laboratory of Medical Physics, Faculty of Medicine, School of Health Sciences, University of Ioannina, Ioannina, Greece

Correspondence should be addressed to Georgios Gaitanis; ggaitan@cc.uoi.gr

Academic Editor: Alireza Firooz

Bowen's disease (BD) is a relatively rare *in situ* squamous cell carcinoma (SCC) with a limited potential of becoming invasive. Ingenol mebutate (IM) was relatively successful for the treatment of BD lesions in small case series. Optical coherence tomography (OCT) is a promising method for the diagnosis of cutaneous keratinocytic carcinomas, including BD. Herein we report the treatment of BD with the combination of cryosurgery and IM and the application of OCT imagining in treatment monitoring. Patients treated within a period of 12 months are retrospectively compiled. Treatment consisted of a mild cryosurgery session (liquid N_2, open spray, and 2 freeze-thaw cycles of 15 sec each) of a field including the BD lesion and a 0.5cm rim and IM application for 4 consecutive days starting at the cryosurgery day. Four patients (3 females; average age: 76.5 years) with 4 lesions (20-70mm maximal diameter; average 36.2mm) were included. Healing was excellent and no relapse was observed at 12 months' follow-up. Baseline OCT revealed a disarranged, thickened epidermis, while a normally layered epidermis overlying a hyperreflective dermis was present after treatment. Conclusively, the combination of cryosurgery followed by IM is a feasible, effective treatment for BD that should be evaluated in further studies.

1. Introduction

Bowen's disease (BD) is a relatively rare *in situ* cutaneous squamous cell carcinoma (SCC) with the potential of becoming invasive in a small fraction of cases [1, 2]. BD can acquire extensive dimensions or present in poor healing sites challenging treatment selection [1]. Photodynamic therapy is currently considered the treatment of choice, yet it has been associated with increased relapse rates, the need for repeated treatments [3], and still an appreciable risk of developing an invasive SCC within the treated region [4, 5]. Up to now, ingenol mebutate (IM) has been used in small case series for the treatment of Bowen's disease lesions with relative success [6–11].

Optical coherence tomography (OCT) is a promising imaging modality for the noninvasive evaluation of cutaneous keratinocytic neoplasms, including BD [12]. Preliminary findings in the literature claim the identification of architectural disorganization of the epidermis with a prominent wide spindle layer as the principal OCT diagnostic sign of this latter condition [12].

Herein, we retrospectively report on the feasibility of BD treatment with a 4-day short combination scheme of a cryosurgery session at day 0 followed by 4 daily topical ingenol mebutate applications (days 0-3) and the potential of OCT imaging in treatment monitoring.

2. Case Series

All patients included in this study had biopsy-proven BD and gave informed consent according to the principles of the Declaration of Helsinki prior to treatment. This retrospective study was approved by the Institutional Review Board of the University Hospital of Ioannina. The period under evaluation ranged from 1 September 2016 to 31 August 2017 and the files

TABLE 1: Patients, tumors, and treatment characteristics. Patients 1 and 3 required half a tube per application of the commercially available ingenol mebutate gel (Picato® Gel, 500MCG/G), while patients 2 and 4 applied the whole tube per application.

Patient/Tumor Number	Gender	Age	Co-morbidities	Concomitant medication	Tumor Localization	Maximal diameter (mm)
1	F	79	Pacemaker, arterial hypertension, diabetes mellitus, hypothyroidism	Aminosalycilic acid, propranol, amlodipine, ramipril, atorvastin, dapagliflozin, vildagliptin, glycazide, thiamazole	Nose	20
2	F	81	Asthma, atrial fibrillation	Flixotide, budesonide, formoterol, aminosalycilic acid, isoprenaline	Preauricular	70
3	F	68	Diabetes	Sitagliptin	Mandible	22
4	M	78	Atrial fibrillation, arterial hypertension,	Carvedilol, propafenone, rivaroxaban, olmesartan	Chest	33

were assessed for last follow-up information at 14 September 2018. BD lesions were imaged prior to biopsy with OCT (NITID, DermaLumics, Madrid, Spain). At least 5 scans of the lesion and of proximal or contralateral healthy skin were acquired. OCT scanning of the treated area was additionally followed up at 3, 6, and 12 months after treatment. All authors evaluated the scans independently in the monitor of the OCT device in a darkened room.

A four-day treatment protocol was administered combining one cryosurgery session and 4 daily ingenol mebuate (Picato® Gel, 500MCG/G) applications. Treatment started with a relatively mild cryosurgery session (liquid N_2, open spray, 2 freeze-thaw cycles of 15 sec each) of a skin area including the BD lesion and a 0.5cm rim around it (day 0 of treatment). For larger BD lesions, freezing was performed in slightly overlying 2x2cm skin sections. The patient was instructed to apply ingenol mebutate once daily on the cryosurgery pretreated area starting already at the evening of the same day 0 of the treatment and for the 3 following days: 1-3 (4 once daily applications in 4 consecutive days in total). The patients were evaluated 1 week after the cryosurgery session and at 1, 3, 6, and 12 months after treatment. Primary treatment target was clearance of the lesions (clinical complete response); residual disease <25% of the initial lesion was considered as partial response.

A total of 4 patients (3 females and 1 male; average age: 76.5 years) with 4 BD lesions (20-70mm maximal diameter; average: 36.2mm) were treated with cryosurgery followed by ingenol mebutate according to the above combination scheme (Table 1 and Figure 1). All patients experienced vivid local inflammation with redness, blistering, and scabbing which intensified during treatment with ingenol mebuate. However, the local tissue reaction was reported to peak at day 7 of treatment (Figure 1(b)) and subsequently started to subside. At 1-month follow-up, some redness was evident at the site of treatment, with concomitant hypopigmentation. Scaring was minimal and gradually improved during further follow-up. Taking treatment outcomes together, clearance (complete response) was achieved in all 4 BD cases and no relapses were observed at 12 months' follow-up (Figure 1(c)).

In accordance with findings by other authors [12], however with different OCT devices, OCT imaging of the BD lesions at baseline revealed a thickened epidermis without a prominent granular layer in all cases (Figure 2(c)). Early

after treatment, a normally layered hyporeflective epidermis was present overlying a hyperreflective dermis. Residual, clinically not evident edema could probably account for this finding. At 12 months' follow-up, the posttreatment hyperreflectiveness of the dermis had subsided, leaving behind a pattern almost indistinguishable from normal skin (Figure 2(d)).

3. Discussion

We presently report the feasible and efficacious treatment of relatively large BD lesions (20 – 70mm in maximal diameter) with 4-day cryosurgery-ingenol mebutate combination consisting of an initial cryosurgery session followed by 4 daily ingenol mebutate applications. In addition, the observations of OCT monitoring of the treated sites are presented. Cryosurgery monotherapy is considered a suitable treatment modality for selected BD lesions [1]. Its mode of action is not restricted to the direct destruction of the malignant tissues, but it also addresses the induction of a proapoptotic state in malignant cells, the destruction of tumor vasculature, and antitumoral immune stimulation [13]. We suggest that the pathophysiological effects of the cryoablation may synergize with the cellular and tissue sequels of the concomitant ingenol mebutate application on the skin [14, 15] which might predict an enhanced therapeutic efficacy of the above combination. Also, physical disruption of the epidermal barrier with cryosurgery definitely increases ingenol mebutate penetration into the skin and probably enhances efficacy. We have previously evaluated in our department alternative combination therapeutic modalities for BD with overall satisfactory results, however, of substantially protracted application time in comparison to the present proposal. In an overview of BD treatment with immunocryosurgery, that is, the 5 weeks combination of daily imiquimod and a session of relatively mild cryosurgery at day 14 of the cycle [16, 17], sustained clearance was achieved in >95% of 35 BD lesions in 29 patients, including some particularly large BD sites (>100mm in maximal diameter) or lesions in poor healing sites like the shins. However, with the accumulation of extensive experience in the treatment of BCC [18], we acknowledge that lengthy topical treatment protocols (e.g., 35 days of a typical immunocryosurgery cycle) may limit the compliance particularly of the usually older patients with BD. Therefore,

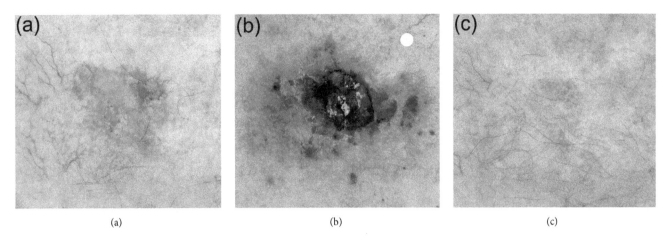

FIGURE 1: A 33 mm Bowen's disease lesion of the sternum (Patient 4). Cross-polarized photography is applied to enhance the visualization of the vascular pattern. Panel (a): the lesion at baseline. Panel (b): the area of the lesion at day 7 of treatment (one week after treatment onset with cryosurgery at day 0 and 4 daily applications of ingenol mebutate in days 0-3 of treatment). The white label is included for calibration purposes. Panel (c): the site of the lesion at 12 months follow-up. A slightly hypopigmented shallow scar is evident with excellent skin healing (hair follicle preservation) in a skin location of overall problematic healing features (sternum).

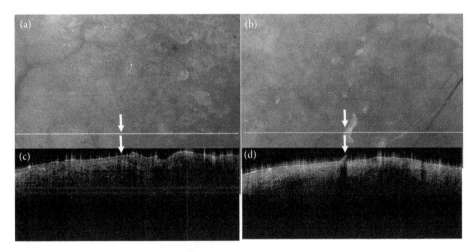

FIGURE 2: Dermoscopic images of the lesion acquired with the digital dermatoscope incorporated to the NITID device and the corresponding OCT image of Bowen's lesion shown in Figure 1. The white line on the dermatoscopic image corresponds to the section scanned by OCT. Panels (a, b): the lesion at baseline. The left half of the OCT scan includes a healthy skin segment (control) featuring a well-defined epidermis (asterisk). At the transition of healthy skin to the lesion, the typical for Bowen's disease thickening and disarrangement of the epidermis becomes evident (right to the arrow). Panels (b, d): the site of the lesions at the 12th month follow-up. There is normalization of the epidermis in the dermoscopic and the OCT images (asterisk). The focal hyperkeratosis evident in the dermatoscopic image (Panel (b), arrow) is also evident in the OCT image as a disruption in the epidermis (Panel (d), arrow) which, however, causes no concern as the epidermis is homogenous throughout the scanned section.

highly effective minimally invasive treatment modalities of shortened application periods are anticipated to further improve overall effectiveness of nonsurgical modalities for skin malignancies. In published cases of ingenol mebutate-treated Bowen's diseases, there is an effort to increase efficacy through the combination with prior laser ablation [10] or ingenol mebutate application under occlusion even in transplanted patients [9, 11] without entailing safety issues in this special setting. Our present findings confirm the feasibility of the proposed topical combination modality for BD, as it seems to combine promising efficacy and acceptable side effects profile. It is worth noting that a similar to the

present combination modality of cryosurgery and IM has been evaluated in the treatment of actinic keratosis on the dorsal hands and was compared to cryosurgery monotherapy. The authors confirmed increased efficacy in addition to the feasibility of the proposed approach [19].

The OCT features of the treated area include a well-defined homogenous epidermis band over a normal dermis, findings that constitute an unequivocal background for the monitoring for BD relapses after efficient tissue sparring treatment modalities.

In conclusion, the present case series demonstrates the feasibility of a 4-day combination modality of cryosurgery and ingenol mebutate for BD as well as the potential of OCT imaging to improve the noninvasive monitor of treatment outcomes. Both goals should be evaluated in further studies.

Conflicts of Interest

The authors state that there are no conflicts of interest.

Acknowledgments

The OCT device was a generous donation from the "S. Niarchos" foundation. Georgios Gaitanis and Ioannis D. Bassukas have received Travel Grants from LEO Hellas.

References

[1] C. A. Morton, A. J. Birnie, and D. J. Eedy, "British Association of Dermatologists' guidelines for the management of squamous cell carcinoma in situ (Bowen's disease) 2014," *British Journal of Dermatology*, vol. 170, no. 2, pp. 245–260, 2014.

[2] V. Lai, W. Cranwell, and R. Sinclair, "Epidemiology of skin cancer in the mature patient," *Clinics in Dermatology*, vol. 36, no. 2, pp. 167–176, 2018.

[3] O. Zaar, J. Fougleberg, A. Hermansson, M. Gillstedt, A.-M. Wennberg-Larkö, and J. Paoli, "Effectiveness of photodynamic therapy in Bowen's disease: a retrospective observational study in 423 lesions," *Journal of the European Academy of Dermatology and Venereology*, vol. 31, no. 8, pp. 1289–1294, 2017.

[4] J.-Y. Park, S. K. Kim, K. H. Cho, and Y. C. Kim, "Huge Bowen's disease: A pitfall of topical photodynamic therapy," *Photodiagnosis and Photodynamic Therapy*, vol. 10, no. 4, pp. 546–548, 2013.

[5] C. Ratour-Bigot, M. Chemidling, C. Montlahuc et al., "Squamous cell carcinoma following photodynamic therapy for cutaneous Bowen's disease in a series of 105 patients," *Acta Dermato-Venereologica*, vol. 96, no. 5, pp. 658–663, 2016.

[6] M. Salleras Redonnet and M. Quintana Codina, "Ingenol mebutate gel for the treatment of Bowen's disease: a case report of three patients," *Dermatologic Therapy*, vol. 29, no. 4, pp. 236–239, 2016.

[7] S. A. Braun, B. Homey, and P. A. Gerber, "Successful treatment of Bowen disease with ingenol mebutate," *Der Hautarzt*, vol. 65, no. 10, pp. 848–850, 2014.

[8] M. T. Mohanna and G. F. L. Hofbauer, "Bowenoid Actinic Keratosis and Bowen's Disease Treated Successfully with Ingenol Mebutate," *Dermatology*, vol. 232, no. 1, pp. 14–16, 2016.

[9] A. Alkhalaf and G. F. L. Hofbauer, "Ingenol Mebutate 150 mg as Physician-Directed Treatment of Bowen's Disease under Occlusion," *Dermatology*, vol. 232, no. 1, pp. 17–19, 2016.

[10] D. W. Lee, H. H. Ahn, Y. C. Kye, and S. H. Seo, "Clinical experience of ingenol mebutate gel for the treatment of Bowen's disease," *The Journal of Dermatology*, vol. 45, no. 4, pp. 425–430, 2018.

[11] M. Mohanna and G. Hofbauer, "Pronounced local skin reaction to ingenol mebutate against actinic keratosis in kidney transplant recipient without systemic adverse events," *JAAD Case Reports*, vol. 1, no. 6, pp. S19–S22, 2015.

[12] S. Batz, C. Wahrlich, A. Alawi, M. Ulrich, and J. Lademann, "Differentiation of Different Nonmelanoma Skin Cancer Types Using OCT," *Skin Pharmacology and Physiology*, vol. 31, no. 5, pp. 238–245, 2018.

[13] J. G. Baust, J. C. Bischof, S. Jiang-Hughes et al., "Re-purposing cryoablation: A combinatorial 'therapy' for the destruction of tissue," *Prostate Cancer and Prostatic Diseases*, vol. 18, no. 2, pp. 87–95, 2015.

[14] S. Emmert, H. A. Haenssle, J. R. Zibert et al., "Tumor-Preferential Induction of Immune Responses and Epidermal Cell Death in Actinic Keratoses by Ingenol Mebutate," *PLoS ONE*, vol. 11, no. 9, p. e0160096, 2016.

[15] S. N. Freiberger, P. F. Cheng, G. Iotzova-Weiss et al., "Ingenol mebutate signals via PKC/MEK/ERK in keratinocytes and induces interleukin decoy receptors IL1R2 and IL13RA2," *Molecular Cancer Therapeutics*, vol. 14, no. 9, pp. 2132–2142, 2015.

[16] G. Gaitanis and I. D. Bassukas, "Immunocryosurgery - an effective combinational modality for Bowen's disease," *Dermatologic Therapy*, vol. 29, no. 5, pp. 334–337, 2016.

[17] G. Gaitanis, G. Mitsou, G. Tsiouri, I. Alexis, and I. D. Bassukas, "Cryosurgery during imiquimod cream treatment ("immunocryosurgery") for Bowen's disease of the skin: A case series," *Acta Dermato-Venereologica*, vol. 90, no. 5, pp. 533-534, 2010.

[18] G. Gaitanis and I. D. Bassukas, "Immunocryosurgery for non-superficial basal cell carcinomas ≤ 20 mm in maximal diameter: Five-year follow-up," *Journal of Geriatric Oncology*, 2018.

[19] P. W. Hashim, J. K. Nia, S. Singer, and G. Goldenberg, "An investigator-initiated study to assess the safety and efficacy of ingenol mebutate 0.05% gel when used after cryosurgery in the treatment of hypertrophic actinic keratosis on dorsal hands," *Journal of Clinical and Aesthetic Dermatology*, vol. 9, no. 7, pp. 16–22, 2016.

Perianal Comedones: A Rare Incidental Finding

Priscilla R. Powell,[1] Juana Irma Garza-Chapa,[2] Joseph S. Susa,[3] and Stephen E. Weis[4]

[1]Medical City Weatherford, 713 East Anderson St., Weatherford, TX 76086, USA
[2]Medipiel, Centro Dermatológico y Clínica Laser, Av. Vasconcelos 405 Ote., Col. Residencial San Agustín,
  66260 Garza García, NL, Mexico
[3]Cockerell Dermatopathology, University of Texas Southwestern Medical Center, 2110 Research Row, Suite 100, Dallas, TX 75235, USA
[4]University of North Texas Health Science Center, 855 Montgomery St., Floor 5, Fort Worth, TX 76107, USA

Correspondence should be addressed to Priscilla R. Powell; priscilla_powell@alumni.baylor.edu

Academic Editor: Ioannis D. Bassukas

Comedones occur when an overproliferation of keratinocytes blocks sebum secretion in a pilosebaceous duct. Comedones have multiple possible etiologies and contributing factors. While comedones are common to acne, they are also seen in occupational exposures and are associated with certain syndromes. We describe a particularly rare case of comedones at the perianus that is not associated with any known exposure or disease and is a rare incidental finding.

1. Introduction

Comedones represent pilosebaceous ductal hyperkeratinization that begins at the junction of the isthmus and the infundibulum [1, 2]. Within the duct, the proliferation of keratinocytes blocks sebaceous secretion with ensuing accumulation of abnormal levels of sebaceous lipids [1, 3]. The etiology of comedone formation is not concretely established but formation mechanisms include hyperproliferation and abnormal desquamation of ductal keratinocytes [1]. The transformation from a normal pilosebaceous duct into a comedone occurs when the sebaceous gland progenitor cells or leucine-rich repeats and immunoglobulin-like domain 1 cells (LRIG1 cells) differentiate into epithelial type cells due to comedogenic factors [2]. Multiple contributing factors to comedone formation have been identified including abnormal levels of lipids such as linoleate and squalene, androgenic factors, the proinflammatory cytokine interleukin-1α (IL-1α), vitamin A deficiency, and possibly bacteria [1, 2]. The oxidation of lipids and squalene is specifically associated with comedone formation as the oxidized sebaceous materials instigate the release of IL-1α and keratin hyperproliferation. In regard to squalene, its oxidation may be precipitated by cigarette smoke [4]. Comedones can also arise with use of ingredients seen in skin care products such as cocoa butter and esters like isopropyl myristate and isopropyl isostearate that have varying levels of comedogenicity [5]. Leptin, which regulates sebum lipogenesis, has also been identified as a contributor to the comedogenic process. Leptin is mTORC1 pathway dependent, and when mTORC1 is overactivated and upregulated, sebum production and proinflammatory sebum lipids increase [6]. Thus, comedone formation is multifactorial. We describe a case of a 57-year-old female with focal, perianal open comedones with no associated illness. To the best of our knowledge, there has only been three reports of perianal comedones to date.

2. Case Presentation

A 57-year-old female presented to the clinic for a skin exam. She had a long-term history of heavy sun exposure and a family history of both melanoma and nonmelanoma skin cancer. She had a personal history of nodular basal cell carcinoma. She had a history of alcohol abuse and 40 pack-year tobacco use. Other medical conditions included cerebral aneurysm, diffuse atherosclerosis of the carotids, bilateral peripheral artery disease, and alcoholic peripheral neuropathy. Her BMI was 21 and her blood pressure was 126/74. On full-skin exam

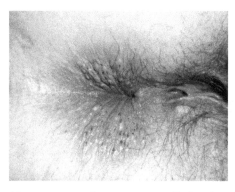

FIGURE 1: Numerous comedones symmetrically distributed around the perianus at the anal verge.

she had numerous comedones symmetrically distributed around the perianus at the anal verge. She had no comedones in the axilla, below breasts, groin, or other stigmata of hidradenitis suppurativa (Figure 1). No comedones were seen on the face, shoulders, or neck. She was unaware of lesions at the anus and had no gastrointestinal or anal symptoms. She denied application of any topical products or medications to her perianus. She did not have any of the environmental exposures that would predispose her to comedone formation in an unusual location. During several follow-up exams for her skin cancer over 18 months the comedones have remained asymptomatic and stable in size and number.

Histopathological examination from a biopsy specimen of the perianal skin revealed multiple open comedones, characterized by a dilated follicular infundibulum with a wide patulous opening and a thin epithelial lining. The comedones were filled with keratinous material and debris as well as multiple hair shaft fragments (Figures 2(a) and 2(b)).

3. Discussion

There are only three prior reports of perianal comedones. The first case was associated with chronic topical steroid application to the anus. The patient had applied 0.025% flurandrenolide 3 to 5 times per day for three years for intractable pruritus ani associated with chronic diarrhea. He was unaware of any perianal lesions. The authors proposed that the distribution of the comedones was secondary to topical steroid application and the occlusive effect of the perianus [7]. The second report occurred in a correspondence letter to the first case. Silver remarked that it was assumed that the comedones were not present before steroid use. He reported having seen patients with perianal comedones in conjunction with pruritus ani without steroid treatment but did not add further details about specific patients [8]. The third report of perianal comedones was an incidental finding on an 84-year-old male. That patient, as was our patient, was unaware of the lesions. He had not applied any topical steroid or used mineral oil-based suppositories. The comedones were surrounding the anal orifice and were confirmed by biopsy [9]. These reports attribute the origin of perianal comedones to either steroids or pruritus ani or as an incidental finding. These cases, while differing as to their attribution, reinforce

the rarity of the condition. In summary, two of the prior reports of the perianal comedones were pruritic, though in the first report the pruritus may have been preceded by the chronic diarrhea rather than the lesions themselves. The third report and our patient were asymptomatic. Only one patient had a history of topical agent application to the area. We believe that comedones in the perianal area do not require topical agents to arise nor do they necessarily indicate disease. Perianal comedones, as illustrated by our patient, do not require treatment as they can be asymptomatic and do not progress.

When faced with comedone-like lesions, both the location and symptoms should be considered when establishing a diagnosis. Comedones, as part of disease, are commonly seen in acne vulgaris, Favre-Racouchot syndrome, and cases of nevus comedonicus [1, 10]. Infrequently, comedones are seen with occupational and chemical exposures. Rarely, open comedones are seen in Birt-Hogg-Dube (BHD) syndrome [11–13]. Comedones as part of acne vulgaris are typically found on the forehead, the shoulders, and the neck. Our patient only had comedones at the perianal area. She also would not have cosmetic acne as described in the introduction as she does not apply products to the perianal area. Favre-Racouchot syndrome is an environmental exposure in which comedones are found in the lateral periorbital part of the face corresponding to areas of solar elastosis. Recently, there was a case of elastosis-related comedone formation associated with unilateral cigarette smoking [10]. Comedones are also part of nevus comedonicus and hidradenitis suppurativa (HS). In nevus comedonicus, they are often distributed in a linear pattern, most commonly on the face, neck, upper arm, and trunk; they can be present at birth or appear by 15 years of age [1, 14]. As for HS, comedones are usually double-headed and present over nodules and/or scars, together with abscesses and sinus tracts located on axillae, groin, buttocks, and breasts [14]. Our patient was asymptomatic and had findings in a single location, with no associated inflammatory nodular lesions, sinus tracts, or scarring. In occupational exposures to dioxin, open comedones are seen on the malar cheeks, postauricular area, axilla, and scrotum. Those chronically exposed to pitch or coal tar can get periorbital comedones. Lastly, oil acne presents with comedones on the dorsal hands and the extensors of the arms [12, 13]. Our patient had no history of chemical exposure to the perianal area.

When a patient presents with comedones in an unusual distribution, it is appropriate to consider other conditions. One such example is Birt-Hogg-Dube syndrome, an autosomal dominant disease characterized by hair follicle hamartomas and an increased risk for renal cell carcinoma. The open comedones in Birt-Hogg-Dube are found on the face, neck, chest, and abdomen; on histopathology they represent comedonal or cystic fibrofolliculomas, demonstrating a dilated hair follicle with proliferation of the perifollicular fibrous sheath and thin epithelial strands emanating from the infundibular portion of the hair follicle [11]. While considering all of these, from common to uncommon, our patient did not meet the description of any of these syndromes.

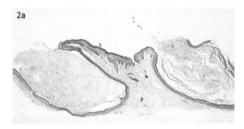
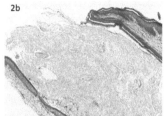

FIGURE 2: (a) A shave biopsy demonstrating two open comedones, note the wide opening and the thin epithelial lining (40x). (b) A close-up view of one lesion, showing the keratinous material and the multiple hair shaft fragments (100x).

A possible explanation for the unusual location of the comedones is the occlusive effect of the perianus which may be sufficient for the comedone formation process, perhaps in combination with her smoking history [4, 7, 10]. The determination to see if there is a correlation with perianal comedones and cigarette smoking may be of interest for future studies as smoking history was not included in the prior reports. Another potential cause is the intrinsically unique environment of the perineum. The perineal skin is a common site for irritant dermatitis. In addition to occlusion, the skin is more prone to irritating factors such as maceration and irritation from fecal contact that may expose the skin to greater bacterial exposures, bile acids, and local pH alteration from spicy or acidic foods [15, 16]. While we may not have cosmetic or toxic chemical exposures in this site there can be other contacts that could lead to local irritation.

4. Conclusion

We describe perianal comedones as a rare incidental finding. This report serves to provide reassurance of the benignity of the lesion which is not necessarily related to medication use or other gastrointestinal disease. As described by Oliet, this finding may be underreported due to the infrequency of full-skin exams. Lastly, we would like to call for the "first do no harm principle" in patient care. The lesions were asymptomatic and incidental and do not necessitate treatment. The three prior reports and our report attributed perianal open comedones to chronic topical steroids or pruritus ani or as an incidental finding. Therefore, there are no reported associations of perianal comedones with systemic disease.

Abbreviations

BHD: Birt-Hogg-Dube
RCC: Renal cell carcinoma
IL: Interleukin
HS: Hidradenitis suppurativa
LRIG-1: Leucine-rich repeats and immunoglobulin-like domain 1 or sebaceous gland progenitor cell.

Conflicts of Interest

The authors declare that they have no conflicts of interest.

References

[1] W. J. Cunliffe, D. B. Holland, and A. Jeremy, "Comedone formation: etiology, clinical presentation, and treatment," *Clinics in Dermatology*, vol. 22, no. 5, pp. 367–374, 2004.

[2] J.-H. Saurat, "Strategic targets in acne: the comedone switch in question," *Dermatology*, vol. 231, no. 2, pp. 105–111, 2015.

[3] J. Q. Del Rosso and L. H. Kircik, "The sequence of inflammation, relevant biomarkers, and the pathogenesis of acne vulgaris: what does recent research show and what does it mean to the clinician?" *Journal of Drugs in Dermatology: JDD*, vol. 12, no. 8, pp. s109–s115, 2013.

[4] B. Capitanio, V. Lora, M. Ludovici et al., "Modulation of sebum oxidation and interleukin-1α levels associates with clinical improvement of mild comedonal acne," *Journal of the European Academy of Dermatology and Venereology*, vol. 28, no. 12, pp. 1792–1797, 2014.

[5] S. H. Nguyen, T. P. Dang, and H. I. Maibach, "Comedogenicity in rabbit: some cosmetic ingredients/vehicles," *Cutaneous and Ocular Toxicology*, vol. 26, no. 4, pp. 287–292, 2007.

[6] B. C. Melnik, "Is sebocyte-derived leptin the missing link between hyperseborrhea, ductal hypoxia, inflammation and comedogenesis in acne vulgaris?" *Experimental Dermatology*, vol. 25, no. 3, pp. 181-182, 2016.

[7] E. J. Oliet and S. A. Estes, "Perianal comedones associated with chronic topical fluorinated steroid use," *Journal of the American Academy of Dermatology*, vol. 7, no. 3, pp. 405–407, 1982.

[8] S. E. Silver, "Perianal comedones and topical corticosteroids," *Journal of the American Academy of Dermatology*, vol. 8, no. 6, article 912, 1983.

[9] M. C. Lurati and D. Hohl, "Multiple comedonelike lesions encircling the anal orifice—quiz case," *JAMA Dermatology*, vol. 145, no. 12, pp. 1447–1452, 2009.

[10] J. Dyer, M. Mitchell, J. Gapp, and M. Greenfield, "Unilateral, perioral Favre-Racouchot syndrome associated with cigarette smoking: case and discussion," *Journal of the American Academy of Dermatology*, vol. 74, supplement 1, no. 5, p. AB76, 2016.

[11] O. Aivaz, S. Berkman, L. Middelton, W. M. Linehan, J. J. DiGiovanna, and E. W. Cowen, "Comedonal and cystic fibrofolliculomas in Birt-Hogg-Dube syndrome," *JAMA Dermatology*, vol. 151, no. 7, pp. 770–774, 2015.

[12] J. P. Tindall, "Chloracne and chloracnegens," *Journal of the American Academy of Dermatology*, vol. 13, no. 4, pp. 539–558, 1985.

[13] B. B. Adams, V. B. Chetty, and D. F. Mutasim, "Periorbital comedones and their relationship to pitch tar: a cross-sectional analysis and a review of the literature," *Journal of the American Academy of Dermatology*, vol. 42, no. 4, pp. 624–627, 2000.

[14] T. Ergun, "Hidradenitis suppurativa and the metabolic syndrome," *Clinics in Dermatology*, vol. 36, no. 1, pp. 41–47, 2018.

[15] L. Y. McGirt and C. R. Martins, "Dermatologic diagnoses in the perianal area," *Clinics in Colon and Rectal Surgery*, vol. 17, no. 4, pp. 241–245, 2004.

[16] C. M. White, R. A. Gailey, and S. Lippe, "Cholestyramine ointment to treat buttocks rash and anal excoriation in an infant," *Annals of Pharmacotherapy*, vol. 30, no. 9, pp. 954–956, 1996.

3

Development of Asymmetric Facial Depigmentation in a Patient Treated with Dasatinib with New-Onset Hypovitaminosis D

Kirsten C. Webb,[1] **Magdalena Harasimowicz,**[2] **Monica Janeczek,**[2] **Jodi Speiser,**[3] **James Swan,**[1] **and Rebecca Tung**[1]

[1]*Department of Dermatology, Loyola University Chicago, Chicago, IL, USA*
[2]*Stritch School of Medicine, Loyola University Chicago, Chicago, IL, USA*
[3]*Department of Pathology, Loyola University Chicago, Chicago, IL, USA*

Correspondence should be addressed to Kirsten C. Webb; kcarlywebb@gmail.com

Academic Editor: Kowichi Jimbow

Dasatinib is a second-generation tyrosine kinase inhibitor (TKI) used to treat imatinib-resistant chronic myelogenous leukemia (CML), as well as other Philadelphia chromosome-positive lymphoproliferative disorders. While the most commonly reported cutaneous side effects with this therapy include a morbilliform eruption, skin exfoliation, and skin irritation, pigmentary abnormalities have also been observed, albeit much more rarely. We present the case of a 72-year-old South Asian male with CML who presented with new-onset hypopigmentation of his face and scalp three years after a dose increase of dasatinib therapy, in the setting of newly discovered borderline hypovitaminosis D. Dasatinib and the other TKIs are believed to induce dyschromias via modulation of the c-kit receptor and its associated signaling pathway, which is involved in melanocyte survival, proliferation, and migration.

1. Introduction

Dasatinib is a second-generation tyrosine kinase inhibitor (TKI) used to treat imatinib-resistant chronic myelogenous leukemia (CML), other Philadelphia chromosome-positive lymphoproliferative disorders, and certain solid tumors [1]. The most commonly reported cutaneous side effects with this therapy include morbilliform eruptions, skin exfoliation, and skin irritation [2]. While hypopigmentation can affect up to 41% of patients treated with imatinib [3], it is much more rarely reported in patients treated with second-generation TKIs, such as dasatinib. We present a case of dasatinib-associated dyschromia in the setting of newfound borderline hypovitaminosis D and review those cases in the literature.

2. Case

A 72-year-old South Asian male presented with new-onset hypopigmented patches on his frontal scalp, cheeks, and forehead of four weeks' duration. He had a past medical history significant for imatinib-resistant CML, currently being treated with dasatinib. There was no personal or family history of autoimmune diseases, pigmentary disorders, or melanoma. Of note, the patient had been diagnosed with CML 13 years priorly and was successfully treated with imatinib 400 mg po daily for 10 years. However, over nine months' time, the patient's quantitative Bcr-Abl fusion transcript product serum level subsequently rose from an undetectable amount (zero) to 1.443. This prompted a repeat bone marrow biopsy, which revealed a novel heterozygous point mutation, c.1003G>A, within the Abl kinase domain. At this time, the patient underwent a therapeutic switch from imatinib to dasatinib. The patient had noted diffuse skin lightening of the head and neck while treated with imatinib, which subsequently resolved in its entirety after he was transitioned to dasatinib. He was initiated on dasatinib therapy at a dose of 50 mg daily for the first 10 weeks, and then his dose was increased to 100 mg daily. Three years after this dose escalation, the patient presented to dermatology clinic with new-onset hypopigmented and depigmented macules

TABLE 1: Summary of cases reporting dasatinib-induced hypopigmentation.

Age (years)	Malignancy	Dasatinib dose (mg)	Time to onset of depigmentation (weeks)	Time to repigmentation (weeks)	Ref
52	Metastatic hemangiopericytoma	70 (twice daily)	8	4–6	[1]
29	Chronic myelogenous leukemia	70 (once daily)	6–8	N/A	[4]
16	Acute lymphoblastic leukemia	100 (twice daily)	4	N/A	[5]
27	Chronic myelogenous leukemia	100 (once daily)	24	N/A	[6]
56	Chronic myelogenous leukemia	70 (once daily)	8	8	[7]

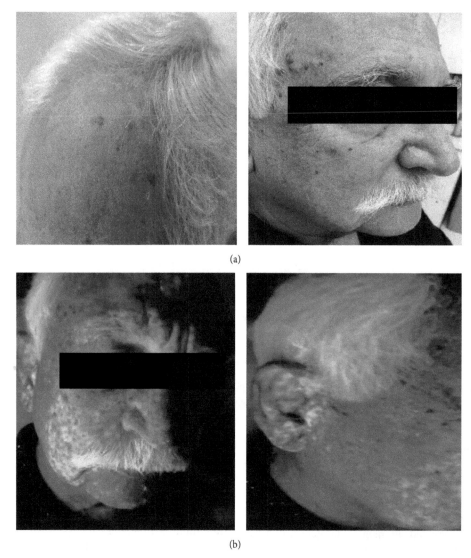

(a)

(b)

FIGURE 1: Hypopigmented and depigmented areas on the (a) face, scalp, and (b) ears, highlighted on Wood's lamp examination.

and patches of varying sizes on his superior forehead, bilateral melolabial cheeks, and chin (Figure 1(a)). Additionally, confetti-like depigmentation was present on the bilateral ears. These achromic lesions were more fully appreciated on Wood's lamp examination (Figure 1(b)). All of the patient's scalp hair and the majority of the facial hair were depigmented. Laboratory workup revealed a low normal serum vitamin D level. Shave biopsy of a representative lesion on the frontal scalp revealed a decreased melanocyte number

on MART-1 staining, and PAS staining was negative for fungal organisms. The patient's hypopigmented lesions were attributed to his dasatinib therapy.

3. Discussion

Dyschromias are rarely reported in patients treated with dasatinib and other second-generation TKIs. In reported cases of dasatinib-associated dyschromias (Table 1), pigmentary changes began four weeks to six months following treatment initiation and appear to have a predilection for the head and neck [1, 4–7]. Our patient's cutaneous pigmentary changes were noted approximately three years (37.5 months) after treatment initiation, which is the longest time to onset reported as of yet. His hair depigmentation predated his treatment with any TKI. Dyspigmentation appears to be dose-dependent, and repigmentation is achievable with cessation of dasatinib therapy. In reported cases, repigmentation began as early as four to eight weeks following withdrawal of therapy [1, 7]. Unfortunately, while effective, this is not a practical treatment approach in most cases, including our own patient's case, as patients' underlying malignancies often necessitate continued treatment with the offending TKI.

Dasatinib targets multiple mutant forms of the Bcr-Abl protein, as well as the SRC family of kinases, c-kit, and Platelet-Derived Growth Factor Receptor β (PDGFR-β) tyrosine kinases [8]. Dasatinib and other TKIs are thought to induce dyschromias via inhibition of the protooncogene, c-kit. C-kit encodes a class III transmembrane tyrosine kinase receptor found on the surface of melanocytes and hematopoietic stem cells [1, 9–11]; its ligand is stem cell factor (SCF). Upon binding with SCF, c-kit undergoes dimerization and autophosphorylation, which activates downstream pathways involved in melanocyte proliferation, migration, and survival [9–11].

There is ample support for c-kit's role in melanocyte survival and functioning. C-kit's role in melanocyte migration is highlighted by the clinical disorder, piebaldism [12]. Affected patients have c-kit mutations, resulting in failed proliferation or migration of melanoblasts from the neural crest during embryonic development to their appropriate destination in the skin [12]. This results in the clinical findings of white skin patches and white hair, most commonly on the forehead, trunk, and extremities [13]. C-kit's role in melanocyte proliferation is demonstrated in a study in which human skin xenografts treated with KIT inhibitory antibodies resulted in a decrease in melanocyte number [9]. C-kit also appears to play a role in melanocyte functioning. Skin samples from mice treated with sunitinib, a TKI which inhibits c-kit, showed no change in the number of KIT-positive melanocytes; however, these mice exhibited dose-dependent and reversible hair depigmentation [14]. Clearly, c-kit plays an integral role in melanocyte biology. Thus, it is not surprising that interference with this pathway results in the clinical pigmentary anomalies observed in patients treated with TKIs.

While hypopigmentation and depigmentation are the most commonly observed pigmentary anomalies with TKIs, hyperpigmentation has also been reported. In one series, 3.6% of patients treated with imatinib experienced hyperpigmentation [3]. Moreover, one patient treated with dasatinib initially experienced widespread hypopigmentation. Upon withdrawal of dasatinib, she experienced transient hyperpigmentation before her baseline pigment was restored [1]. These latter observations suggest that, rather than inducing true absolute inhibition of c-kit, TKIs may instead act as c-kit modulators, resulting in a spectrum of possible pigmentary abnormalities. Interestingly, the ability of TKIs to inhibit c-kit activity and signaling may depend on the conformation of

c-kit ligand (SCF) present in the tissues, namely, whether SCF is spliced into a membrane-bound or soluble form. Indeed, a recent study showed that membrane-bound c-kit ligand was capable of inducing c-kit mediated signaling independent of kinase functioning and rendered membrane-bound SCF/c-kit receptors insensitive to imatinib. This was found in contrast to their soluble SCF/c-kit receptor counterparts, which were sensitive to this therapy [15].

The reason dyschromias are much more frequently observed with first-generation TKIs compared to second-generation TKIs is not fully understood. There also appears to be a disparity between members of the same TKI generation in terms of their likelihood of inducing pigmentary anomalies. This is demonstrated in a report by Fujimi et al., in which a CML patient experienced reversible dasatinib-induced skin and hair depigmentation and then did not experience any depigmentation when subsequently treated with bosutinib [7]. Bosutinib is a tyrosine kinase inhibitor which targets multiple Bcr-Abl mutant forms but, in contrast to dasatinib and other second-generation TKIs, has little to no affinity for the c-kit and PDGF receptors [16–18]. Variations in receptor affinities afford a possible explanation for the differing frequencies of observed dyschromias between different TKI generations and between individual members of each TKI generation. On a similar note, variations in patients' receptor sequencing and structure may play an important role in determining which patients ultimately develop pigmentary anomalies when treated with TKI therapies. Indeed, the necessity of possessing a certain genetic predisposition and/or having certain environmental exposures could explain why only certain patients are afflicted with these side effects and may also explain the observed differences in time to onset of depigmentation and doses of TKIs required to elicit pigmentary anomalies.

Another important consideration in this case is the role of vitamin D in cutaneous disorders of hypopigmentation. Its various biologic properties have different implications depending upon the dermatologic condition in question. For example, its immunomodulatory properties, including inhibition of the inflammatory and proapoptotic cytokines, IL-6, IL-8, TNF-α, and TNF-γ [19], inhibition of antigen presentation [20, 21], and its observed depletion (low serum levels) in patients with various autoimmune diseases [22], sparked investigations into its potential role in vitiligo pathogenesis. Although a causative role for vitamin D deficiency in vitiligo has not yet been established [23], topical and systemic vitamin D formulations are often employed in vitiligo treatment given its known immunomodulatory effects. More relevant to our own patient's case are vitamin D's effects on melanocyte biology and survival. Vitamin D plays a role in melanocyte differentiation, maturation, proliferation, migration, and melanogenesis [24]. Importantly, vitamin D has also been shown to have protective effects against melanocyte apoptosis [25, 26]. It exerts these effects via interaction with the nuclear vitamin D receptor (VDR) on melanocytes [27–29]. Our patient experienced only minimal improvement with administration of topical and systemic vitamin D supplementation, suggesting that dasatinib therapy was the main driver of his pigment loss. However, given vitamin

D's recognized melanocytic effects as discussed above, it is possible that his borderline hypovitaminosis D led to more pronounced depigmentation at presentation than might have been observed if he had higher baseline serum vitamin D levels.

Since our patient's underlying CML necessitated continued treatment with dasatinib and he declined procedural treatments, we treated his dyschromia topically with mometasone 0.1% and calcipotriene 0.005% creams. We also initiated over-the-counter therapy with oral vitamin D3 (2000 IU) supplementation. These interventions produced modest improvement in his skin findings. Interestingly, the patient's reported remote past history of diffuse skin lightening was probably attributable to his prior treatment with imatinib. Although he never sought treatment at that time, it fully resolved with therapy cessation, as expected. We present this case to highlight a rare cutaneous side effect of a medication that is being utilized with increasing frequency for treatment-resistant hematological malignancies and certain solid tumors. We encourage clinicians to consider this cutaneous side effect in the differential diagnosis of vitiligo, postinflammatory hypopigmentation, and pityriasis versicolor in patients undergoing treatment with dasatinib. Additionally, continued research exploring how the SCF/c-kit pathway and tyrosine kinase receptors impact melanocyte biogenesis and survival could afford further insight into management of patients suffering from vitiligo and other pigmentary disorders.

Conflicts of Interest

The authors declare that there are no conflicts of interest regarding the publication of this paper.

References

[1] K. Boudadi and R. Chugh, "Diffuse hypopigmentation followed by hyperpigmentation in an African American woman with hemangiopericytoma treated with dasatinib," *Journal of Clinical and Diagnostic Research*, vol. 8, no. 11, pp. QD01–QD02, 2014.

[2] I. Amitay-Laish, S. M. Stemmer, and M. E. Lacouture, "Adverse cutaneous reactions secondary to tyrosine kinase inhibitors including imatinib mesylate, nilotinib, and dasatinib," *Dermatologic Therapy*, vol. 24, no. 4, pp. 386–395, 2011.

[3] B. Arora, L. Kumar, A. Sharma, J. Wadhwa, and V. Kochupillai, "Pigmentary changes in chronic myeloid leukemia patients treated with imatinib mesylate," *Annals of Oncology*, vol. 15, no. 2, pp. 358–359, 2004.

[4] A. Sun, R. S. Akin, E. Cobos, and J. Smith, "Hair depigmentation during chemotherapy with dasatinib, a dual Bcr-Abl/Src family tyrosine kinase inhibitor," *Journal of Drugs in Dermatology*, vol. 8, no. 4, pp. 395–398, 2009.

[5] V. Brazzelli, V. Grasso, V. Barbaccia et al., "Hair depigmentation and vitiligo-like lesions in a leukaemic paediatric patient during chemotherapy with dasatinib," *Acta Dermato-Venereologica*, vol. 92, no. 2, pp. 218–219, 2012.

[6] S. Samimi, E. Chu, J. Seykora et al., "Dasatinib-induced leukotrichia in a patient with chronic myelogenous leukemia," *JAMA Dermatology*, vol. 149, no. 5, pp. 637–639, 2013.

[7] A. Fujimi, S. Ibata, Y. Kanisawa et al., "Reversible skin and hair depigmentation during chemotherapy with dasatinib for chronic myeloid leukemia," *Journal of Dermatology*, vol. 43, no. 1, pp. 106–107, 2016.

[8] S. Shayani, "Dasatinib, a multikinase inhibitor: therapy, safety, and appropriate management of adverse events," *Therapeutic Drug Monitoring*, vol. 32, no. 6, pp. 680–687, 2010.

[9] J. M. Grichnik, J. A. Burch, J. Burchette, and C. R. Shea, "The SCF/KIT pathway plays a critical role in the control of normal human melanocyte homeostasis," *Journal of Investigative Dermatology*, vol. 111, no. 2, pp. 233–238, 1998.

[10] B. Wehrle-Haller, "The role of Kit-ligand in melanocyte development and epidermal homeostasis," *Pigment Cell Research*, vol. 16, no. 3, pp. 287–296, 2003.

[11] A. Galanis and M. Levis, "Inhibition of c-kit by tyrosine kinase inhibitors," *Haematologica*, vol. 100, no. 3, pp. E77–E79, 2015.

[12] L. B. Giebel and R. A. Spritz, "Mutation of the KIT (mast/stem cell growth factor receptor) protooncogene in human piebaldism," *Proceedings of the National Academy of Sciences of the United States of America*, vol. 88, no. 19, pp. 8696–8699, 1991.

[13] K. Ezoe, S. A. Holmes, L. Ho et al., "Novel mutations and deletions of the KIT (steel factor receptor) gene in human piebaldism," *American Journal of Human Genetics*, vol. 56, no. 1, pp. 58–66, 1995.

[14] K. G. Moss, G. C. Toner, J. M. Cherrington, D. B. Mendel, and A. D. Laird, "Hair depigmentation is a biological readout for pharmacological inhibition of KIT in mice and humans," *Journal of Pharmacology and Experimental Therapeutics*, vol. 307, no. 2, pp. 476–480, 2003.

[15] S. Tabone-Eglinger, Z. Calderin-Sollet, P. Pinon et al., "Niche anchorage and signaling through membrane-bound Kit-ligand/c-kit receptor are kinase independent and imatinib insensitive," *The FASEB Journal*, vol. 28, no. 10, pp. 4441–4456, 2014.

[16] M. Puttini, A. M. L. Coluccia, F. Boschelli et al., "In vitro and in vivo activity of SKI-606, a novel Src-Abl inhibitor, against imatinib-resistant Bcr-Abl+ neoplastic cells," *Cancer Research*, vol. 66, no. 23, pp. 11314–11322, 2006.

[17] A. Quintás-Cardama, H. Kantarjian, and J. Cortes, "Flying under the radar: the new wave of BCR-ABL inhibitors," *Nature Reviews Drug Discovery*, vol. 6, no. 10, pp. 834–848, 2007.

[18] L. L. Remsing Rix, U. Rix, J. Colinge et al., "Global target profile of the kinase inhibitor bosutinib in primary chronic myeloid leukemia cells," *Leukemia*, vol. 23, no. 3, pp. 477–485, 2009.

[19] H. Koizumi, A. Kaplan, T. Shimizu, and A. Ohkawara, "1,25-Dihydroxyvitamin D3 and a new analogue, 22-oxacalcitriol, modulate proliferation and interleukin-8 secretion of normal human keratinocytes," *Journal of Dermatological Science*, vol. 15, no. 3, pp. 207–213, 1997.

[20] G. Penna and L. Adorini, "1α,25-Dihydroxyvitamin D3 inhibits differentiation, maturation, activation, and survival of dendritic cells leading to impaired alloreactive T cell activation," *The Journal of Immunology*, vol. 164, no. 5, pp. 2405–2411, 2000.

[21] M. D. Griffin, W. Lutz, V. A. Phan, L. A. Bachman, D. J. McKean, and R. Kumar, "Dendritic cell modulation by 1α,25 dihydroxyvitamin D3 and its analogs: a vitamin D receptor-dependent pathway that promotes a persistent state of immaturity in vitro and in vivo," *Proceedings of the National Academy of Sciences of the United States of America*, vol. 98, no. 12, pp. 6800–6805, 2001.

[22] M. Hewison, "An update on vitamin D and human immunity," *Clinical Endocrinology*, vol. 76, no. 3, pp. 315–325, 2012.

[23] E. Karagün, C. Ergin, S. Baysak, G. Erden, H. Aktaş, and Ö. Ekiz, "The role of serum vitamin D levels in vitiligo," *Advances in Dermatology and Allergology*, vol. 33, no. 4, pp. 300–302, 2016.

[24] R. Doss, A.-A. El-Rifaie, Y. Gohary, and L. Rashed, "Vitamin D receptor expression in vitiligo," *Indian Journal of Dermatology*, vol. 60, no. 6, pp. 544–548, 2015.

[25] R. S. Mason and C. J. Holliday, "1, 25-Dihydroxyvitamin D contributes to photoprotection in skin cells," in *Vitamin D Endocrine System: Structural, Biological, Genetic and Clinical Aspects*, pp. 605–608, University of California, Riverside, Calif, USA, 2000.

[26] B. Sauer, L. Ruwisch, and B. Kleuser, "Antiapoptotic action of 1α,25-dihydroxyvitamin D3 in primary human melanocytes," *Melanoma Research*, vol. 13, no. 4, pp. 339–347, 2003.

[27] Y. Tomita, W. Torinuki, and H. Tagami, "Stimulation of human melanocytes by vitamin D3 possibly mediates skin pigmentation after sun exposure," *Journal of Investigative Dermatology*, vol. 90, no. 6, pp. 882–884, 1988.

[28] H. Watabe, Y. Soma, Y. Kawa et al., "Differentiation of murine melanocyte precursors induced by 1,25-dihydroxyvitamin D3 is associated with the stimulation of endothelin B receptor expression," *Journal of Investigative Dermatology*, vol. 119, no. 3, pp. 583–589, 2002.

[29] K. AlGhamdi, A. Kumar, and N. Moussa, "The role of vitamin D in melanogenesis with an emphasis on vitiligo," *Indian Journal of Dermatology, Venereology and Leprology*, vol. 79, no. 6, pp. 750–758, 2013.

4

Prurigo Pigmentosa: A Clinicopathological Report of Three Middle Eastern Patients

N. Almaani⑩,[1,2] A. H. Al-Tarawneh,[2,3] and H. Msallam[2]

[1]*Department of Dermatology, Faculty of Medicine, The University of Jordan, Amman, Jordan*
[2]*Department of Dermatology, Jordan University Hospital, Amman, Jordan*
[3]*Department of Dermatology, Faculty of Medicine, Mu'tah University, Karak, Jordan*

Correspondence should be addressed to N. Almaani; noor.almaani@nhs.net

Academic Editor: Michela Curzio

Prurigo pigmentosa is a unique cutaneous inflammatory disorder characterized by a sudden onset of pruritic and erythematous macules, urticarial papules, and plaques that may coalesce to form a reticulated pattern. Lesions typically heal within weeks leaving a reticulated and mottled postinflammatory hyperpigmentation. The majority of reported cases originate from Japan with much fewer cases described worldwide without predominant ethnicity. The histopathological features of prurigo pigmentosa can be nonspecific; however, distinct features exist for each stage of the disease. The aetiology of prurigo pigmentosa is not fully understood. However, ketoacidosis has been implicated in the pathogenesis and indeed prurigo pigmentosa has been associated with ketoacidotic states such as diabetes mellitus, fasting, dieting, and anorexia nervosa. In this report, we present 3 Jordanian patients with prurigo pigmentosa and describe their clinicopathological features. One patient developed prurigo pigmentosa while fasting during the month of Ramadan and another was undertaking a strict diet. No associations were identified in the third patient. In view of the largely nonspecific clinical and histological features, a high index of suspicion is required as many cases of prurigo pigmentosa are probably undiagnosed.

1. Introduction

Prurigo pigmentosa (PP) is a unique cutaneous inflammatory disorder first described in Japan by Nagashima *et al.* in 1971 as a "peculiar pruriginous dermatosis with gross reticular pigmentation." [1] The term "prurigo pigmentosa" was later coined in 1978. [2] PP is an under-recognized disorder in countries other than Japan, where hundreds of cases have been reported. On the contrary, much fewer cases have been described worldwide without predominant ethnicity [3–6]. Herein, we present 3 Jordanian patients with PP and describe their clinicopathological features.

2. Case Presentation

Patient 1 is a 31-year-old Jordanian female with a history of a recurrent and itchy eruption involving the mid- to lower back, lateral chest wall, and the nape of the neck. This resolved with net-like pigmentation (Figures 1(a) and 1(b)).

The occurrence of the eruption was linked with fasting in Ramadan, in addition to travels to North America. No other medical problems were identified.

Patient 2 is a 16-year-old Jordanian female who presented with an itchy eruption of new onset. This appeared 3 weeks earlier and affected the upper to mid-back and the "V" of the neck (Figures 1(c) and 1(d)). The occurrence of the eruption followed a 1-month period of strict dieting.

Patient 3 is a 45-year-old Jordanian female with an itchy eruption of 3 months' duration. This affected the nape of the neck and the upper back. No triggers were identified and the patient was otherwise healthy.

The patients' demographics and their clinical features are outlined in Table 1. Clinically, all patients were noted to have erythematous papules that coalesced to form plaques. These were arranged in a reticular pattern that was more prominent peripherally. In addition, patient 1 had associated vesicles and minimal erosions (Figures 1(a) and 1(b)). In all patients, the lesions were symmetrically distributed and had

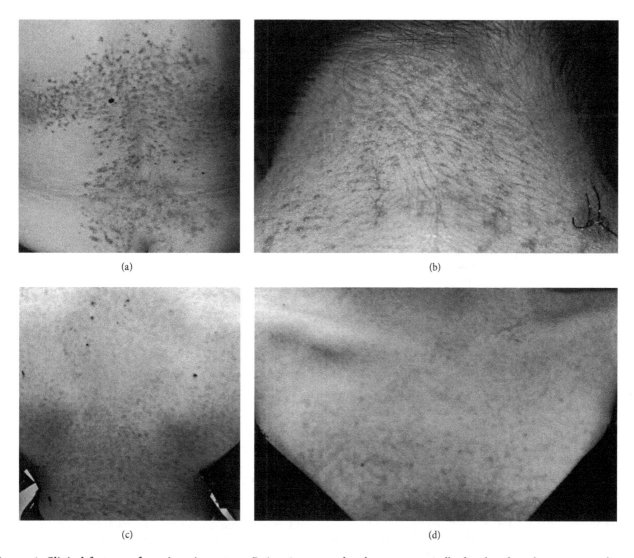

(a)   (b)

(c)   (d)

FIGURE 1: **Clinical features of prurigo pigmentosa.** Patient 1 was noted to have symmetrically distributed erythematous papules and papulovesicules, admixed with postinflammatory and reticulated hyperpigmentation on the middle back, lumbosacral area, lateral chest wall (a), and the nape of the neck (b). In patient 2, there were erythematous papules with postinflammatory hyperpigmentation on the lateral chest wall, the back (c), and the central chest (d). Scattered excoriations were also noted.

a predilection for the trunk. Other involved areas included the lateral and posterior aspects of the neck (patients 1 and 3), the lateral chest wall (patient 1), and the lumbosacral area (patient 1). Different types of lesions coexisted in all patients including papules, patches, and plaques, in addition to vesicles and erosions in patient 1. A clinical diagnosis of PP was suspected clinically in patients 1 and 2.

The main histological findings are summarized in Figure 2 and Table 2. The histopathological features were similar in all cases, showing features consistent with early lesions according to Boer's criteria [7]. The major histological differential diagnoses were impetiginized spongiotic dermatitis, pityriasis lichenoides, and viral exanthem. Periodic acid-Schiff stain was negative in all specimens. Direct immunofluorescence was performed for patients 1 and 2 only and was negative.

The clinical course varied, but all three patients had eventual complete resolution of all lesions. Patient 1 was treated with superpotent topical corticosteroids prior to presentation to our department. However, there was no improvement and new lesions continued to emerge. The patient subsequently reported gradual spontaneous resolution 10 weeks after onset of the eruption, leaving postinflammatory hyperpigmentation. Patient 2 was previously treated with moderately potent topical corticosteroids and antihistamines without any improvement. New lesions continued to emerge. On initiation of doxycycline, the lesions cleared within 1 week. No recurrence was reported during a 10-month follow-up period throughout which the patient avoided strict dieting. Patient 3 reported spontaneous resolution of some lesions before presentation to our department. Doxycycline was subsequently initiated with complete resolution.

TABLE 1: Demographics, clinical features, and outcomes of 3 Jordanian patients with prurigo pigmentosa.

	Patient 1	Patient 2	Patient 3
Age (years)	32	16	45
Gender	Female	Female	Female
Symptoms	Recurrent itchy eruption	Itchy eruption	Itchy eruption
Distribution	Lateral and nape of the neck, mid and lower back, lateral chest wall	Upper and mid back, V-area of the chest	Nape of the neck and upper back
Duration of lesions	1 year, recurrent	3 weeks	1 month
Clinical examination	Reticulated erythematous papulovesicular lesions with focal erosions and crusting, prominent postinflammatory hyperpigmentation	Erythematous maculopapular lesions with faint postinflammatory hyperpigmentation	Erythematous urticarial reticulated papular lesions
Triggers	Ramadan fasting	Strict dieting	No reported association
Treatment	Spontaneous resolution	Doxycycline 100mg po bid for 1 month	Doxycycline 100mg po bid for 1 month
Follow-up	No recurrences during 10 month follow up period	Excellent response within 2 weeks, no recurrences after stopping strict diets	Excellent response, no recurrences after treatment

3. Discussion

Prurigo pigmentosa continues to be described more frequently in Japanese patients, yet reports have emerged from other countries, albeit in much smaller numbers [3, 4, 6]. This might reflect underreporting or misdiagnosis rather than a genetic predilection for the Japanese population [3, 5, 8]. PP most commonly occurs in females in the third decade of life (range: 7-61 years) with a female-to-male ratio of 2-4:1 [3, 4, 9]. This is consistent with the findings in our report, where all patients were female with a mean age of 31 years.

Seasonal clustering is reported in the literature particularly in the spring and summer [3, 4], as in our cases. Reported cases were sporadic with no reported familial clustering [8].

PP is characterized by a sudden onset of pruritic and erythematous macules, urticarial papules, and plaques that may coalesce to form a reticulated pattern [4, 8–10]. Pustular and bullous variants have been reported [3, 4, 10]. Scales and crusts usually appear while the lesions are resolving [3, 4]. Complete resolution might take from one to several weeks [4, 10]. However, lesions typically heal with reticulated and mottled postinflammatory hyperpigmentation that usually persists for months [3, 4, 9, 10].

PP typically has a symmetrical distribution with a predilection for the nape of the neck, central chest, upper back, lumbosacral area, and abdomen [3–5, 11]. However, asymmetric patterns have been described including unilateral [12] and segmental [11] distributions. On the chest, the inter- and submammary areas are most frequently affected [3]. Involvement of the hair, nails, and mucous membranes has not been described [3, 8]. Recurrences are common in

the course of this disease and might occur months or years after initial presentation [8]. The three patients described in this report exhibited clinical features consistent with those described in the literature, with lesions of various stages of development noted at the time of presentation.

The aetiology of PP is not fully understood. However, endogenous and exogenous factors have been implicated including atopic diathesis, Sjogren's disease, and adult onset still's disease [3–5, 13].

A possible hormonal role has been hypothesized as worsening during pregnancy and menstruation has been reported [3, 5]. Multiple infectious agents such as *Helicobacter pylori* and *Borrelia spirochetes* may have associations with PP [3]. Possible aggravating exogenous factors include sweat, summer heat [4, 5], sun light [3, 5], physical trauma, friction [9, 12, 14], and contact allergens [3, 13]. Moreover, due to the recurrent nature of PP, a viral association has been postulated; however, this has not been confirmed [9].

More recently, the role of ketoacidosis in the pathogenesis of PP has gained momentum. This occurs with diabetes mellitus, fasting, dieting, anorexia nervosa, and following bariatric surgery, all of which are associated with PP [3–5, 9, 14]. Many studies documented a high level of ketones in the blood or urine [3, 7, 14]. Ketone bodies are thought to accumulate around blood vessels, leading to a predominantly neutrophilic inflammation [7]. The ketones subsequently enter the cells, leading to alterations in intracytoplasmic cellular processes [7]. In our report, patient 1 developed PP while fasting during Ramadan, while patient 2 was undertaking a strict diet. Unfortunately, ketone levels were not measured. In recent papers, PP cases associated with ketogenic diet were successfully treated with diet correction

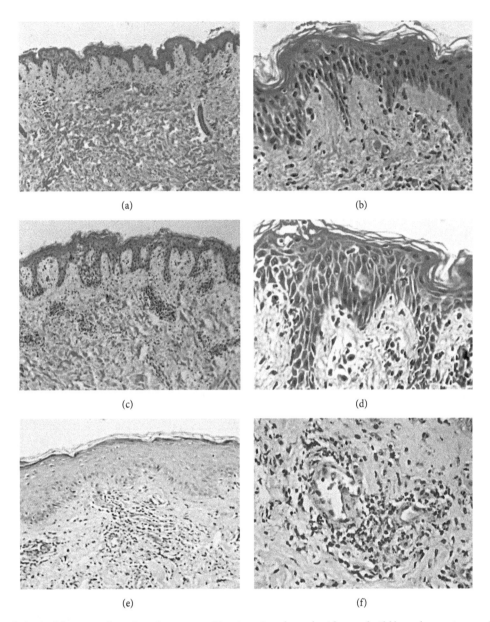

FIGURE 2: **Histopathological features of prurigo pigmentosa.** Biopsies taken showed evidence of mild hyperkeratosis, acanthosis, spongiosis, and mild superficial perivascular inflammatory cell infiltrate on low power in patient 1, patient 2, and patient 3 (a, c, and e, resp.), as well as dyskeratosis and hydropic degeneration of the basal cell layer, papillary dermal oedema, and superficial perivascular lymphoid cell infiltrate containing neutrophils and nuclear dust on high power. High power showed additional features of dyskeratotic hydropic degeneration of the basal cell layer, papillary dermal oedema, and superficial perivascular lymphoid cell infiltrate containing neutrophils and nuclear dust in patient 1, patient 2, and patient 3 (b, d, and f, resp.).

only [15]. In those cases, the efficacy of antibiotic therapy is probably due to the improvement on gut microbiome.

The histopathological features of PP can be nonspecific; however, distinct features exist for each stage of the disease [3–5, 7, 8]. The early stage is characterized by a superficial and perivascular dermal neutrophilic infiltrate along with papillary dermal edema, slight spongiosis, and neutrophilic exocytosis. The following stage, where lesions are fully developed, is characterized by a heavier dermal infiltrate in a lichenoid pattern. Lymphocytes usually predominate over neutrophils and the epidermis shows a variable degree of spongiosis, reticular degeneration of basal cell layer, and numerous necrotic keratinocytes. In the final resolution stage, a sparse lymphocytic dermal infiltrate is found along with upper dermal melanophages. The epidermis becomes hyperplastic with focal parakeratosis and few scattered necrotic keratinocytes. All our three cases showed similar histopathological features as seen in Figure 2. Boer *et al.* proposed that the histopathological changes of prurigo pigmentosa may be specific and transpire rapidly [16]. The histopathological features of our cases concur with this proposal. Therefore,

TABLE 2: The main histologic findings in 3 Jordanian patients with prurigo pigmentosa.

Lesion biopsied	Patient 1 Papulovesicular neck lesion	Patient 2 Erythematous papule on the back	Patient 3 Erythematous urticated plaque on the neck
Epidermal changes			
Orthokeratosis	+	+	+
Parakeratosis	−	−	−
Scale crust	−	+	−
Epidermal hyperplasia	+	+	+
Keratinocyte necrosis	+	+	+
Spongiosis	+	+	+
Vesiculation	−	−	−
Neutrophilic exocytosis	−	+	−
Basal cell vacuolization	+	+	+
Secondary impetiginization	−	−	−
Dermal changes			
Perivascular lymphocyte infiltrate	+	+	+
Perivascular polymorphonuclear infiltrate	+	+	+
Papillary dermal oedema	+	+	+
Pigment incontinence	−	−	−

the histopathological features of prurigo pigmentosa are diagnostic in the appropriate clinical setting.

Histological differential diagnoses include spongiotic dermatitis with secondary impetiginization, early guttate psoriasis, viral exanthem, and acute spongiotic dermatitis in the fully developed stage and postinflammatory hyperpigmentation and chronic spongiotic dermatitis in the late stage [3]. In addition, it has been suggested that both PP and confluent and reticulated papillomatosis of Geougerot and Carteaud lie on a spectrum of one disease [13]. Direct immunofluorescence studies have consistently been reported as either negative or nonspecific [3, 8, 11]. Direct immunofluorescence studies were only done for patients 1 and 2 and were negative.

In view of the largely nonspecific clinical features, the diagnosis of PP requires a high index of suspicion, as well as clinicopathological correlation. Clinical differential diagnoses include acute lupus erythematosus, dermatitis herpetiformis, linear immunoglobulin A disease, pigmented contact dermatitis, confluent and reticulated papillomatosis of Geougerot and Carteaud, Dowling-Degos disease, macular amyloidosis, and ashy dermatosis [3–5, 8].

Multiple therapeutic options exist for PP, yet tetracyclines remain the favoured option. This is thought to be related to their anti-inflammatory effect, particularly in the inhibition of neutrophil migration and function, matrix metalloprotease activity, and proinflammatory cytokine expression [3–5, 8, 10].

Other therapeutic options include macrolide antibiotics, dapsone, sulfamethoxazole, isotretinoin, and potassium iodide [3–5, 8–10, 14]. Corticosteroids and antihistamines have limited, if any, effect on PP [3, 5, 9], helping to differentiate PP from steroid-responsive dermatoses such as eczema.

The two patients who received doxycycline in this report had rapid clearance of the eruption. Patients were followed up for at least 6 months with maintained clearance. However, patients were advised about possible recurrence with future fasting or dieting, as well as other ketotic states.

To our knowledge, this is the first report of PP in Jordanian patients. The paucity of reports outside Japan is likely attributed to lack of awareness and misdiagnosis. Clinicopathological correlation is imperative in making this diagnosis as is the awareness of the possible triggering factors including ketoacidotic states such as fasting and strict diets.

Conflicts of Interest

The authors declare that they have no conflicts of interest.

References

[1] M. Nagashima, A. Ohshiro, and N. Schimuzu, "A peculiar pruriginous dermatosis with gross reticular pigmentation [in Japanese]," *The Japanese Journal of Dermatology*, pp. 81-38, 1971.

[2] M. Nagashima, "PRURIGO PIGMENTOSA: CLINICAL OBSERVATIONS OF OUR 14 CASES," *The Journal of Dermatology*, vol. 5, no. 2, pp. 61–67, 1978.

[3] M. Hijazi, J. Kehdy, A.-G. Kibbi, and S. Ghosn, "Prurigo pigmentosa: A clinicopathologic study of 4 cases from the

middle east," *American Journal of Dermatopathology*, vol. 36, no. 10, pp. 800–806, 2014.

[4] L. C. Gironi, P. Farinelli, A. Giacalone, and E. Colombo, "The efficacy of minocycline in inflammatory dermatoses: A case of prurigo pigmentosa of prepubescent onset in Western world," *Dermatologic Therapy*, vol. 28, no. 4, pp. 239–242, 2015.

[5] E. Satter, C. Rozelle, and L. Sperling, "Prurigo Pigmentosa: An under-recognized inflammatory dermatosis characterized by an evolution of distinctive clinicopathological features," *Journal of Cutaneous Pathology*, vol. 43, no. 10, pp. 809–814, 2016.

[6] T. J. De Sousa Vargas, C. M. Abreu Raposo, R. B. Lima, A. L. Sampaio, A. B. Bordin, and M. A. Jeunon Sousa, "Prurigo Pigmentosa-Report of 3 Cases from Brazil and Literature Review," *American Journal of Dermatopathology*, vol. 39, no. 4, pp. 267–274, 2017.

[7] A. Böer, N. Misago, M. Wolter, H. Kiryu, X. D. Wang, and A. B. Ackerman, "Prurigo pigmentosa: A distinctive inflammatory disease of the skin," *American Journal of Dermatopathology*, vol. 25, no. 2, pp. 117–129, 2003.

[8] S. B. Corley and P. M. Mauro, "Erythematous papules evolving into reticulated hyperpigmentation on the trunk: A case of prurigo pigmentosa," *JAAD Case Reports*, vol. 1, no. 2, pp. 60–62, 2015.

[9] J. D. Michaels, E. Hoss, D. J. Dicaudo, and H. Price, "Prurigo pigmentosa after a strict ketogenic diet," *Pediatric Dermatology*, vol. 32, no. 2, pp. 248–251, 2015.

[10] T. I. Kim, J. W. Choi, K.-H. Jeong, M. K. Shin, and M.-H. Lee, "Pustular prurigo pigmentosa treated with doxycycline," *The Journal of Dermatology*, vol. 43, no. 8, pp. 965-966, 2016.

[11] A. Torrelo, D. Azorín, L. Noguera, A. Hernández-Martín, R. Happle, and L. Requena, "Segmental prurigo pigmentosa," *Pediatric Dermatology*, vol. 31, no. 4, pp. 523–525, 2014.

[12] Y. Teraki and K. Hitomi, "Unilateral prurigo pigmentosa: A report of two cases," *The Journal of Dermatology*, vol. 43, no. 7, pp. 846-847, 2016.

[13] D. Ilkovitch and T. J. Patton, "Is prurigo pigmentosa an inflammatory version of confluent and reticulated papillomatosis?" *Journal of the American Academy of Dermatology*, vol. 69, no. 4, pp. e193–e195, 2013.

[14] M. Abbass, F. Abiad, and O. Abbas, "Prurigo pigmentosa after bariatric surgery," *JAMA Dermatology*, vol. 151, no. 7, pp. 796-797, 2015.

[15] MW. Maco, E. Lee, Y. Wu, and R. Lee, "Treatment of Prurigo Pigmentosa with Diet Modification: A Medical Case Study," *Hawaii Medical Journal*, vol. 77, pp. 114–117, 2018.

[16] A. Böer and A. B. Ackerman, "Prurigo pigmentosa is distinctive histopathologically," *International Journal of Dermatology*, vol. 42, no. 5, pp. 417-418, 2003.

Two Cases of Pachydermodactyly Presenting as Polyarthritis

Roxana Mititelu ⓘ,[1] Sarah Finch,[2] Paul Dancey ⓘ,[3] and Ian Landells ⓘ[4]

[1]*Department of Dermatology, McGill University Health Centre, Montreal, QC, Canada*
[2]*Department of Pathology, Memorial University, St. John's, NL, Canada*
[3]*Department of Rheumatology, Memorial University, St. John's, NL, Canada*
[4]*Department of Dermatology, Memorial University, St. John's, NL, Canada*

Correspondence should be addressed to Paul Dancey; paul.dancey@med.mun.ca

Academic Editor: Alireza Firooz

Pachydermodactyly is characterized by asymptomatic, progressive swelling of the lateral aspects of the 2nd to 4th finger along the proximal interphalangeal (PIP) joint without involving the joint itself. We present 2 interesting cases of patients with periarticular swelling who were initially diagnosed and treated as juvenile idiopathic arthritis (JIA) with subsequent clinical and pathology confirmation of pachydermodactyly. These cases emphasize the importance of considering pachydermodactyly in young patients with development of periarticular swelling and no joint involvement.

1. Introduction

Pachydermodactyly is a rare, benign, acquired digital fibromatosis characterized by asymptomatic, progressive swelling of periarticular soft tissues of the fingers without joint involvement. The diagnosis is usually made clinically; however, histopathology will demonstrate coarse collagen bundles and dermal mucin deposition. The etiology is believed to be mechanical trauma in most cases. Treatment is often not indicated given its benign prognosis.

2. Case Reports

2.1. Case 1. A 17-year-old young man was seen in the pediatric rheumatology clinic for investigation of presumed JIA polyarthritis affecting his hands. The patient described the gradual appearance of discrete "swellings" of his fingers beginning 5 years earlier, without pain, or significant physical limitations. He reported mild morning stiffness of short duration and fatigue in the hands after prolonged writing. He was otherwise well, and a review of systems was unremarkable. Prior to the rheumatology assessment, he was seen by his pediatrician who diagnosed JIA and initiated NSAID treatment. On physical exam, a nodular swelling was noted adjacent to the PIP and to a lesser extent the metacarpophalangeal (MCP) joints of both hands (Figure 1). There was minimal tenderness on palpation and range of motion was preserved.

The radiograph of the hands revealed soft tissue swelling concordant with the clinical presentation, but no joint space narrowing or erosions. Magnetic Resonance Imaging (MRI) with gadolinium of the hands did not reveal signs of synovitis. Complete blood count (CBC), antinuclear antibody (ANA), rheumatoid factor (RF), and inflammatory markers were all normal.

As the presentation was not typical for JIA, a biopsy of a nodule was performed to clarify the diagnosis. Histological examination revealed coarse dermal collagen bundles with perieccrine collagen deposition, increased fibroblasts, reduction in elastic fibers, and scant perivascular lymphocytic inflammation (Figure 2). Furthermore, alcian blue and colloidal iron confirmed increased dermal mucin deposition (Figure 3).

A diagnosis of pachydermodactyly was provided and dermatology was consulted for further management. During the subsequent 4 years, the patient remained well with no change in the condition. As the patient was concerned about the appearance of his hands, a trial of hydroxychloroquine

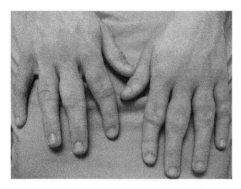

FIGURE 1: Periarticular nodules involving mainly the PIP joints of the 2nd to 4th finger of both hands.

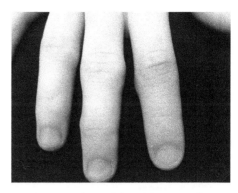

FIGURE 4: Periarticular nodules of the PIP and DIP joints.

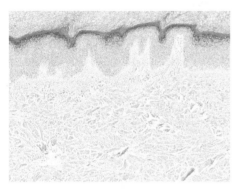

FIGURE 2: Histological examination revealed coarse dermal collagen bundles with perieccrine collagen deposition, increased fibroblasts, reduction in elastic fibers, and scant perivascular lymphocytic inflammation (hematoxylin-eosin stain; original magnification ×10).

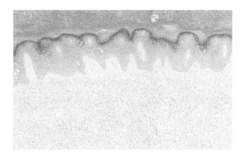

FIGURE 5: Histology examination showed increased collagen bundles, increased fibroblasts, reduction in elastic fibers, and scant perivascular lymphocytic inflammation (hematoxylin-eosin stain; original magnification ×4).

FIGURE 3: Alcian blue stain showing increased dermal mucin deposition (Alcian blue; original magnification ×10).

was then initiated, but discontinued after 1 month due to a side effect of vertigo. One year later, he remained well with no change in the condition.

2.2. Case 2. A 14-year-old girl was referred to pediatric rheumatology for investigation of a one-year history of "joint swelling" of the fingers in her right hand. She described some mild discomfort when opening and closing her hand, but no morning stiffness or other physical limitations. She had occasional arthralgia of her knees with activity, but was otherwise well, and a review of systems was unremarkable.

There was a significant family history of rheumatoid arthritis. Physical exam revealed a nodular prominence, with mild tenderness, in the area of her PIP and DIP joints of the right hand (Figure 4). She had limited active but normal passive flexion of the fingers. The remainder of the musculoskeletal exam and general physical was normal.

Investigations including CBC, ANA, RF, thyroid testing, and inflammatory markers were all normal. The radiograph of the right hand revealed soft tissue swelling, but no joint space narrowing or erosions. A subsequent MRI with gadolinium of the hands was of poor quality due to motion artifact, but was reported as showing possible synovitis, resulting in a preliminary diagnosis of polyarticular JIA. The patient was then started on a NSAID and methotrexate therapy.

Despite six months of treatment, she reported no change in her symptoms or the appearance of her hand, prompting reconsideration of the arthritis diagnosis. Subsequently, a biopsy of one of the nodules was performed. Histology showed increased mucin deposition in the full thickness of the dermis, strongly positive for alcian blue and colloidal iron staining (Figures 5 and 6). There was also evidence of increased collagen bundles, increased fibroblasts, reduction in elastic fibers, and scant perivascular lymphocytic inflammation. The patient was then referred to dermatology for the management of pachydermodactyly. Given the patient's concern about the appearance of her hands, she was offered treatment with hydroxychloroquine. After 6 months

FIGURE 6: Alcian blue stain showed increased mucin deposition in the full thickness of the dermis (Alcian blue; original magnification ×10).

of therapy, her lesions were showing mild improvement but nevertheless persisting. The patient chose to stop further treatment.

3. Discussion

Pachydermodactyly is an uncommon type of digital fibromatosis. Typically, it presents in adolescent boys as swelling of the soft tissue involving the lateral aspects of the PIP joints particularly of the second to the fourth fingers. Involvement of other joints including the DIP and the MCP, consistent with our patients' clinical appearance, has also been described [1]. In certain cases, the disorder is hypothesized to be related to mechanical trauma. In a review of pachydermodactyly, mechanical trauma was found to be a precipitant factor in 44% of patients. Activities which have been implicated include martial arts, rock climbing, and repetitive labour [1]. The histopathology is characterized by hyperkeratosis and acanthosis of the epidermis [2]. The dermis is characterized by coarse collagen bundles with an increase in fibroblasts [2]. There can also be mucin deposition of varying degrees in the interstitium and decreased elastic fibers [2].

The treatment of this condition is not well-defined and few studies examining treatment options have been published. Elimination of mechanical stimulation with occupational therapy has been shown to be helpful [1]. Oral tranilast, intralesional triamcinolone injection, and surgical excision have been used with benefit in some cases [3–5]. Interestingly, in other forms of fibromatoses, such as Dupuytren's contracture, injectable collagenase has been shown to be promising with a response rate of 45–65% [6].

Here, we have described 2 additional cases, who were initially referred for possible JIA prior to clinical and histopathological confirmation of pachydermodactyly. JIA is also a relatively rare condition in which rheumatoid nodules may develop over MCP and PIP joints in polyarticular disease. A key distinguishing feature is joint involvement in JIA. Other differential diagnoses include self-healing juvenile cutaneous mucinosis and acral persistent papular mucinosis. Self-healing juvenile cutaneous mucinosis is less likely given the lesions persisted in our patients. While acral persistent papular mucinosis has similar histopathologic findings, the primary skin lesions are papules rather than the nodules seen

in our patients. While milder cases of pachydermodactyly can be observed and patients can be counselled to avoid any possible aggravating factors, both patients were concerned about the appearance of their hands. Consequently, we proposed treatment with hydroxychloroquine given its anti-inflammatory and antiproliferative actions. As the pathogenesis of pachydermodactyly is driven by fibroblastic proliferation and resultant collagen deposition, we feel there is some rationale to this approach [1]. One of our patients showed some improvement of the lesions during a 6-month course of hydroxychloroquine before stopping. Ideally a longer follow-up will be needed to determine the outcome and possible effectiveness of this treatment approach.

4. Conclusion

Pachydermodactyly is a rare condition which can mimic the appearance of arthritis. Careful attention to the physical exam, particularly to distinguish between an intra-articular and a cutaneous process, is important to facilitate arrival at the correct diagnosis and avoid potentially unnecessary investigations. More research is needed to determine the optimal treatment choice for this rare condition.

Conflicts of Interest

The authors declare no conflicts of interest regarding the publication of this paper.

References

[1] T. Dallos, B. Oppl, L. Kovács, and J. Zwerina, "Pachydermodactyly: a review," *Current Rheumatology Reports*, vol. 16, no. 9, p. 442, 2014.

[2] W. P. James and A. H. Hosler, "Pachydermodactyly," in *Weedons Skin Pathology*, Churchill Livingstone Elsevier, Edinburgh, Scotland, 4th edition, 2016.

[3] A. Plana Pla, J. Bassas Vila, M. A. Toro Montecinos, and C. Ferrandiz Foraster, "Pachydermodactyly successfully treated with triamcinolone injections," *Actas Dermo-Sifiliográficas*, vol. 105, no. 3, pp. 319–321, 2014.

[4] T. B. Fleeter, C. Myrie, and J. P. Adams, "Pachydermodactyly: A case report and discussion of the pathologic entity," *Journal of Hand Surgery*, vol. 9, no. 5, pp. 764–766, 1984.

[5] C. Higuchi, T. Tomita, and H. Yoshikawa, "Pachydermodactyly treated with tranilast in a young girl," *Case Reports in Orthopedics*, vol. 2014, Article ID 132854, 4 pages, 2014.

[6] S. S. Desai and V. R. Hentz, "The treatment of Dupuytren disease," *Journal of Hand Surgery*, vol. 36, no. 5, pp. 936–942, 2011.

Protein C Deficiency Caused by a Novel Mutation in the *PROC* Gene in an Infant with Delayed Onset Purpura Fulminans

Mariam S. Al Harbi[1] and Ayman W. El-Hattab[2]

[1]*Department of Pediatrics, Tawam Hospital, P.O. Box 15258, Al-Ain, UAE*
[2]*Division of Clinical Genetic and Metabolic Disorders, Tawam Hospital, P.O. Box 15258, Al-Ain, UAE*

Correspondence should be addressed to Ayman W. El-Hattab; elhattabaw@yahoo.com

Academic Editor: Alireza Firooz

Protein C is an anticoagulant that is encoded by the *PROC* gene. Protein C deficiency (PCD) is inherited in an autosomal dominant or recessive pattern. Autosomal dominant PCD is caused by monoallelic mutations in *PROC* and often presents with venous thromboembolism. On the other hand, biallelic *PROC* mutations lead to autosomal recessive PCD which is a more severe disease that typically presents in neonates as purpura fulminans. In this report, we describe an 8-month-old infant with autosomal recessive PCD who presented with multiple lumps on his lower extremities at the age of 2 months and later developed purpura fulminans after obtaining a muscle biopsy from the thigh at the age of 5 months. Protein C level was less than 10% and *PROC* gene sequencing identified a novel homozygous missense mutation, c.1198G>A (p.Gly400Ser). Autosomal recessive PCD typically presents with neonatal purpura fulminans which is often fatal if not recognized and treated early. Therefore, early recognition is critical in preventing morbidity and mortality associated with autosomal recessive PCD.

1. Introduction

Protein C, a vitamin K-dependent factor synthesized in the liver, plays a significant role in regulating the coagulation cascade. It circulates as a zymogen and exerts its anticoagulant function after being activated on endothelial surfaces following binding to the endothelial protein C receptor. The inhibitory effect of activated protein C is enhanced by protein S. Protein C primarily inactivates factors V and VIII, hence preventing thrombin generation and thrombosis formation. *PROC*, the gene encoding protein C, is located on chromosome 2q14.3 and contains 9 exons [1].

Similar to other inherited thrombophilias, a deficiency in protein C can predispose to thrombosis. Protein C deficiency (PCD) can be classified into type I, where there is a decrease in protein C concentration, and type II, where there is a decreased activity with normal level of protein C. Type I deficiency results from defective synthesis or secretion of the protein, whereas type II results from impaired binding to substrate, calcium, or receptor. Type I deficiency is the most common type, whereas type II accounts for 10–15% of cases [2].

PCD can be an autosomal dominant or recessive disease. Autosomal dominant PCD is caused by heterozygous (monoallelic) mutations in *PROC* and has an incidence of 1 in 200–500. Individuals with this form have a plasma protein C level around 50% of normal values. Affected individuals with autosomal dominant PCD are typically asymptomatic; however, some may develop venous thromboembolism during childhood or later as young adults [1]. Biallelic (homozygous or compound heterozygous) *PROC* mutations lead to the autosomal recessive PCD which occurs in 1 in 40,000–250,000 individuals. Autosomal recessive PCD, which is more severe than autosomal dominant PCD, is associated with very low level of protein C and typically presents in neonatal period with neonatal purpura fulminans [3].

Herein, we describe an infant who presented with delayed onset purpura fulminans and was found to have autosomal recessive PCD caused by a novel homozygous *PROC* mutation.

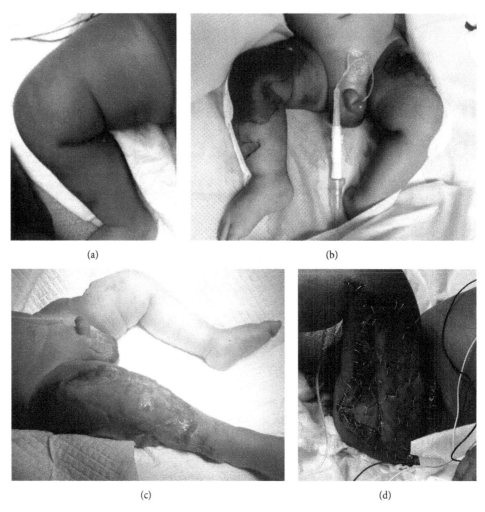

(a)

(b)

(c)

(d)

FIGURE 1: Skin changes at various stages: (a) on the 6th day of hospitalization showing discoloration after the muscle biopsy; (b) on the 8th day of hospitalization showing hemorrhagic necrosis; (c) on the 12th day of hospitalization after fasciotomy and debridement; (d) on the 12th day showing Integra application.

2. Case Presentation

An 8-month-old male infant developed a perianal mass during the first week of life which was treated as an abscess. The infant at that time had a full septic work-up that was negative and it was decided to treat him conservatively with antibiotic without incision and drainage. At the age of 2 months, he started having recurrent subcutaneous lumps on the lower extremities. At 5 months of age, he was provisionally diagnosed to have panniculitis and was hospitalized at that time for a muscle biopsy from the right thigh to confirm the diagnosis of panniculitis and evaluate other possible etiologies. After the muscle biopsy, he developed rapidly progressive bluish discolorations and indurations in the upper thighs which extended to the buttocks and scrotum over a period of 2 days (Figure 1(a)). The skin lesions progressed to hemorrhagic necrosis on the 8th day of hospitalization (Figure 1(b)). When the hemorrhagic necrosis developed, purpura fulminans was considered and protein C deficiency was suspected. He was started on regular fresh frozen plasma transfusion and later started on protein C

concentrate and low-molecular-weight heparin. His course was complicated by compartment syndrome that required bilateral lower extremity fasciotomy followed by extensive debridement with artificial dermis (Integra®) application (Figures 1(c) and 1(d)). Additionally, he developed anemia requiring multiple blood transfusions, thrombocytopenia, consumptive coagulopathy (prolonged prothrombin time (PT), activated partial thromboplastin time (aPTT), and low fibrinogen), and fibrinolysis (increased D-dimer) which were consistent with disseminated intravascular coagulation (DIC). His illness was further complicated by Gram-negative sepsis (Klebsiella oxytoca and Enterobacter cloacae), hypertension, and respiratory failure requiring ventilatory support. The infant was hospitalized for 3 months during which he gradually improved while receiving protein C concentrate. He was transferred to another facility for further care and skin grafting at the age of 8 months.

His growth parameters were appropriate for the age. His parents were cousins and they had 6 other older children who were reportedly healthy and there was no family history of any hematological diseases.

Protein C level was found to be very low (less than 10%, normal: 68–143%) consistent with autosomal recessive PCD. The *PROC* gene was sequenced at PreventionGenetics LLC, Marshfield, Wisconsin, USA, and a novel homozygous missense mutation (c.1198G>A; p.Gly400Ser) was identified, confirming the diagnosis of autosomal recessive PCD. Protein C level was 56% in the mother and 73% in the father (normal: 68–143%), suggesting that both parents are carriers and have autosomal dominant PCD. Genetic testing showed that both parents are heterozygous for the p.Gly400Ser mutation in *PROC*, confirming the diagnosis of autosomal dominant PCD in both parents. Both parents were healthy with no history suggestive of thrombophilia.

3. Discussion

Purpura fulminans describes microvascular thrombosis associated with DIC and perivascular hemorrhage. It usually presents with cutaneous purpuric lesions that start as dark-red and then become purple-black indurated lesions. It occurs at sites of previous traumas like intravenous cannula sites. There is a predilection to limbs but the lesions can also occur on the buttocks and thighs. With time, these lesions become gangrenous and can result in the loss of extremities. There are both congenital and acquired causes of purpura fulminans. Inherited causes are due to an autosomal recessive PCD or protein S deficiency [4]. Acquired causes are more common and are often associated with severe infections causing a consumptive coagulopathy and a relative deficiency of protein C and/or S. The clinical severity may vary depending on the underlying cause; however, the condition is often fatal if not recognized and treated early. The onset of symptoms in severe congenital causes is usually within the first days of life [5].

The suspicion of PCD in the infant presented here appeared after the infant developed severe hemorrhagic necrotic skin lesions and DIC consistent with purpura fulminans. The skin lesions in purpura fulminans usually start after a trauma. In the infant described here, the muscle biopsy was the trauma that precipitated the development of purpura fulminans. Although purpura fulminans due to severe congenital causes usually occurs within the first few days of life, infants presenting with a delayed onset purpura fulminans, between 6 and 12 months of age, were reported [6, 7]. The infant in this report had a delayed purpura fulminans which appeared at the age of 5 months. Purpura fulminans is often fatal if not recognized and treated early [5]. The clinical presentation of hemorrhagic skin necrosis and DIC in the infant reported here raised the suspicion of this condition and treatment was immediately started. Early recognition is critical in preventing morbidity and mortality associated with this disease.

Individuals with autosomal recessive PCD carry biallelic *PROC* mutations and have very low level of protein C, whereas individuals carrying heterozygous *PROC* mutations have protein C level at about 50% of reference values [1]. The infant in this report had very low protein C level consistent with autosomal recessive PCD and his parents exhibited low protein C levels consistent with heterozygous carrier status.

Molecular studies have further confirmed the diagnosis as the affected infant was found to have a homozygous mutation in the *PROC* gene and both parents were found to be heterozygous for this mutation. The identified *PROC* novel mutation c.1198G>A (p.Gly400Ser) was not previously reported. This mutation is located in a highly conserved region of the enzyme and the amino acid substitution prediction programs (PolyPhen-2, SIFT, and MutationTaster) predicted that this variant is deleterious. These *in silico* data along with the biochemical and clinical phenotypes support that p.Gly400Ser is indeed a disease causing mutation that is responsible for PCD in this infant.

In conclusion, the classic presentation of autosomal recessive PCD is neonatal purpura fulminans. Early recognition is critical in preventing morbidity and mortality associated with autosomal recessive PCD. Although the identified p.Gly400Ser mutation in *PROC* was not previously reported, its pathogenicity is supported by different *in silico* prediction programs and the biochemical and clinical phenotypes that are consistent with autosomal recessive PCD. Therefore, p.Gly400Ser in *PROC* is a novel mutation causing autosomal recessive PCD that presented in this infant with late onset purpura fulminans.

Conflicts of Interest

The authors declare that there are no conflicts of interest regarding the publication of this paper.

References

[1] P. C. Cooper, M. Hill, and R. M. Maclean, "The phenotypic and genetic assessment of protein C deficiency," *International Journal of Laboratory Hematology*, vol. 34, no. 4, pp. 336–346, 2012.

[2] K. B. Kovács, I. Pataki, H. Bárdos et al., "Molecular characterization of p.Asp77Gly and the novel p.Ala163Val and p.Ala163Glu mutations causing protein C deficiency," *Thrombosis Research*, vol. 135, no. 4, pp. 718–726, 2015.

[3] E. Chalmers, P. Cooper, K. Forman et al., "Purpura fulminans: recognition, diagnosis and management," *Archives of Disease in Childhood*, vol. 96, no. 11, pp. 1066–1071, 2011.

[4] V. E. Price, D. L. Ledingham, A. Krümpel, and A. K. Chan, "Diagnosis and management of neonatal purpura fulminans," *Seminars in Fetal and Neonatal Medicine*, vol. 16, no. 6, pp. 318–322, 2011.

[5] Y. Dogan, D. Aygun, Y. Yilmaz et al., "Severe protein S deficiency associated with heterozygous factor V Leiden mutation in a child with purpura fulminans," *Pediatric Hematology and Oncology*, vol. 20, no. 1, pp. 1–5, 2003.

[6] E. G. Tuddenham, T. Takase, A. E. Thomas et al., "Homozygous protein C deficiency with delayed onset of symptoms at 7 to 10 months," *Thrombosis Research*, vol. 53, no. 5, pp. 475–484, 1989.

[7] R. A. Marlar, R. R. Montgomery, A. W. Broekmans, and the Working Party, "Diagnosis and treatment of homozygous protein C deficiency. Report of the working party on homozygous protein C deficiency of the subcommittee on protein C and protein S, international committee on thrombosis and haemostasis," *The Journal of Pediatrics*, vol. 114, no. 4, pp. 528–534, 1989.

7

Sporotrichoid-Like Spread of Cutaneous *Mycobacterium chelonae* in an Immunocompromised Patient

Daria Marley Kemp,[1] Anusha G. Govind,[2] Jun Kang,[1]
Caroline C. Brugger,[2] and Young C. Kauh[1]

[1]Department of Dermatology and Cutaneous Biology, Thomas Jefferson University, Philadelphia, PA, USA
[2]Department of Infectious Disease, Thomas Jefferson University, Philadelphia, PA, USA

Correspondence should be addressed to Anusha G. Govind; anusha.govind@jefferson.edu

Academic Editor: Kowichi Jimbow

Mycobacterium chelonae is a rapidly growing mycobacterium found in water and soil that can cause local cutaneous infections in immunocompetent hosts but more frequently affects immunocompromised patients. Typically, patients will present with painful subcutaneous nodules of the joints or soft tissues from traumatic inoculation. However, exhibiting a sporotrichoid-like pattern of these nodules is uncommon. Herein, we report a case of sporotrichoid-like distribution of cutaneous *Mycobacterium chelonae* in a patient with systemic lupus erythematosus on significant immunosuppressive medications. Clinicians treating immunocompromised patients should be cognizant of their propensity to develop unusual infections and atypical presentations.

1. Case Presentation

A 54-year-old female, with a history of systemic lupus erythematosus on mycophenolate mofetil (3 g daily), prednisone (10 mg daily), and cyclosporine (50 mg twice a day), presented with a 4-month duration of unilateral painful well-circumscribed erythematous to violaceous subcutaneous nodules extending from her 2nd finger web space to her dorsal wrist and forearm in a sporotrichoid-like pattern (Figure 1(a)). She denied exposure to fish tanks, swimming pools, tattoo needles, gardening, fresh or brackish waters, or nail salons.

Dorsal wrist nodule biopsy revealed suppurative granulomatous inflammation (Figures 2(a) and 2(b)). Both acid-fast bacilli (AFB) and Fite's acid-fast stains (Figure 2(c)) showed bacilli in the dermis, consistent with a mycobacterial infection. AFB culture and stain were positive for the rapid grower, *Mycobacterium chelonae*. Initially, she was started on dual antibiotic regimen of linezolid 600 mg twice daily and azithromycin 250 mg daily. Subsequently, she was converted to linezolid 600 mg and clarithromycin 250 mg twice daily once susceptibilities returned and also due to gastrointestinal

upset from azithromycin. Although the patient had no adverse reaction to linezolid, the dose was decreased to 600 mg daily to ensure tolerability and continued normal blood counts. Given her active infection, rheumatology decreased her mycophenolate mofetil dose and discontinued cyclosporine. Improvement of her skin lesions was evident on follow-up within three months (Figure 1(b)). At four months, her nodules had fully resolved and therapy was discontinued.

2. Discussion

Mycobacterium chelonae is a rapidly growing mycobacterium commonly found in water and soil. The name *chelonae* is derived from the Greek word for turtle, chelōnē, as it was initially isolated in 1903 from sea turtles [1]. It can cause local cutaneous infections in immunocompetent patients, but infections are more frequently identified in patients taking immunosuppressive medications. Patients can develop painful subcutaneous nodules involving joints or soft tissue [2]. These skin nodules, as well as deeper and more disseminated infections, are usually from traumatic introduction. However, preceding trauma may not always be

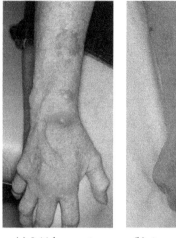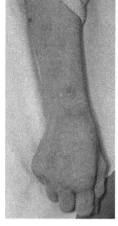

(a) Initial encounter   (b) 4-month follow-up

FIGURE 1: Clinical photos.

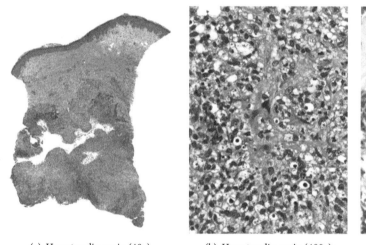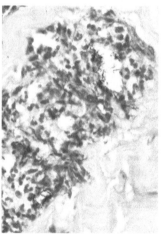

(a) Hematoxylin-eosin (40x)   (b) Hematoxylin-eosin (400x)   (c) Fite's acid-fast stain (400x)

FIGURE 2: Pathologic findings from a right wrist skin nodule: suppurative granulomatous dermatitis in deep dermis (a & b) and numerous acid-fast bacilli highlighted by Fite's acid-fast stain (c).

readily apparent. Sporotrichoid spread is a linear ascending extension along lymphatic chains, generally found with deep fungal infections but can also be present in other organisms. [3]. In 1992, Wallace et al. presented a series of 53 cases of *M. chelonae* disseminated cutaneous infections (>5 lesions), which were either well-circumscribed lesions or a "confluent mass of cellulitis with multiple draining fistulas." They were generally at the distal end of an extremity but did not form a linear or sporotrichoid pattern [4]. Differential diagnosis for skin nodules in a sporotrichoid-spread pattern includes *Sporothrix schenckii*, *M. marinum*, other nontuberculous mycobacteria, *Nocardia*, *Leishmania*, and Tularemia [5].

Clinical presentation of *Mycobacterium chelonae* is often influenced by the immunological status of the patient. Approximately 10 cases have been described in the literature with a sporotrichoid-like pattern of *M. chelonae* involving an immunosuppressed patient [1, 3, 5–10] and at least two cases

in a presumably immunocompetent patient [11]. Mycobacteria are referred to as AFB for the complex that forms during the histological staining process between the mycolic acid in the mycobacterial cell wall and dye, which is resistant to the decolorizing mineral acid. Compared to classic AFB staining, Fite's acid-fast stain uses a milder destaining acid, as well as less alcohol during the staining process, which it suitable for more delicate mycobacterium, such as *leprosy bacillus* [12].

Although clarithromycin was initially the drug of choice in treatment, increasing drug resistance makes it an unsuitable single agent. Treatment generally involves two antibacterial agents, particularly in immunocompromised patients. Linezolid has been shown to be an effective second medication; however, its adverse effects of bone marrow suppression warrant close monitoring [2]. Once daily dosing of linezolid 600 mg has demonstrated a potential benefit of decreasing the risk of toxicity over a prolonged course of treatment.

However, a recent retrospective study found that the efficacy and safety profile of linezolid 600 mg once daily and 300 mg once daily in the treatment of multidrug and extensively drug-resistant tuberculosis showed potentially fewer neurotoxicities than a lower dose of linezolid [13].

Given the large number of immunocompromised patients clinicians serve, one must be mindful of their increased susceptibility to unusual infections and atypical presentations. It is vital that patients with suspicious sporotrichoid cutaneous lesions should have a biopsy with routine bacterial culture, mycobacterial culture, fungal culture, prolonged culture hold, molecular testing for *Nocardia*, and pathology. Only a few literature cases reported of *M. chelonae* present with sporotrichoid-like spread, typically in immunocompromised patients.

Abbreviations and Acronyms

AFB: Acid-fast bacilli
M. chelonae: *Mycobacterium chelonae*
M. marinum: *Mycobacterium marinum*.

Disclosure

This case has been presented at the 2017 AAD Annual Meeting Gross & Microscopic Symposium on Saturday, March 4, 2017.

Conflicts of Interest

The authors declare that there are no conflicts of interest regarding the publication of this paper.

Acknowledgments

Jason B. Lee, M.D., Department of Dermatology and Cutaneous Biology, Thomas Jefferson University Hospital, provided the histopathological photos.

References

[1] E. Orrin, F. Worsnop, and J. Natkunarajah, "Sporotrichoid *Mycobacterium chelonae*," *Australasian Journal of Dermatology*, vol. 57, no. 3, pp. 244-245, 2016.

[2] P. Parize, A. Hamelin, N. Veziris et al., "Induction therapy with linezolid/clarithromycin combination for *Mycobacterium chelonae* skin infections in immunocompromised hosts," *Journal of the European Academy of Dermatology and Venereology*, vol. 30, no. 1, pp. 101–105, 2016.

[3] E. M. Higgins and C. M. Lawrence, "Sporotrichoid spread of *Mycobacterium chelonei*," *Clinical and Experimental Dermatology*, vol. 13, pp. 234–236, 1988.

[4] R. J. Wallace, B. A. Brown, and G. O. Onyi, "Skin, soft tissue, and bone infections due to *Mycobacterium chelonae* chelonae: importance of prior corticosteroid therapy, frequency of disseminated infections, and resistance to oral antimicrobials other than clarithromycin," *Journal of Infectious Diseases*, vol. 166, no. 2, pp. 405–412, 1992.

[5] M. N. Schwendiman, R. P. Johnson, and J. S. Henning, "Subcutaneous nodules with sporotrichoid spread," *Dermatology Online JournaL*, vol. 15, no. 5, p. 11, 2009.

[6] T. Demitsu, H. Nagato, T. Inoue et al., "Cutaneous *Mycobacterium chelonae* infection with bilateral sporotrichoid involvement," *International Journal of Dermatology*, vol. 40, no. 9, pp. 597–599, 2001.

[7] W. Godard, N. Cordier, A. Kazmierczak, and D. Lambert, "Sporotrichosis-like skin infection caused by *Mycobacterium chelonei* and cured by minocycline," *Presse Medicale*, vol. 15, no. 3, p. 120, 1986.

[8] K. E. Greer, G. P. Gross, and S. H. Martensen, "Sporotrichoid Cutaneous Infection due to *Mycobacterium chelonei*," *Archives of Dermatology*, vol. 115, no. 6, pp. 738-739, 1979.

[9] A. G. Jopp-McKay and P. Randell, "Sporotrichoid cutaneous infection due to *Mycobacterium chelonei* in a renal transplant patient," *Australasian Journal of Dermatology*, vol. 31, no. 2, pp. 105–109, 1990.

[10] M. E. Murdoch and I. M. Leigh, "Sporotrichoid spread of cutaneous *Mycobacterium chelonei* infection," *Clinical and Experimental Dermatology*, vol. 14, pp. 309–312, 1989.

[11] E. Rosón, I. García-Doval, A. De la Torre, A. Losada, C. Feal, and M. Cruces, "Sporotrichoid spread of *Mycobacterium chelonae* in a presumably immunocompetent patient," *Acta Dermato-Venereologica*, vol. 82, no. 2, pp. 142-143, 2002.

[12] N. Wengenack, Mycobacteria part 1: Stains and culture. Mayo Medical Laboratories, http://www.mayomedicallaboratories.com/articles/hot-topic/2014/10-15-mycobacteria-pt-1/index.html.

[13] W.-J. Koh, Y. R. Kang, K. Jeon et al., "Daily 300 mg dose of linezolid for multidrug-resistant and extensively drug-resistant tuberculosis: Updated analysis of 51 patients," *Journal of Antimicrobial Chemotherapy*, vol. 67, no. 6, Article ID dks078, pp. 1503–1507, 2012.

8

Palliative Radiotherapy for Disfiguring Mycosis Fungoides Lesion: A Key Treatment to Reduce Psychological and Social Impact

Axel Egal [ID],[1] Caroline Ram-Wolf,[2] Laurent Quero,[3] Martine Bagot,[2] Marie-Dominique Vignon-Pennamen,[4] Christophe Hennequin,[3] and Basma M'Barek[1,3]

[1]Department of Radiotherapy, Montfermeil Hospital, France
[2]Department of Dermatology, Saint Louis Hospital, AP-HP, Paris, France
[3]Department of Radiotherapy, Saint Louis Hospital, AP-HP, Paris, France
[4]Department of Pathology, Saint Louis Hospital, AP-HP, Paris, France

Correspondence should be addressed to Axel Egal; axelegal1@hotmail.com

Academic Editor: Ioannis D. Bassukas

Mycosis Fungoides (MF) is a rare disease with a relatively good prognosis at early stage. However, skin lesions can impair quality of life due to extensive skin lesions. In some cases, skin lesions, and especially those of the face, become visible and change the physical appearance of the patients. This aspect can deeply affect patients psychologically and can impact their social life. Here, we report the case of a patient with multiple lesions including a disfiguring lesion arising from the nose. The extent of his skin lesions gave a palliative intent to his treatment project. The patient underwent several lines of chemotherapy and immunotherapy with poor results. He was then referred to our radiotherapy and received localized radiotherapy. Lesions disappeared completely within a few weeks. The patient reported a psychological relief. This case highlights the fact that radiotherapy can be done in a "palliative" intent in order to improve esthetic aspects of lesions that can dramatically impact the psychosocial side of patient's life. Clinicians can consider radiotherapy as treatment of some MF lesions as far as they impair the patient's comfort from a psychological and social point of view.

1. Introduction

Mycosis Fungoides (MF) is the most common form of cutaneous T-cell lymphoma. It typically affects patients with a median age of 55 to 60 years, mostly men [1]. The disease is traditionally indolent at early stage and progresses slowly. However, both folliculotropic variant and large cell transformation are known to have worse outcomes.

Skin involvement is classically presenting as pruritic erythematous patches in nonsun exposed areas that can evolve toward infiltrative plaques and tumors. Overall survival is usually very good at early stage with reported rates of 5-year survival approaching 90% [2] and thus treatment is primarily determined by disease extent and impact on quality of life. Multiple treatments exist for early MF such as topical corticosteroids, topical chlormethine, or phototherapy [3]. In case of extensive or more aggressive disease, systemic treatments can be introduced such as retinoids, interferon, methotrexate, histone deacetylase inhibitors, monoclonal antibodies, systemic chemotherapy, total skin electron beam therapy (TSEBT), and sometimes even allogeneic stem cell transplantation [4, 5]. Local radiation therapy may be useful in selected patients with localized infiltrative and/or ulcerating cutaneous lesions. Complete and long-lasting response rates reported in the literature are often higher than 90 percent [6–9]. Several treatment schedules are possible with multifractionated doses being the most used. At the opposite, low-dose radiation with a single or 2 fractions of 7 or 8 Gy are also possible [8, 10]. Compared to TSEBT, local radiotherapy presents less toxicities and better tolerance [11].

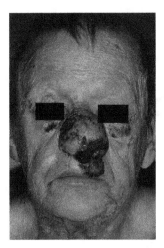

FIGURE 1: Exophytic lesion of the nose before radiotherapy (front view).

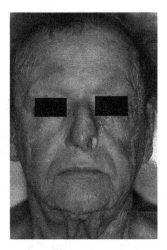

FIGURE 3: Aspect after radiotherapy (front view).

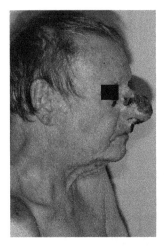

FIGURE 2: Exophytic lesion of the nose before radiotherapy (side view).

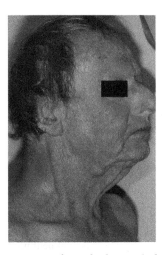

FIGURE 4: Aspect after radiotherapy (side view).

2. Case Report

A Folliculotropic Mycosis Fungoides was diagnosed in a 58-year-old male patient in 1997 and treated with local chlormethine between 1998 and 2006.

In 2006, MF progressed toward a tumoral form with infiltrating plaques and nodules all over his body, the most important being an exophytic one arising from the nasal region. No Sezary cell was noted in the blood smear. A biopsy of cutaneous tumor was performed and the pathologist confirmed a localization of tumoral nontransformed MF.

Between 2006 and 2014 the patient received several systemic treatment lines including methotrexate, PUVA therapy, pegylated liposomal doxorubicin, polychemotherapy, histone deacetylase inhibitors, and anti-CCR4 monoclonal antibody. All these drugs were without long-lasting effect and tumoral lesions progressed including the tumoral lesion of the nose (Figures 1 and 2).

The extent, progression, and resistance of his skin lesions gave a palliative intent to his treatment project. The patient reported that the aspect of his nose refrained him from interacting with people, which led him progressively to get socially isolated. He reported difficulties in interacting with his family members especially with his young grandchildren. Histology from the nasal lesion was obtained and showed classical Mycosis Fungoides of granulomatous type without transformation.

He was then referred to our radiotherapy unit in August 2014. We opted for a conventional radiotherapy with 12 MeV electrons and 6 MV and 18 MV photons. The patient received 36 Gy in 18 fractions (2 Gy per fraction, 5 fractions per week).

Lesions disappeared completely within a few weeks (Figures 3 and 4). The patient presented acute grade I radiodermatitis (NCI CTCAE Version 4.03) which resolved spontaneously. No clinical relapse had been noted 3 years after the treatment.

As the physical appearance of the irradiated nose got better the patient reported a psychological relief. The recovery of the normal aspect of his nose helped him resume some of his social activities, use public transportation, and better interact with friends and family members.

3. Discussion

Radiotherapy is a highly effective treatment option of MF, which can lead to excellent response rates when used in both curative and palliative intent. The high radio sensitivity of the MF lesions makes this treatment option possible in palliative intent because of the limited treatment options. The international lymphoma radiation group as well as the European Organization for Research and Treatment of Cancer (EORTC) includes radiotherapy as a key treatment option in both curative and palliative intent for MF skin lesions [11, 12].

This patient's case report highlights the fact that radiotherapy can also be done in a "palliative" intent, in order to improve quality of life in its psychological and social dimension. Lesions of the uncovered skin, especially lesions located on the face, may impact the patient's social life. Taking into account the psychological and social impacts of the disease is important. Radiotherapy can be of great help as it comes to improve the local aspect of the skin lesions. Indeed, most of the skin lesions have an excellent response rate to radiotherapy even if in the literature, lower responses rate are common in transformed MF and/or in lesions associated with poor circulation and wound healing located on the lower extremities. Moreover, radio-sensitizing agents, such as histone deacetylase inhibitors, are thought to work synergistically with low-dose local radiation therapy [13, 14].

Required dose varies with the intent of the treatment and tends to be more important in isolated unique lesion of MF. It has been reported a dose-dependent response with better local control with delivered doses around 30 Gy [7]. Irradiation is delivered to the macroscopic gross tumor volume with 1 cm margins. In patients treated with curative intent, margins tend to be larger (2 cm) for isolated unique lesion of MF. The European society for treatment and research for cancer advises to deliver doses around 24 Gy [12]. The international lymphoma radiotherapy oncology group suggests dose range between 24 and 30 Gy, as local recurrences seem to be rare when a minimal dose of 24 Gy is delivered [11]. Electron beam therapy is well adapted as well as orthovoltage radiation therapy (100 kV). For thicker lesions, as for the case we have reported, the use of higher energy photons (6 MeV) may be needed. Low-dose and short-course irradiation lead to better patient convenience even in a palliative setting.

Both the European consensus on the treatment and the international lymphoma radiation oncology group consider the treatment by total skin electron beam therapy as a treatment option. This radiotherapy technique consists in delivering low doses irradiation (10-12 Gy) to larger volumes, which has the benefits of being shorter in duration, with fewer side effects. Retreatment is even feasible if required. This treatment option is unfortunately not widely available and could not be delivered on a routine basis by most radiotherapy teams.

We used a 36 Gy total dose irradiation delivered in a classical regimen of 2 Gy/fraction, 5 fractions a week in order to ensure the best possible chances of local control while assuring a good treatment tolerance. Electron beam therapy is the most frequent way of doing described in the literature but in our case, nasal infiltration was so important that we added photons in order to achieve better lesion coverage. It is of interest to note that side effects were low despite the dose and that a major efficacy was obtained. As it is notable in the figures below, wounds of the nose healed and the nose walls got thinner offering a normal aspect for the nose's skin and mucosa.

Multidisciplinary boards with participation of psychologists, social workers as well as radiation oncologists, and palliative care actors are important in the comprehensive patient care of advanced stage of MF.

4. Conclusion

In conclusion, local radiotherapy is an effective treatment in infiltrated or tumoral lesions of MF and can be considered with a "palliative" intent in order to improve quality of life in patients with disfiguring lesions impacting their psychosocial life. Radiotherapy induces a high response rate with little toxicity and can be done concomitantly with other systemic treatments.

Conflicts of Interest

The authors have no conflicts of interest to declare.

References

[1] P. T. Bradford, S. S. Devesa, W. F. Anderson, and J. R. Toro, "Cutaneous lymphoma incidence patterns in the United States: a population-based study of 3884 cases," *Blood*, vol. 113, no. 21, pp. 5064–5073, 2009.

[2] S. I. Jawed, P. L. Myskowski, S. Horwitz, A. Moskowitz, and C. Querfeld, "Primary cutaneous T-cell lymphoma (mycosis fungoides and Sézary syndrome): part I. Diagnosis: clinical and histopathologic features and new molecular and biologic markers," *Journal of the American Academy of Dermatology*, vol. 70, no. 2, pp. 205.e1–205.e16, 221–222, 2014.

[3] S. Whittaker, R. Hoppe, and H. M. Prince, "How I treat mycosis fungoides and Sézary syndrome," *Blood*, vol. 127, no. 25, pp. 3142–3153, 2016.

[4] G. W. Jones, D. Rosenthal, and L. D. Wilson, "Total skin electron radiation for patients with erythrodermic cutaneous T-cell lymphoma (mycosis fungoides and the sezary syndrome)," *Cancer*, vol. 85, no. 9, pp. 1985–1995, 1999.

[5] C. E. Introcaso, B. Micaily, S. K. Richardson et al., "Total skin electron beam therapy may be associated with improvement of peripheral blood disease in Sézary syndrome," *Journal of the American Academy of Dermatology*, vol. 58, no. 4, pp. 592–595, 2008.

[6] L. D. Wilson, B. M. Kacinski, and G. W. Jones, "Local superficial radiotherapy in the management of minimal stage IA cutaneous T-cell lymphoma (mycosis fungoides)," *International Journal of Radiation Oncology, Biology, Physics*, vol. 40, no. 1, pp. 109–115, 1998.

[7] G. W. Cotter, R. T. Baglan, T. H. Wasserman, and W. Mill, "Palliative radiation treatment of cutaneous mycosis fungoides—a dose response," *International Journal of Radiation Oncology, Biology, Physics*, vol. 9, no. 10, pp. 1477–1480, 1983.

[8] K. J. Neelis, E. C. Schimmel, M. H. Vermeer, N. J. Senff, R. Willemze, and E. M. Noordijk, "Low-dose palliative radiotherapy for cutaneous B- and T-cell lymphomas," *International Journal of Radiation Oncology, Biology, Physics*, vol. 74, no. 1, pp. 154–158, 2009.

[9] L. Esposito, R. Piccinno, L. Marchese, and E. Berti, "Results of radiotherapy in minimal stage mycosis fungoides: a reappraisal after ten years," *Giornale Italiano di Dermatologia e Venereologia*, 2018.

[10] T. O. Thomas, P. Agrawal, J. Guitart et al., "Outcome of patients treated with a single-fraction dose of palliative radiation for cutaneous T-cell lymphoma," *International Journal of Radiation Oncology, Biology, Physics*, vol. 85, no. 3, pp. 747–753, 2013.

[11] L. Specht, B. Dabaja, T. Illidge, L. D. Wilson, and R. T. Hoppe, "Modern radiation therapy for primary cutaneous lymphomas: field and dose guidelines from the International Lymphoma Radiation Oncology Group," *International Journal of Radiation Oncology, Biology, Physics*, vol. 92, no. 1, pp. 32–39, 2015.

[12] F. Trautinger, J. Eder, C. Assaf et al., "European Organisation for Research and Treatment of Cancer consensus recommendations for the treatment of mycosis fungoides/Sézary syndrome – Update 2017," *European Journal of Cancer*, vol. 77, pp. 57–74, 2017.

[13] K. Camphausen and P. J. Tofilon, "Inhibition of histone deacetylation: A strategy for tumor radiosensitization," *Journal of Clinical Oncology*, vol. 25, no. 26, pp. 4051–4056, 2007.

[14] O. E. Akilov, C. Grant, R. Frye, S. Bates, R. Piekarz, and L. Geskin, "Low-dose electron beam radiation and romidepsin therapy for symptomatic cutaneous T-cell lymphoma lesions," *British Journal of Dermatology*, vol. 167, no. 1, pp. 194–197, 2012.

Topical Imiquimod for the Treatment of Relapsed Cutaneous Langerhans Cell Histiocytosis after Chemotherapy in an Elderly Patient

Shinsaku Imashuku ⓘ,[1] **Miyako Kobayashi,**[2] **Yoichi Nishii,**[3] **and Keisuke Nishimura**[4]

[1]*Department of Laboratory Medicine, Uji-Tokushukai Medical Center, Uji 611-0042, Japan*
[2]*Department of Internal Medicine, Uji-Tokushukai Medical Center, Uji 611-0042, Japan*
[3]*Division of Plastic Surgery, Uji-Tokushukai Medical Center, Uji 611-0042, Japan*
[4]*Department of Pathology, Uji-Tokushukai Medical Center, Uji 611-0042, Japan*

Correspondence should be addressed to Shinsaku Imashuku; shinim95@mbox.kyoto-inet.or.jp

Academic Editor: Ioannis D. Bassukas

Diagnosis and treatment of Langerhans cell histiocytosis (LCH) in elderly patients are often difficult. We report here a 61-year-old female suffering from a refractory axillary ulcer for nearly a year, whose biopsy revealed LCH. It was also noted that the patient had other cutaneous papulovesicular eruptions of LCH as well as central diabetes insipidus. The patient was first successfully treated with multiagent chemotherapy (cytosine arabinoside/vinblastine/prednisolone). DDAVP also well controlled diabetes insipidus; however, the axillary ulcer and cutaneous LCH relapsed. Thereafter, we found topical imiquimod to be effective in the treatment of relapsed cutaneous LCH lesions.

1. Introduction

Langerhans cell histiocytosis (LCH) is a rare disease characterized by granulomatous lesions consisting of clonal CD1a+/CD207+/S100+ immature dendritic cells and various inflammatory cells. Currently, LCH is defined as inflammatory myeloid neoplasia [1]. Approximately two-thirds of LCH cases occur in pediatric patients, while the remaining one-third occur in adult patients. In an analysis of 275 adults with LCH, involvement of the lungs was the highest (58.4%), followed by bone (57.3%), skin (36.9%), and central diabetes insipidus (29.6%) [2]. However, LCH in adults is often misdiagnosed because of its rarity, particularly cutaneous lesions, which affect the scalp, neck, axilla, groin, and trunk with various forms from papules to vesicles; thus, if not biopsied, cutaneous LCH is overlooked as nonspecific eruptions. In terms of treatment of LCH, multiagent chemotherapy is employed for systemic multifocal lesions [3, 4]. On the other hand, for isolated cutaneous LCH, oral or topical steroids are considered as first-line treatment [5]; however, the appropriate therapy for refractory cutaneous LCH cases remains controversial. To date, various therapies such as topical nitrogen mustard [6] or thalidomide [7] and systemic low-dose methotrexate [8] or interferon- (IFN-) alpha [9] were reported. In addition, although numbers are limited, the effectiveness of topical imiquimod treatment was described [10–13]. Here, we report on an elderly patient whose relapsed, postchemotherapy cutaneous LCH lesions were successfully treated with topical imiquimod.

2. Case Report

The case described here is a 61-year-old Japanese female who had been treated for diabetes mellitus and a refractory large ulcer (2.0 cm × 2.6 cm) at her right axilla (Figure 1(a)) for nearly a year. Eventually, the ulcer was biopsied, revealing a typical LCH pathology, with dermal infiltrate of morphologically characteristic Langerhans cells extending into the epidermis, which were positive for S100, CD1a, and CD207, with other inflammatory cells (Figure 2). Prior to

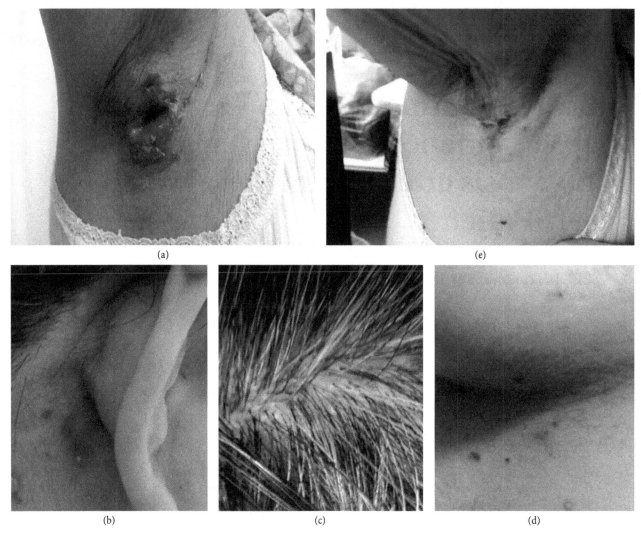

FIGURE 1: Photos of pretreatment right-axillary ulcer (a); cutaneous eruptions of LCH at the retroauricular area (b), scalp (c), and under the breast (d); posttreatment (after 4.5 months of imiquimod) status at the right axilla (e).

the diagnosis, cutaneous eruptions, such as erythematous papules/vesicles at retroauricular regions, crusted papules at the scalp, and reddish-brown papules at the lower chest under the breasts, were present (Figures 1(b), 1(c), and 1(d)). These cutaneous lesions remained undiagnosed until a biopsy of the retroauricular papule was performed which also revealed an LCH pathology. It was thought that one of such cutaneous eruptions caused a deep ulcer in the axillary. Thereafter, we examined whether the patient had systemic LCH lesions in the lungs, bones, and other organs. None was found except for abnormal brain MRI findings showing a thickened pituitary stalk and absent high signal at the posterior lobe of pituitary on T1WI (figure not shown). Based on her symptoms of polyuria/polydipsia, she was diagnosed with LCH-related central diabetes insipidus. Serum levels of antidiuretic hormone were undetectable (<0.8; reference value: >4.2 pg/mL). The reason for the delayed diagnosis of central diabetes insipidus was because her physician had been so concerned about treating axillary ulcer and her occasional

complaints of polyuria/polydipsia were thought to be due to diabetes mellitus. After the diagnosis of LCH, we chose to treat this patient systematically, because the axillary ulcer was so deep and enlarged (see Figure 1(a)) along with the presence of CNS lesion. The patient underwent treatment with DDAVP for central diabetes and systemic chemotherapy consisting of (I) vinblastine (VBL; 8 mg/day, intravenous infusion) and prednisolone (PSL; 30 mg/day, intravenous infusion) on Day 1 and (II) cytosine arabinoside (AraC; 200 mg/day, intravenous infusion) and PSL (30 mg/day, intravenous infusion) on Day 2 every 4 weeks. After 8 cycles of chemotherapy, the axillary ulcer healed and cutaneous lesions disappeared; however, the thickened pituitary stalk in the CNS was unchanged. Three months later, the axillary ulcer relapsed and cutaneous eruptions reappeared, and diagnosis of LCH was again confirmed by a biopsy (Figure 3). Central diabetes insipidus did not exacerbate and no increase of DDAVP dose was required. This time, considering the adverse effects of the previous systemic chemotherapy (glucose intolerance in the

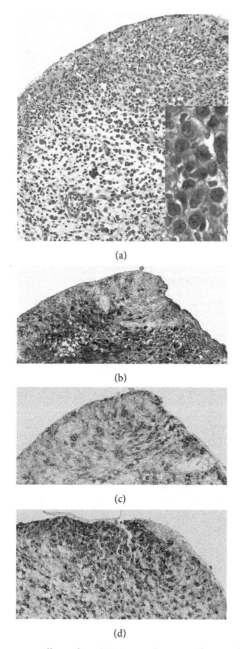

(a)

(b)

(c)

(d)

FIGURE 2: Pathology of the biopsied pretreatment axillary ulcer. H&E stain (a; original magnification ×200 with magnified photo showing LCH cells with folded coffee bean-like nucleus, ×400) and immunostaining of S100-positive (b), CD1a-positive (c), and CD207-positive (d) LCH cells (original magnification: ×200).

presence of diabetes mellitus and progressive dementia), we chose to employ topical imiquimod to treat the relapsed axillary ulcer and cutaneous LCH lesions, in addition to continuation of DDAVP for central diabetes insipidus. In this case, imiquimod (5%) cream was applied 5 days a week to the right axilla, scalp, and retroauricular areas and lower chest lesions, according to the instructions of the manufacturer. Following treatment for 4 months, the relapsed axillary ulcer as well as other cutaneous lesions improved significantly (Figure 1(e)). During the total 6.5 months of imiquimod treatment, no adverse effects such as fever or cutaneous redness, sore, and exfoliation were noted. At the

time of writing this paper, more than 8 months after stopping the imiquimod treatment, no further relapse of the axilla and other cutaneous lesions was noted. We assessed the therapeutic results as a clinical remission, since no biopsy was performed to confirm the complete loss of LCH cells, as summarized in Table 1.

3. Discussion

Imiquimod, a cytokine inducer and a modifier of the innate immune response [14], is approved in Japan for the treatment of genital warts and actinic keratosis. Imiquimod is believed

TABLE 1: Report of topical imiquimod trials for cutaneous LCH.

References	Case (age/gender)	Disease	Previous Rx		Topical imiquimod; duration (response)	Follow-up/outcome after finishing imiquimod
			Systemic chemotherapy	Topical Rx for skin LCH		
Dodd and Hook [13]	16 mo/F	Isolated skin LCH alone	None	Corticosteroids/tacrolimus.	5 months (CR)	>2 yrs No relapse
Aubert-Wastiaux et al. [12]	4 yr/M	Simultaneous skin LCH with T-ALL	For T-ALL	None	1 month (CHR)	Aggressive LCH Died in <2 months
O'Kane et al. [11]	53 yr/F	Breast carcinoma, followed by isolated skin LCH	For breast carcinoma	None	6 weeks (CHR)	Relapse after 6 months and then repeat imiquimod CR for 12 months
Taverna et al. [10]	74 yr/F	Isolated skin LCH alone	None	Ketoconazole/hydrocortisone	2 months (CR)	Relapse after 6 months and then repeat imiquimod
Current	61 yr/F	Skin LCH/CDI	For LCH ulcer	None	6.5 months (CR)	>8 months No relapse

LCH: Langerhans cell histiocytosis; ALL: acute lymphocytic leukemia; CDI: central diabetes insipidus; Rx: treatment; CR: clinical remission (not confirmed by biopsy after treatment); CHR: complete histological remission (confirmed by biopsy after treatment).

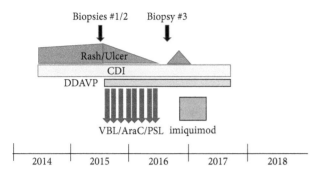

FIGURE 3: Clinical course and treatment. Biopsies #1/2 were done on the axillary ulcer and the retroauricular cutaneous lesions and biopsy #3 was done on the relapsed retroauricular cutaneous lesion. Diagnosis of LCH was made after biopsy #1. Pathological findings of #2 and #3 were almost identical to those of #1 shown in Figure 2. Details of the chemotherapy (VBL/AraC/PSL) and imiquimod regimens are described in the text. Symptoms of central diabetes insipidus were controlled by DDAVP.

to function as a potent stimulator of T-helper-1 cytokines causing local release of IFN-alfa, tumor necrosis factor-alpha, interleukin-1, interleukin-6, and others [15]. In LCH, it was postulated that topical imiquimod might be effective through IFN-alpha, but sparing patients the systemic side effects of IFN treatment [10]. Although imiquimod cream was not approved as an agent for LCH, we employed it in this case because its efficacy was reported in the past in the treatment of cutaneous LCH [10–13]. Including our case, topical imiquimod was employed for the duration of 1 month to 6.5 months in two pediatric and three adult patients, in whom no significant side effects were reported, and all showed complete histological or clinical remission, although two showed a relapse after 6 months (see Table 1).

This case illustrates the difficulty of diagnosing LCH in elderly patients and the usefulness of topical imiquimod for relapsed cutaneous LCH after chemotherapy. The good outcome in this case may have been the result of the additive effect of the initial systemic chemotherapy and later imiquimod treatment; however, it is emphasized that the rapid response of relapsed cutaneous LCH to topical imiquimod was obtained after short-term administration. Although the patient's condition has been stable, considering previous reports, she may still have a risk of relapse in the future after imiquimod treatment. In view of the risk of recurrence and subsequent malignancy in adult LCH [16], it is recommended that this case requires further long-term follow-up. Finally, we think that it is worth testing more this topical imiquimod in the future in the treatment of cutaneous LCH, particularly in elderly patients who are not tolerable to chemotherapy, considering its easy availability and effectiveness without significant side effects.

Conflicts of Interest

The authors declare that they have no conflicts of interest.

References

[1] M. L. Berres, M. Merad, and C. E. Allen, "Progress in understanding the pathogenesis of Langerhans cell histiocytosis: back to Histiocytosis X?" *British Journal of Haematology*, vol. 169, no. 1, pp. 3–13, 2015.

[2] M. Aricò, M. Girschikofsky, T. Généreau et al., "Langerhans cell histiocytosis in adults. Report from the International Registry of the Histiocyte Society," *European Journal of Cancer*, vol. 39, no. 16, pp. 2341–2348, 2003.

[3] M. Minkov, N. Grois, A. Heitger, U. Potschger, T. Westermeier, and H. Gadner, "Treatment of multisystem Langerhans cell histiocytosis. Results of the DAL-HX 83 and DAL-HX 90 studies," *Klinische Pädiatrie*, vol. 212, no. 4, pp. 139–144, 2000.

[4] A. Morimoto, Y. Shioda, T. Imamura et al., "Intensified and prolonged therapy comprising cytarabine, vincristine and prednisolone improves outcome in patients with multisystem Langerhans cell histiocytosis: results of the Japan Langerhans Cell Histiocytosis Study Group-02 Protocol Study," *International Journal of Hematology*, vol. 104, no. 1, pp. 99–109, 2016.

[5] L. Park, C. Schiltz, and N. Korman, "Langerhans cell histiocytosis," *Journal of Cutaneous Medicine and Surgery*, vol. 16, no. 1, pp. 45–49, 2012.

[6] L. M. Lindahl, M. Fenger-Grøn, and L. Iversen, "Topical nitrogen mustard therapy in patients with Langerhans cell histiocytosis," *British Journal of Dermatology*, vol. 166, no. 3, pp. 642–645, 2012.

[7] C. S. Sander, M. Kaatz, and P. Elsner, "Successful treatment of cutaneous langerhans cell histiocytosis with thalidomide," *Dermatology*, vol. 208, no. 2, pp. 149–152, 2004.

[8] A. E. Steen, K. H. Steen, R. Bauer, and T. Bieber, "Successful treatment of cutaneous Langerhans cell histiocytosis with low-dose methotrexate," *British Journal of Dermatology*, vol. 145, no. 1, pp. 137–140, 2001.

[9] S. E. Chang, G. J. Koh, J. H. Choi et al., "Widespread skin-limited adult Langerhans cell histiocytosis: Long-term follow-up with good response to interferon alpha," *Clinical and Experimental Dermatology*, vol. 27, no. 2, pp. 135–137, 2002.

[10] J. A. Taverna, C. M. Stefanato, F. D. Wax, and M.-F. Demierre, "Adult cutaneous Langerhans cell histiocytosis responsive to topical imiquimod," *Journal of the American Academy of Dermatology*, vol. 54, no. 5, pp. 911–913, 2006.

[11] D. O'Kane, H. Jenkinson, and J. Carson, "Langerhans cell histiocytosis associated with breast carcinoma successfully treated with topical imiquimod," *Clinical and Experimental Dermatology*, vol. 34, no. 8, pp. e829–e832, 2009.

[12] H. Aubert-Wastiaux, S. Barbarot, F. Mechinaud et al., "Childhood Langerhans cell histiocytosis associated with T cell acute lymphoblastic leukemia," *European Journal of Dermatology*, vol. 21, no. 1, pp. 109-110, 2011.

[13] E. Dodd and K. Hook, "Topical Imiquimod for the Treatment of Childhood Cutaneous Langerhans Cell Histiocytosis," *Pediatric Dermatology*, vol. 33, no. 3, pp. e184–e185, 2016.

[14] D. Vidal, "Topical imiquimod: Mechanism of action and clinical applications," *Mini-Reviews in Medicinal Chemistry*, vol. 6, no. 5, pp. 499–503, 2006.

[15] L. M. Imbertson, J. M. Beaurline, A. M. Couture et al., "Cytokine induction in hairless mouse and rat skin after topical application of the immune response modifiers imiquimod and S-28463," *Journal of Investigative Dermatology*, vol. 110, no. 5, pp. 734–739, 1998.

[16] J. R. Edelbroek, M. H. Vermeer, P. M. Jansen et al., "Langerhans cell histiocytosis first presenting in the skin in adults: Frequent association with a second haematological malignancy," *British Journal of Dermatology*, vol. 167, no. 6, pp. 1287–1294, 2012.

10

Atypical Histiocyte-Rich Sweet's Syndrome

Sharon Chi,[1] Marcia Leung,[2] Mark Carmichael,[3] Michael Royer,[4] and Sunghun Cho[5]

[1]*Internal Medicine Residency Program, Tripler Army Medical Center, 1 Jarrett White Road, Honolulu, HI 96859, USA*
[2]*John A. Burns School of Medicine, University of Hawaii, Honolulu, HI, USA*
[3]*Hematology-Oncology Service, Tripler Army Medical Center, Honolulu, HI, USA*
[4]*Department of Pathology, Walter Reed National Military Medical Center, Bethesda, MD, USA*
[5]*Dermatology Service, Tripler Army Medical Center, Honolulu, HI, USA*

Correspondence should be addressed to Sharon Chi; sharonwchi@gmail.com

Academic Editor: Jacek Cezary Szepietowski

Sweet's Syndrome is a rare neutrophilic dermatosis thought to be a result of immune dysregulation occurring in the setting of drug exposure, recent infection, pregnancy, and underlying malignancy or idiopathic with specific and widely accepted diagnostic criteria established in the literature. Other organ systems can be involved with varying degrees of severity. An unusual case of Sweet's Syndrome associated with myopericarditis, acral involvement, and atypical histological findings with predominance of histiocytes is described here.

1. Introduction

Sweet's Syndrome is characterized by neutrophilic dermal infiltration that is idiopathic (classical Sweet's) or drug-induced or is attributed to a predisposing condition such as malignancy, preceding infection, or pregnancy [1]. Its pathogenesis has been hypothesized as a manifestation of cytokine dysregulation or autoimmunity [1]. In addition to the skin, other organs can be involved, including the heart on rare occasions [2, 3].

The widely used diagnostic criteria for Sweet's Syndrome include the presence of the two major criteria (acute painful erythematous plaques or nodules and dense neutrophilic infiltrate without vasculitis on histological evaluation) and four minor criteria (fever, associated condition such as malignancy, response to steroid or potassium iodide treatment, and lab abnormalities); both major criteria and at least two minor criteria are required for a diagnosis to be made [4]. However, several histologic and clinical variants exist, including histiocytoid and acral Sweet's Syndrome [5]. Furthermore, there are previously published reports of lymphocyte and histiocyte abundance in cases of Sweet's Syndrome [6–9]. A description of an unusual case of Sweet's Syndrome associated with myopericarditis, acral involvement, and atypical histiocyte-rich histologic findings on skin biopsy is presented

herein. Informed consent was obtained from the patient for publication of his case.

2. Case Presentation

A 41-year-old previously healthy nonsmoking male was admitted for non-ST-segment-elevation myocardial infarction after sudden substernal chest pain. Three weeks earlier, bilateral knee, elbow, wrist, and hand pain with multiple erythematous papules and plaques on his neck, forehead, and forearms abruptly developed without response to naproxen (Figure 1). He did not take any other medications. Painful erythema and edema of the fingertips with splinter hemorrhages of the nails appeared at two weeks (Figure 1). Review of systems revealed night sweats, nausea, and nonbloody diarrhea three days before initial presentation. Lab studies revealed a troponin I level of 10.2 ng/mL (0–0.034 ng/mL), WBC count of $15.05 \times 10^3/\mu L$ (4.4–$9.4 \times 10^3/\mu L$) with elevated neutrophils, elevated hepatic enzymes, ESR of 84 mm/h (0–15 mm/h), and CRP of 524 mg/L (<10.0 mg/L). Coronary angiography was unremarkable. Cardiac MRI revealed myopericarditis.

A diagnosis of Sweet's Syndrome was suspected based on clinical presentation and skin findings. Skin biopsy was performed and systemic steroids were initiated. The skin lesions and joint pain significantly improved within 24 hours

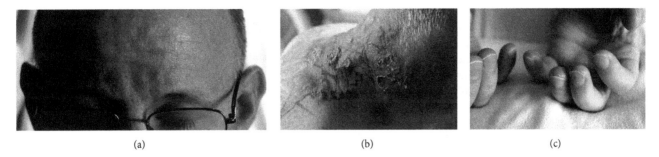

(a)   (b)   (c)

FIGURE 1: *Skin findings.* (a) Edematous papules and plaques of acute lesions of Sweet's Syndrome. (b) Well-established lesions of Sweet's Syndrome consisting of annual papules and plaques with scale and crust. (c) Finger changes seen in our patient with subungual inflammation splinter hemorrhages and inflammation and scaling of several fingertips.

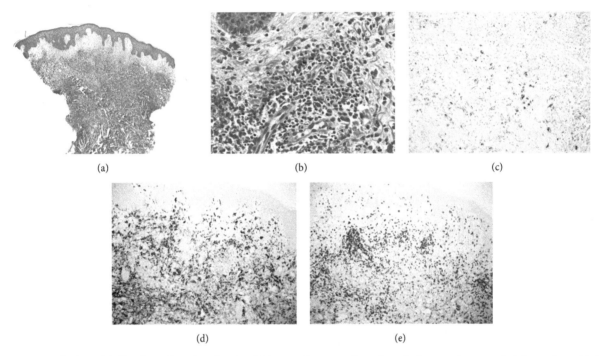

(a)   (b)   (c)

(d)   (e)

FIGURE 2: *Biopsy findings.* (a) Histological section showing fairly prominent papillary dermal edema and a somewhat dense dermal infiltrate comprised of mixed inflammatory cells (hematoxylin-eosin, original magnification: ×40). (b) Many large histiocytic cells are present as well as lymphocytes and scattered neutrophils (hematoxylin-eosin, original magnification: ×400). Leukocytoclastic debris is noted, but evidence of vasculitis is lacking. (c) Myeloperoxidase immunohistochemical stain reveals scattered neutrophils but is negative in the histiocytic cells (original magnification: ×200). (d) Histiocytic cells are confirmed to be histiocytes and not mononuclear myelocytes (CD163 immunohistochemical stain, original magnification: ×100). (e) Background T lymphocytes (CD3 immunohistochemical stain, original magnification: ×100).

of high-dose 1 mg/kg prednisone treatment. Analysis of the skin biopsy from a 22-day-old lesion is shown in Figure 2. A 30-day course of prednisone plus colchicine was prescribed, followed by an aspirin taper. Extensive workup for infectious, rheumatological, and malignant associations was unrevealing and included multiple blood cultures, viral studies, imaging, esophagogastroduodenoscopy, and colonoscopy.

3. Discussion

The diagnosis of Sweet's Syndrome was initially suspected clinically with abrupt onset of skin lesions, leukocytosis, and elevated inflammatory markers, as well as a preceding viral-like illness. Histological findings of papillary dermal edema, karyorrhexis, and the presence of neutrophils within the inflammatory infiltrate without evidence of leukocytoclastic vasculitis supported Sweet's Syndrome. However, the infiltrate was composed predominantly of histiocytes and lymphocytes. Immunohistochemical analysis did not show clonality. The diagnosis was based on the clinical morphology and distribution of the lesions, acute onset, inflammatory markers, abrupt response to steroids, preceding illness, and supportive biopsy.

Cardiac involvement is rare in Sweet's Syndrome. Various cardiac sequelae are described in the literature including myopericarditis, valvular disease, coronary artery occlusion, and aneurysm [1–3]. In this case, high-dose prednisone therapy was initiated early due to concern for worsening myopericarditis. A course of colchicine plus prednisone was followed by high-dose aspirin and colchicine due to concern for myopericarditis relapse with glucocorticoid monotherapy.

Another unique feature was fingertip and nail involvement (Figure 1(c)). Neutrophilic dermatosis of the hand is a variant of Sweet's Syndrome with skin lesions isolated to the hands [5]. In our patient, hand involvement occurred two weeks after initial symptoms.

This case illustrates the presence of atypical histological findings in a case of Sweet's Syndrome associated with myopericarditis and acral involvement. These findings challenge the currently accepted diagnostic criteria for Sweet's Syndrome based on the predominance of histiocytes and lymphocytes over neutrophils. This is in line with prior observations also noting a predominance of histiocytic infiltrates in established lesions of Sweet's Syndrome.

Disclosure

The views expressed in this manuscript are those of the authors and do not reflect the official policy or position of the Department of the Army, Department of Defense, or the US Government.

Conflicts of Interest

The authors declare that there are no conflicts of interest regarding the publication of this paper.

References

[1] P. R. Cohen, "Sweet's syndrome—a comprehensive review of an acute febrile neutrophilic dermatosis," *Orphanet Journal of Rare Diseases*, vol. 2, no. 1, article 34, 2007.

[2] W. Y.-H. Yu, E. Manrriquez, T. Bhutani et al., "Sweet heart: A case of pregnancy-associated acute febrile neutrophilic dermatosis with myopericarditis," *JAAD Case Reports*, vol. 1, no. 1, pp. 12–14, 2015.

[3] S. Acikel, M. Sari, and R. Akdemir, "The relationship between acute coronary syndrome and inflammation: A case of acute myocardial infarction associated with coronary involvement of Sweet's syndrome," *Blood Coagulation & Fibrinolysis*, vol. 21, no. 7, pp. 703–706, 2010.

[4] P. von den Driesch, "Sweet's syndrome (acute febrile neutrophilic dermatosis)," *Journal of the American Academy of Dermatology*, vol. 31, no. 4, pp. 535–560, 1994.

[5] R. Wolf and Y. Tüzün, "Acral manifestations of Sweet syndrome (neutrophilic dermatosis of the hands)," *Clinics in Dermatology*, vol. 35, no. 1, pp. 81–84, 2017.

[6] M.-D. Vignon-Pennamen, C. Juillard, M. Rybojad et al., "Chronic recurrent lymphocytic sweet syndrome as a predictive marker of myelodysplasia: A report of 9 cases," *JAMA Dermatology*, vol. 142, no. 9, pp. 1170–1176, 2006.

[7] A. V. Evans, R. A. Sabroe, K. Liddell, and R. Russell-Jones, "Lymphocytic infiltrates as a presenting feature of Sweet's syndrome with myelodysplasia and response to cyclophosphamide," *British Journal of Dermatology*, vol. 146, no. 6, pp. 1087–1090, 2002.

[8] J. Delabie, C. De Wolf-Peeters, M. Morren, K. Marien, T. Roskams, and V. Desmet, "Histiocytes in Sweet's syndrome," *British Journal of Dermatology*, vol. 124, no. 4, pp. 348–353, 1991.

[9] J. F. Bourke, J. L. Jones, A. Fletcher, and R. A. C. Graham-Brown, "An immunohistochemical study of the dermal infiltrate and epidermal staining for interleukin 1 in 12 cases of Sweet's syndrome," *British Journal of Dermatology*, vol. 134, no. 4, pp. 705–709, 1996.

11

Anogenital Ulcers: An Unusual Manifestation of Invasive Aspergillosis

Pablo Vargas [iD],[1] **Fernando Valenzuela,**[1] **Viera Kaplan,**[1] **Jacob Yumha,**[2] **Montserrat Arceu,**[1] **and Claudia Morales**[3]

[1]*Department of Dermatology, Faculty of Medicine, University of Chile, Santiago, Chile*
[2]*Faculty of Medicine, University of Chile, Santiago, Chile*
[3]*Pathology Service, University of Chile Clinical Hospital, Santiago, Chile*

Correspondence should be addressed to Pablo Vargas; pablovargas.med@gmail.com

Academic Editor: Alireza Firooz

Aspergillus spp. is one of the most ubiquitous fungi but generally does not cause disease in immunocompetent patients. It is the second most frequent agent of opportunistic fungal infections, after *Candida albicans*, with a rise in its incidence on recent years. Invasive fungal diseases represent an important cause of morbidity and mortality. Its origin can be primary, in relation to a cutaneous injury, or secondary, by extension from contiguous tissues, or by hematogenous spread, usually in the context of pulmonary aspergillosis. In this report, we describe the case of an elderly woman with invasive aspergillosis that manifested with anogenital and skin ulcers, with unfavorable outcome, despite intensive therapy and intravenous antifungals.

1. Introduction

Invasive fungal diseases represent an important cause of morbidity and mortality, mainly in immunocompromised patients. *Aspergillus* spp., after *Candida albicans*, is the second most frequent agent of opportunistic fungal infections, with an increase in its incidence on recent years [1, 2]. It is one of the most ubiquitous fungi but generally does not cause disease in immunocompetent patients [3]. Its most frequent portal of entry is the airway; therefore, pulmonary aspergillosis has been well characterized in the literature; however, the cutaneous form has not been that well characterized, probably because of its lower prevalence. Its origin can be primary, in relation to a cutaneous injury, or secondary, by extension from contiguous tissues, or by hematogenous spread, usually in the context of pulmonary aspergillosis [4]. We present the case of an elderly woman with invasive aspergillosis that manifested with anogenital and skin ulcers.

2. Case Report

An 82-year-old female patient is with a history of chronic arterial hypertension, ischemic stroke without sequelae, and hypothyroidism. She is hospitalized in our institution with a diagnosis of nephrotic syndrome, for study and management. Prednisone 1 mg/kg/day is started at admission. There was a torpid progression with multiple intercurrent infections, right renal infarction, and a progressive deterioration of kidney function, requiring the initiation of hemodialysis. In this context, after 3 weeks of hospitalization, she manifested multiple painful genital and inguinal ulcers, the largest one on the skin of the left labia majora, 1.5 cm in diameter, with a well-defined erythematous border and base with scarce fibrin. There was a rapid progression of the ulcers, with an increase in their size, number, and the extension to the perianal region, thighs, and right leg (Figure 1). Dermatology department was consulted, and polymerase chain reaction (PCR) for *herpes simplex viruses 1 and 2*, *Varicella zoster virus*, *Epstein barr virus*, and *Cytomegalovirus*, in addition to *HIV* serology and *VDRL*, were performed, with negative results. Biopsies of the vulvar and right leg lesions were taken and, on the PAS staining of the latter, septate hyphae were found, some with ramifications at acute angles and with invasion of blood vessels (Figure 2). Cultures of the lesions were negative. The patient presented with respiratory distress, and chest

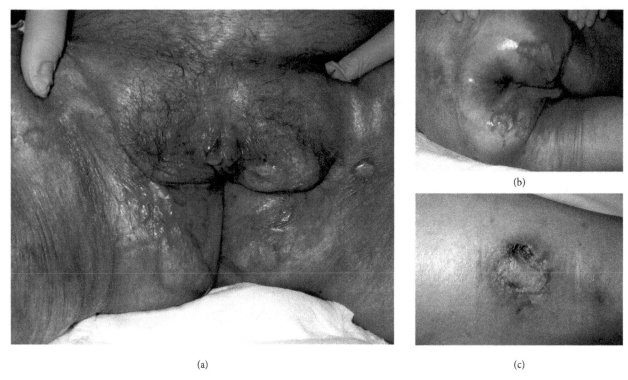

FIGURE 1: (a) Multiple painful genital and inguinal ulcers. (b) Ulcers extension to perianal region. (c), Ulcer in the right leg.

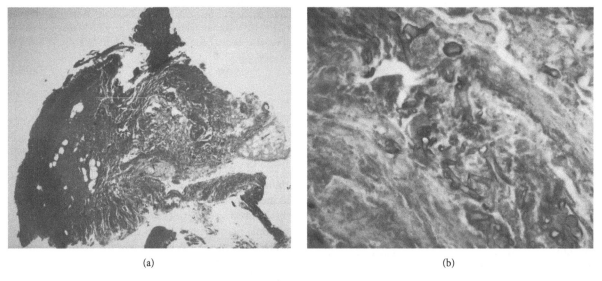

FIGURE 2: (a) 20x H/E. Skin and subcutaneous adipose tissue with ulcer and tissue necrosis. (b) 400x PAS. Septate and fragmented hyphaes of medium thickness in dermis with invasion of blood vessels.

computed tomography showed a cavitated lesion in the upper segment of the left lower lobe, suggestive of aspergilloma. Galactomannan blood test came back positive, thus confirming the diagnosis of invasive aspergillosis. Intravenous antifungal therapy with voriconazole and caspofungin was initiated; however, the patient deteriorated rapidly, with multiorgan failure, and died despite intensive care and twenty days of antifungal treatment.

3. Discussion

Invasive aspergillosis affects the skin in 1 to 10% of cases, according to some retrospective series, and it is the second most frequent site after the lung [5, 6]. It usually manifests with papules and nodules on the trunk and limbs. It can evolve with necrosis and ulceration [6], the latter being more frequent in cases of primary aspergillosis. In the main retrospective series, no cases of aspergillosis with anogenital involvement have been reported [5–7], and only one case is described, which corresponds to a primary cutaneous form [8]. The development of this fungal infection usually occurs in immunocompromised patients, mainly in hemato-oncological patients. Other independent risk factors are recognized, among which advanced age stands out and also leads to higher mortality [9]. Our patient was elderly and, in addition, immunocompromised by the use systemic corticosteroids due to the nephrotic syndrome. Considering the low sensitivity of culture techniques, it is necessary to integrate the clinic with diagnostic tools. For some authors, histopathological study represents the gold standard for diagnosis, even though microscopic differentiation from other filamentous fungi can be difficult. There are some diagnostic clues, such as the branching of hyphae at acute angles, vascular invasion, or thrombosis [8, 9]. There is high quality evidence to recommend serum galactomannan in the diagnosis and follow up of invasive aspergillosis in adult and pediatric patients. Also, PCR techniques are controversial and their use should be evaluated according to the conditions of each patient [8]. Voriconazole is the first-line treatment for invasive aspergillosis, and it is suggested that it should be used along with caspofungin in the case of pulmonary compromise [9, 10].

We present this case given the unusual presentation of invasive aspergillosis with anogenital ulcers, and it should be considered in the differential diagnosis of these kinds of lesions in the immunocompromised.

Conflicts of Interest

The authors declare that they have no conflicts of interest.

References

[1] K. C. Furlan, P. Kakizaki, N. Y. S. Valente, M. C. Pires, and J. C. N. Chartuni, "Primary cutaneous aspergillosis and idiopathic bone marrow aplasia," *Anais Brasileiros de Dermatologia*, vol. 91, no. 3, pp. 381–383, 2016.

[2] Z. Erjavec, H. Kluin-Nelemans, and P. E. Verweij, "Trends in invasive fungal infections, with emphasis on invasive aspergillosis," *Clinical Microbiology and Infection*, vol. 15, no. 7, pp. 625–633, 2009.

[3] C. Ajith, S. Dogra, B. Radotra, A. Chakrabarti, and B. Kumar, "Primary cutaneous aspergillosis in an immunocompetent individual," *Journal of the European Academy of Dermatology and Venereology*, vol. 20, no. 6, pp. 738-739, 2006.

[4] J. van Burik, R. Colven, and D. Spach, "Itraconazole Therapy for Primary Cutaneous Aspergillosis in Patients with AIDS," *Clinical Infectious Diseases*, vol. 27, no. 3, pp. 643-644, 1998.

[5] A. Burgos, T. E. Zaoutis, C. C. Dvorak et al., "Pediatric invasive aspergillosis: a multicenter retrospective analysis of 139 contemporary cases," *Pediatrics*, vol. 121, no. 5, pp. e1286–e1294, 2008.

[6] C. Bernardeschi, F. Foulet, S. Ingen-Housz-Oro et al., "Cutaneous invasive aspergillosis: Retrospective multicenter study of the French invasive-aspergillosis registry and literature review," *Medicine (United States)*, vol. 94, no. 26, Article ID e1018, 2015.

[7] A. Fernandez-Flores, M. Saeb-Lima, and R. Arenas-Guzman, "Morphological findings of deep cutaneous fungal infections," *American Journal of Dermatopathology*, vol. 36, no. 7, pp. 531–556, 2014.

[8] C. Tahir, M. Garbati, H. A. Nggada, E. H. T. Yawe, and A. M. Abubakar, "Primary cutaneous aspergillosis in an immunocompetent patient," *Journal of Surgical Technique and Case Report*, vol. 3, no. 2, pp. 94–96, 2011.

[9] M. Karthaus and D. Buchheidt, "Invasive aspergillosis: New insights into disease, diagnostic and treatment," *Current Pharmaceutical Design*, vol. 19, no. 20, pp. 3569–3594, 2013.

[10] T. F. Patterson, G. R. Thompson, D. W. Denning et al., "Practice guidelines for the diagnosis and management of aspergillosis: 2016 update by the infectious diseases society of America," *Clinical Infectious Diseases*, vol. 63, no. 4, pp. e1–e60, 2016.

12

Unusual Sites of Cutaneous Tuberculosis

Dimple Chopra,[1] Vishal Chopra,[2] Aastha Sharma,[1] Siddharth Chopra,[3] Shivali Aggarwal,[1] and Deepak Goyal[2]

[1]*Department of Dermatology, Government Medical College, Patiala, Punjab, India*
[2]*Department of Pulmonary Medicine, Government Medical College, Patiala, Punjab, India*
[3]*Government Medical College, Patiala, Punjab, India*

Correspondence should be addressed to Vishal Chopra; drvishalchopra@hotmail.com

Academic Editor: Ioannis D. Bassukas

Cutaneous tuberculosis (CTB) is an uncommon small subset of extrapulmonary tuberculosis, comprising 1–1.5% of all extrapulmonary tuberculosis manifestations, which manifests only in 8.4–13.7% of all tuberculosis cases. Lupus vulgaris (LV) and tuberculosis verrucosa cutis (TBVC) are forms of reinfection tuberculosis and often occur in presensitized patients, by exogenous inoculation. We report two cases of cutaneous tuberculosis at unusual sites. A 35-year-old female having a forehead lesion for 2 years was diagnosed as having tuberculosis verrucosa cutis and another 16-year-old girl with lesion in left axilla for 10 years was proven to have lupus vulgaris. The delayed diagnosis was possibly due to lower clinical suspicion due to the presentation of CTB at unusual sites. This highlights the importance of keeping TB as an important differential as misdiagnosis or delayed diagnosis of this entity can lead to prolonged morbidity.

1. Introduction

Cutaneous tuberculosis (CTB) comprises a small fraction (2%) of incident cases of TB [1] and the incidence has decreased from 2% to 0.5% [2]. It can present in many different manifestations. The potentiality of skin to react in many different ways to a single agent is nowhere better illustrated than in tuberculosis [3]. The site and clinical picture of CTB can at times be confusing leading to a delay in diagnosis of the disease as happened in these two cases. We report a case of tuberculosis verrucosa cutis (TBVC) presenting as a warty lesion on the forehead and of lupus vulgaris (LV) in the axilla which is a rare presentation.

2. Case Report

2.1. Case 1. 35-year-old female presented with a hyperkeratotic plaque on the left side of forehead. Lesion started as a small papule after 3 months following a roadside fall 2 years back, gradually increased in size, and spread in an annular fashion to form a plaque with warty surface [Figure 1], which

started showing ulceration in last 3 months. Lupus vulgaris and leprosy were kept as the differential diagnosis. A detailed history and clinical examination were not in favour of leprosy. She had no history of visit to/residence in known endemic areas for leprosy, no family history of leprosy, no hypo/anaesthesia, tingling, or numbness of hands or feet, and no reduced sweating, loss of hair, dryness of eyes, or epistaxis. On clinical examination an erythematous annular hyperkeratotic plaque with a warty surface measuring 4 × 5 cm was present on the left side of forehead. The lesion showed some crusting and a small scar at the periphery. There was no lymphadenopathy. On clinical examination there were no hypopigmented lesions on body, there was no loss of sensations, and there was no nerve enlargement. Systemic examination also did not reveal any abnormalities. Routine investigations and X-ray chest were normal. Tuberculin skin test was positive with an induration of 20 mm.

A punch biopsy from the lesion showed pseudoepitheliomatous hyperplasia with hyperkeratosis, acanthosis [Figure 2(a), H and E (40x), and Figure 2(b), H and E (400x)], and dense inflammatory infiltrates with epithelioid cells and

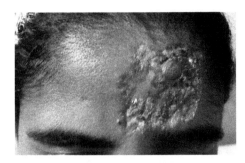

FIGURE 1: Plaque with warty surface on forehead.

giant cells in the dermis with few acid fast bacilli (AFB) [Figure 2(c), H and E (400x), and Figure 2(d), ZN Staining (1000x)]. PAS staining was not performed.

A small scar was evident in the plaque, possibly secondary to an earlier biopsy. Also the histopathology was more in favour of TBVC than lupus vulgaris. A diagnosis of tuberculosis verrucosa cutis was made, and the patient was started on category 1 treatment as per Revised National TB Control Programme (RNTCP) with which the lesions improved.

2.2. Case 2. A 16-year-old girl presented to our OPD with a lesion in left axilla [Figure 3] which started 10 years back as a small papule in axilla which turned into a pustule within a week which crusted and spread slowly over years.

Patient did not give any history of trauma, prolonged cough, sputum production, fever, night sweats, and weight loss. No family member had cough or sputum production or history of treatment for tuberculosis.

On examination the lesion was sharply demarcated 10 × 6 cm erythematous scaly annular plaque showing peripheral extension and central clearing with atrophic scarring. The plaque extended up to upper inner arm. On diascopy apple jelly nodules were appreciated. No BCG scar was present. There was no axillary or peripheral lymphadenopathy. Tinea corporis was considered as a differential diagnosis, but the lesion was asymptomatic and other flexures and nails were normal. PAS staining was not performed.

Routine investigations and X-ray chest were normal. Tuberculin skin test was positive with an induration of 18 mm.

Biopsy revealed well-formed granulomas with epithelioid cells and Langhans giant cells surrounded by chronic inflammatory cells and central necrosis without AFB [Figure 4, H and E (400x)]. PAS staining was not performed.

Diagnosis of lupus vulgaris was made and she was put on category 1 treatment as per Revised National TB Control Programme (RNTCP) with which the lesions improved.

3. Discussion

Cutaneous tuberculosis is a rare form of TB and presents with nonspecific and varied clinical presentations. Estimated incidence of this disease is about 0.1% of total patients attending the dermatology outpatient department [4]. Scrofuloderma is the most common form of cutaneous TB in India (50% cases) followed by lupus vulgaris in 42.86%, tuberculosis verrucosa cutis in 4.76%, and lichen scrofulosorum in 2.38% cases [5].

Other than *Mycobacterium TB* the infection can rarely be caused by *Mycobacterium bovis* or other atypical mycobacteria. Pulmonary TB, at present or in the past, is an important risk factor though it was absent in both of the cases. It is more at the sites with trauma as was in the first case though the site was rare. Limbs are the more common sites for cutaneous TB in India [6, 7] whereas neck sites followed by face and trunk are common sites of involvement in the western world.

Various classifications have been proposed to classify cutaneous tuberculosis. Earlier classification was based on the morphology of the lesions. Lai-Cheong et al. later proposed a classification based on the route of infection whether exogenous or endogenous [8, 9]. Now the recent classification based on bacterial load was proposed [10]. It was classified into paucibacillary forms (e.g., lupus vulgaris, tuberculosis verrucosa cutis, and tuberculids) and multibacillary forms (e.g., scrofuloderma, tuberculous chancre, and acute military tuberculosis).

Tuberculosis verrucosa cutis, a paucibacillary form of cutaneous tuberculosis, occurs in those individuals who have already had tuberculosis and have developed a moderate-to-high degree of immunity against these organisms. It is also known as warty tuberculosis, Prosector's wart, butcher's wart, and verrucous tuberculosis [11]. Tuberculosis verrucosa cutis results from inoculation and has an exogenous route. The sites commonly involved are hands in adults and lower extremities in children [12]. The involvement of forehead in this entity is extremely rare. It is usually solitary but multiple lesions may occur. The lesion typically starts with a painless, dusky red, firm, indurated nodule or papule that expands peripherally and is surrounded by inflammation. Spontaneous central resolution with areas of atrophy surrounded by a verrucous keratotic surface or an annular plaque with a warty advancing border is seen. Occasionally pus and keratinous material may be expressed from fissures in the warty areas. Lymphadenopathy is usually absent and, if seen, indicates secondary infection [13].

Histopathology shows pseudoepitheliomatous hyperplasia with marked hyperkeratosis, acanthosis, and dense inflammatory infiltrates with epithelioid cells and giant cells in the mid-dermis. Typical tuberculosis granulomas with characteristic caseation are not common [10]. Mantoux reaction is markedly positive as also in this case. Diagnosis is usually confirmed by typical clinical appearance, histopathological pattern, and a positive response to antitubercular treatment. The differential diagnoses include blastomycosis, chromomycosis, fixed sporotrichosis, lesions caused by nontubercular mycobacteria, lupus vulgaris, and tertiary syphilis.

Lupus vulgaris is the commonest, chronic, progressive, paucibacillary form of secondary cutaneous tuberculosis [12]. It develops in a previously sensitized host having a high degree of tuberculin sensitivity. Lupus vulgaris results both from inoculation and from endogenous spread through hematogenous or lymphatic route from an underlying infective focus [14]. Rarely, it may develop following direct inoculation of the bacilli into skin or at the site of Bacille Calmette-Guerin (BCG) vaccination [15].

Clinically it is characterized by soft reddish-brown plaques with apple jelly nodules on diascopy. The lesions

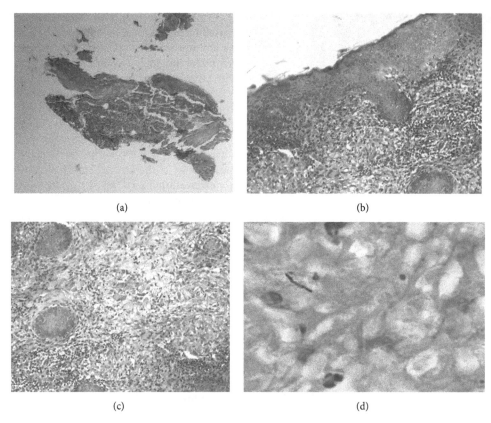

(a)   (b)

(c)   (d)

FIGURE 2: (a) Pseudoepitheliomatous hyperplasia with hyperkeratosis and acanthosis [H and E (40x)]. (b) Pseudoepitheliomatous hyperplasia with hyperkeratosis and acanthosis [H and E (400x)]. (c) Dense inflammatory infiltrates with epithelioid cells and giant cells in the dermis [H and E (400x)]. (d) Ziehl-Neelsen Staining showing scant AFB [ZN Staining (1000x)].

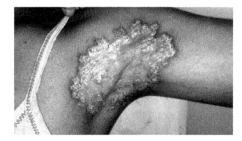

FIGURE 3: Erythematous scaly annular plaque in left axilla extending up to upper inner arm.

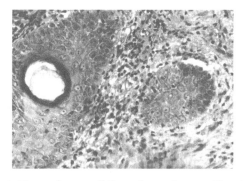

FIGURE 4: Biopsy shows well-formed granulomas with epithelioid cells and Langhans giant cells surrounded by chronic inflammatory cells and central necrosis [H and E (400x)].

pursue a chronic course over several years and grow by peripheral extension and central scarring. The diverse clinical forms of lupus vulgaris include papular, nodular, plaque, ulcerative, vegetative, and tumour-like lesions. In India, trunk, buttocks, and extremities are the predominant sites affected; in the West the lesions favour head and neck. In this case the lesion was present in the axilla without any history of trauma or any lymphadenopathy which delayed the diagnosis of the lesion. Atrophic scarring of lesions and apple jelly colour on diascopy are characteristic. Histopathologically, it is associated with nonnecrotizing granulomas in which acid fast bacilli are usually not found [16].

The treatment of cutaneous tuberculosis is as per RNTCP guidelines in India.

4. Conclusion

Awareness of varied clinical presentations especially at rarer sites with a high index of clinical suspicion of CTB, as in these two cases, is the key to early diagnosis and treatment, thus reducing the morbidity.

Competing Interests

The authors declare that they have no competing interests.

References

[1] B. Kumar and S. Kaur, "Pattern of cutaneous tuberculosis in North India," *Indian Journal of Dermatology, Venereology and Leprology*, vol. 52, pp. 203–207, 1986.

[2] V. N. Sehgal, G. Srivastava, V. K. Khurana, V. K. Sharma, P. Bhalla, and P. C. Beohar, "An appraisal of epidemiologic, clinical, bacteriologic, histopathologic, and immunologic parameters in cutaneous tuberculosis," *International Journal of Dermatology*, vol. 26, no. 8, pp. 521–526, 1987.

[3] D. M. Pillsbury, W. B. Shelley, and A. M. Kligman, *Dermatology*, WB Saunders, Philadelphia, Pa, USA, 1956.

[4] N. Yasmeen and A. Kanjee, "Cutaneous tuberculosis: a three year prospective study," *Journal of the Pakistan Medical Association*, vol. 55, no. 1, pp. 10–12, 2005.

[5] B. K. Thakur, S. Verma, and D. Hazarika, "A clinicopathological study of cutaneous tuberculosis at Dibrugarh district, Assam," *Indian Journal of Dermatology*, vol. 57, no. 1, pp. 63–65, 2012.

[6] B. Dwari, A. Ghosh, R. Paudel, and P. Kishore, "A clinicoepidemiological study of 50 cases of cutaneous tuberculosis in a tertiary care teaching hospital in Pokhara, Nepal," *Indian Journal of Dermatology*, vol. 55, no. 3, pp. 233–237, 2010.

[7] N. Puri, "A clinical and histopathological profile of patients with cutaneous tuberculosis," *Indian Journal of Dermatology*, vol. 56, no. 5, pp. 550–552, 2011.

[8] J. E. Lai-Cheong, A. Perez, V. Tang, A. Martinez, V. Hill, and H. D. P. Menagé, "Cutaneous manifestations of tuberculosis," *Clinical and Experimental Dermatology*, vol. 32, no. 4, pp. 461–466, 2007.

[9] J. Barbagallo, P. Tager, R. Ingleton, R. J. Hirsch, and J. M. Weinberg, "Cutaneous tuberculosis: diagnosis and treatment," *American Journal of Clinical Dermatology*, vol. 3, no. 5, pp. 319–328, 2002.

[10] F. Tigoulet, V. Fournier, and E. Caumes, "Clinical forms of the cutaneous tuberculosis," *Bulletin de la Societe de Pathologie Exotique*, vol. 96, no. 5, pp. 362–367, 2004.

[11] M. K. Pomeranz, O. Philip, S. Jerone, and B. Rena, *Mycobacteria and Skin*, Edited by W. M. Rom and S. Garay, Little Brown Company, London, UK, 1st edition, 1996.

[12] B. Kumar and S. Muralidhar, "Cutaneous tuberculosis: a twenty-year prospective study," *International Journal of Tuberculosis and Lung Disease*, vol. 3, no. 6, pp. 494–500, 1999.

[13] V. N. Sehgal, R. Sehgal, P. Bajaj, G. Sriviastava, and S. Bhattacharya, "Tuberculosis verrucosa cutis (TBVC)," *Journal of the European Academy of Dermatology and Venereology*, vol. 14, no. 4, pp. 319–321, 2000.

[14] V. N. Sehgal and S. A. Wagh, "Cutaneous tuberculosis. Current concepts," *International Journal of Dermatology*, vol. 29, no. 4, pp. 237–252, 1990.

[15] A. J. Kanwar, S. Kaur, R. Bansal, B. D. Radotra, and R. Sharma, "Lupus vulgaris following BCG vacconation," *International Journal of Dermatology*, vol. 27, no. 7, pp. 525–526, 1988.

[16] G. Tappeiner, *Fitzpatrick's Dermatology in General Medicine*, Edited by A. Goldsmith, K. Wolff, S. I. Kalz, A. S. Paller, and S. Gilchrest, McGraw Hill, New York, NY, USA, 6th edition, 2003.

A Rare Case of Vancomycin-Induced Linear Immunoglobulin A Bullous Dermatosis

Pinky Jha,[1] Kurtis Swanson,[2] Jeremiah Stromich,[2] Basia M. Michalski,[2] and Edit Olasz[3]

[1]Section of Hospital Medicine, Division of General Internal Medicine, Medical College of Wisconsin, Milwaukee, WI, USA
[2]Medical College of Wisconsin, Milwaukee, WI, USA
[3]Department of Dermatology, Medical College of Wisconsin, Milwaukee, WI, USA

Correspondence should be addressed to Pinky Jha; pjha@mcw.edu

Academic Editor: Ichiro Kurokawa

Linear IgA bullous dermatosis (LABD) is an autoimmune vesiculobullous disease, which is typically idiopathic but can also rarely be caused by medications or infections. Vancomycin is the most common drug associated with LABD. Lesions typically appear 24 hours to 15 days after the first dose of vancomycin. It is best characterized pathologically by subepidermal bulla (blister) formation with linear IgA deposition at the dermoepidermal junction. Here we report an 86-year-old male with a history of left knee osteoarthritis who underwent a left knee arthroplasty and subsequently developed a prosthetic joint infection. This infection was treated with intravenous vancomycin as well as placement of a vancomycin impregnated joint spacer. Five days following initiation of antibiotic therapy, he presented with a vesiculobullous eruption on an erythematous base over his trunk, extremities, and oral mucosa. The eruption resolved completely when intravenous vancomycin was discontinued and colchicine treatment was begun. Curiously, complete resolution occurred despite the presence of the vancomycin containing joint spacer. The diagnosis of vancomycin-induced linear IgA bullous dermatosis was made based on characteristic clinical and histopathologic presentations.

1. Introduction

Linear IgA bullous dermatosis (LABD) is a rare immune-mediated vesiculobullous disease. The clinical presentation is variable and may simulate bullous pemphigoid, cicatricial pemphigoid, or dermatitis herpetiformis [1, 2]. It is best characterized pathologically by subepidermal bulla (blister) formation, dermal neutrophilic infiltrate and homogeneous linear IgA deposition at the dermoepidermal junction. The diagnosis of linear IgA bullous dermatosis is confirmed by direct immunofluorescence, which reveals the presence of linear deposition of IgA at the basement membrane zone (BMZ) [2–4]. Linear IgA bullous dermatosis is usually idiopathic but may be rarely related to medications or infections.

Vancomycin is the most common drug to cause linear IgA bullous dermatosis, followed by amiodarone, cephalosporins, and diuretics [1, 3]. While drug-induced cases typically resolve in weeks with medication cessation, treatment in severe or nondrug induced cases requires dapsone, sulfonamides, colchicine, topical or systemic steroids, or IVIG [1–3].

We describe a patient with vancomycin-induced linear IgA bullous dermatosis in whom the eruption was documented clinically, histopathologically, and immunologically.

2. Case Presentation

An 86-year-old Caucasian gentleman with a past medical history of dilated cardiomyopathy, aortic insufficiency, and left knee osteoarthritis status after total knee arthroplasty complicated by prosthetic joint infection treated with parenteral vancomycin as well as placement of a vancomycin impregnated joint spacer presented with a chief complaint of diffuse nonpruritic bullous rash involving skin and oral mucosa. The rash appeared nine days after vancomycin spacer placement and five days after starting intravenous vancomycin, first appearing as yellow peri-incisional, but then progressing to the more classical diffuse polymorphic, erythematous vesiculobullous rash two days later. The patient denied any other systemic symptoms. Vitals signs were stable on presentation. On examination, the patient was found

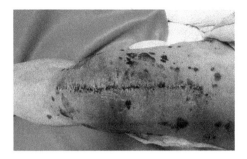

FIGURE 1: Left knee with peri-incisional crusting, coalescing, salmon-colored plaques.

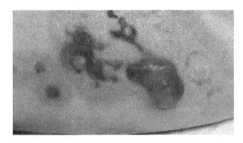

FIGURE 2: Tense bulla with perilesional vesicles on right thigh.

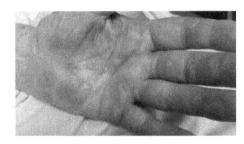

FIGURE 3: Left hand with tense bulla, target lesion, and coalescing, salmon-colored plaques.

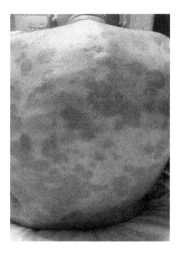

FIGURE 4: Back with extensive annular erythematous coalescing lesions.

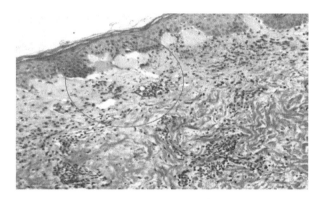

FIGURE 5: H&E, upper chest punch biopsy. Focal subepidermal blistering with dermal PMN infiltrate.

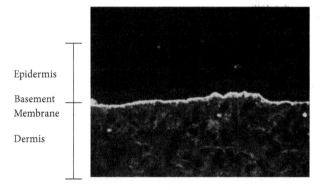

FIGURE 6: Direct immunofluorescence, upper chest punch biopsy. Linear IgA deposition along the basement membrane.

to have multiple eruptions including 1–4 cm tense bulla (blisters) filled with serous and hemorrhagic fluid, superficial erythematous erosions, 0.2–2 cm targetoid macules and papules with perilesional vesicles, and some coalescing in a herpetiform distribution. In addition he had a 2 cm oral mucosal ulcer. Lesions were located along the extensor surfaces of his arms and legs, as well as his back and palms of hands (Figures 1, 2, 3, and 4). He had periorbital erythema as well as conjunctival injection of the left eye. Laboratory results revealed a white blood cell count of 12,000/microliter, creatinine of 1.5 mg/dL (near baseline), and a vancomycin trough level within normal limits.

Other results were unremarkable and included negative anti-nuclear antibodies and anti-double-stranded DNA antibodies. Dermatology was consulted and biopsy of a lesion over the chest showed focal subepidermal blistering with numerous neutrophils and some eosinophils as well as neutrophil collections within the dermal papillae (Figure 5).

The differential diagnosis included linear IgA bullous dermatosis, bullous systemic lupus erythematosus, or dermatitis herpetiformis. Direct immunofluorescence microscopic examination of perilesional tissue showed linear deposits of IgA at the basement membrane zone (Figure 6). Based on the history and correlation of events to the initiation of vancomycin, physical examination, and light and immunofluorescence microscopic examination, the diagnosis of linear IgA bullous dermatosis secondary to vancomycin was made. Prior to admission, Infectious disease was consulted and empirically switched his vancomycin to daptomycin based on organism susceptibilities and a timeline suggesting a drug reaction. Orthopedic Surgery was consulted and recommended keeping the antibiotic spacer to optimize future joint mobility. Ophthalmology was asked to weigh in on the patient's ocular findings and recommended conservative compress therapy given lack of concerning eye involvement. Colchicine therapy was utilized instead of dapsone as the patient was anemic.

The patient was discharged on colchicine 0.6 mg twice daily for fourteen days to a subacute rehabilitation facility. Two weeks following discharge, the patient was seen in the Dermatology clinic. He had complete resolution of his linear IgA bullous dermatosis at that time.

3. Discussion

Linear IgA bullous dermatosis is a rare immune-mediated vesiculobullous disease [2, 3]. It is usually idiopathic but may be related to infection or medication. The incidence globally of all types of linear immunoglobulin A bullous dermatosis is estimated to be 0.5–2.3 cases/million/year. This disease occurs in a bimodal distribution, manifesting in patients ages 6 months and 10 years old and over 60.

Drug-induced linear IgA bullous dermatosis is a rarer subclassification of the disease. Multiple medications have been implicated as potential etiologies leading to this condition. Of the known drug causes of linear IgA bullous dermatosis, vancomycin is the most common. Other implicated medications include penicillins, cephalosporins, angiotensin converting enzyme inhibitors, and nonsteroidal anti-inflammatory drugs. Rarely, furosemide, atorvastatin, and angiotensin receptor blockers can cause linear immunoglobulin A bullous dermatosis [1].

Vancomycin use has been increasing steadily due to the recent rise in the rate of methicillin-resistant Staphylococcus aureus infection, emphasizing the importance of recognizing adverse effects from this medication. While Red Man Syndrome, Type I hypersensitivity reactions, drug reaction with eosinophilia and systemic symptoms (DRESS) and other drug eruptions can occur in the setting of vancomycin, linear IgA bullous dermatosis is another important eruption to recognize.

The first case of vancomycin-induced linear IgA bullous dermatosis was reported in 1988 [5, 6]. Subsequently, 48 cases have been reported (Table 1). Among the 48 reported patients 20 (42%) had recent history of cardiac procedure, cardiac infection, congestive heart failure, or aortic aneurism. The mean age of the 48 patients was 67.5 years (range 32–91) with no gender difference (22 female and 26 male patients). Our patient presented here has history of dilated cardiomyopathy and aortic insufficiency. Further investigation is needed to ascertain the association between LABD, vancomycin, and heart disease [5, 7]. Lesions develop within 24 hours to 15

days after the first dose of vancomycin and new lesions usually cease to appear within one to three days after discontinuation of drug [1, 3, 8, 9]. Lesions vary in nature ranging from tense serous/hemorrhagic bulla (blister), string of pearl "herpetiform" configurations to targetoid/erythema multiforme-like eruptions. Vancomycin-induced linear IgA bullous dermatosis commonly involves extremities and the palms and soles. Mucosal involvement is rare [3, 10, 11]. Our patient had eruptions in oral cavity, trunk, and extremities including palms and soles. Based on clinical presentation and light and direct immunofluorescence microscopy testing, the diagnosis of linear IgA bullous dermatosis was made.

Due to heterogeneous clinical features, linear IgA bullous dermatosis must be differentiated from a number of diseases including pemphigus vulgaris, bullous pemphigoid, dermatitis herpetiformis, and erythema multiforme [12]. Linear deposition of IgA at the dermoepidermal junction seen on direct immunofluorescence exam is a key feature of linear IgA bullous dermatosis [1–4, 12]. Diagnosis centers on the absence of gluten enteropathy or systemic lupus erythematosus as these entities may be difficult to distinguish from linear IgA bullous dermatosis grossly or based on light microscopy exam.

At the current time, there is no gold standard criteria that define this disease. Rather the diagnosis is based upon expert opinion. While linear IgA deposition along the basement membrane zone is considered essential, expert opinion is varied regarding whether or not immunoglobulin deposition must solely consist of immunoglobulin A or if predominant immunoglobulin A is sufficient for diagnosis. Complicating this matter is the fact that linear IgA deposition occurs in many subepidermal eruptions.

Some experts utilize broader diagnostic criteria incorporating serologic antibody testing and/or skin immunoblotting. Uncertainty undermines the usefulness of these criteria for several reasons. One reason is the lack of sensitivity and specificity relative to direct immunofluorescence. For example, autoantibody serologic testing has been cited to be positive in less than 80% of patients with linear IgA deposits at the basement membrane zone. Again complicating the picture is the heterogeneity of serologic findings, that is, circulating IgA antibodies against basement membrane zone antigen are nonspecific to linear IgA bullous dermatosis. Likewise IgG antibodies targeted to BMZ antigen are commonly found in this disease. Similarly, indirect immunofluorescence testing in patients with linear IgA deposition along the BMZ has been reported as low as 30% positive in human skin and less than 50% on NaCl-split skin [7].

In this case, history, physical examination, timing corresponding to drug reaction, and the generally agreed upon criteria of linear IgA deposition along the basement membrane zone were conditions met by the patient. Given the degree of ambiguity surrounding serologic, indirect immunofluorescence testing, as well as the time-consuming, costly nature of further testing, we and our Dermatology colleagues felt that sufficient testing had been performed to achieve diagnosis and that appropriate treatment should be initiated.

Polymorphous clinical and immunopathologic features of this dermatosis can be partially explained by the different

TABLE 1: Vancomycin induced LABD cases reported between 1988 and 2016.

Case	Paper (first author, year)	Gender	Age	Hospitalization history
(1)	Gameiro, 2016	M	72	CABG and aortic valve replacement
(2)	Gameiro, 2016	M	50	CABG and aortic valve replacement
(3)	Nasr J., 2014	M	76	Pneumonia and bacteremia
(4)	Zenke, 2014	M	62	Endocarditis
(5)	Kakar, 2014	F	91	Acute cholecystitis, sepsis
(6)	Tashima, 2014	M	84	Osteomyelitis
(7)	Selvaraj, 2013	F	70	Orthopedic surgery, sepsis
(8)	Jawitz, 2011	F	NR	NR
(9)	Bustillo, 2011	M	77	Endocarditis
(10)	Jheng Wei, 2011	F	41	Meningitis
(11)	Le MEricuett, 2011	F	77	Bacteremia
(12)	MacDonald, 2010	M	32	Accident, ventilator associated pneumonia
(13)	Walsh, 2009	M	76	Bacteremia
(14)	Walsh, 2009	M	77	Endocarditis
(15)	Billet, 2008	M	70	Obesity surgery, hepatic abscess, sepsis
(16)	Billet, 2008	F	61	Sigmoidectomy, wound infection
(17)	Eisendle, 2006	M	65	Arterial popliteal reconstruction, sepsis
(18)	Navi, 2006	M	73	CHF, ICD, Pleural effusion
(19)	Coelho, 2006	F	67	Pneumonia
(20)	Waldman, 2004	F	77	CABG, pneumonia, sepsis
(21)	Joshi, 2004	F	48	Hysterectomy, pelvic abscess
(22)	Armstrong, 2004	M	81	Aortic aneurysm surgery, sternal wound drainage
(23)	Solky, 2004	M	46	Pneumonia
(24)	Dellavalle, 2003	M	74	CVA, UTI, pneumonia
(25)	Palmer, 2001	F	75	Infection of varicose ulcer
(26)	Palmer, 2001	F	86	Femur fracture
(27)	Palmer, 2001	F	78	CABG, sternotomy wound infection
(28)	Wiadrowski, 2001	F	69	Endocarditis, pneumonia
(29)	Hughes, 2001	M	77	Intracranial hemorrhage
(30)	Klein, 2000	F	65	CABG
(31)	Klein, 2000	M	70	CHF, gangrene
(32)	Nousari, 1999	F	74	Endocarditis
(33)	Nousari, 1999	F	41	Endocarditis
(34)	Bernstein, 1998	F	60	Enterocutaneous infected fistula
(35)	Bernstein, 1998	F	71	Pneumonia
(36)	Nousari, 1998	M	65	Subarachnoid hemorrhage
(37)	Bitman, 1996	F	NR	Leg ulcer
(38)	Whitworth, 1996	M	63	Cardiac cath, UTI, bladder cancer
(39)	Richards, 1995	F	72	Bladder cancer
(40)	Geissmann, 1995	F	79	Leg ulcer infection
(41)	Kuechle, 1994	M	69	CABG, sternal wound infection
(42)	Kuechle, 1994	M	74	CABG, sternal wound infection
(43)	Kuechle, 1994	M	67	CABG, sternal wound infection
(44)	Piketty, 1994	M	53	Dissecting aortic aneurysm, groin cellulitis
(45)	Carpenter, 1992	M	54	Bowel perforation
(46)	Carpenter, 1992	F	72	Ovarian cancer, abdomen abscess
(47)	Carpenter, 1992	M	54	Osteomyelitis
(48)	Baden, 1988	M	68	CABG, bacteremia

Adapted from [5].

target antigens identified on Western blotting, including collagen type VII and the 97 kDa and 230 kDa antigens [2, 4, 5, 9, 12]. One study reported two cases of vancomycin-induced LABD with autoantibodies against BP180 and LAD 285 [5, 9, 11]. In addition to immune-mediated process, some have suggested that other clinical conditions may serve as cofactors in the pathogenesis of drug-induced LABD. Triggering events such as infection may initiate an immunologic response [1]. The severity of the reaction does not appear to correlate with serum vancomycin levels.

The usual treatment for drug-induced linear IgA bullous dermatosis is withdrawal of the suspected agent. In nearly all the reported cases of vancomycin-induced LABD, the bullous eruption resolved after discontinuing vancomycin. Other accepted treatments for LABD are dapsone, sulfonamides (sulfapyridine and sulfamethoxypyridazine), colchicine, and topical and oral corticosteroids [1–4, 12].

Our patient represents a case of vancomycin-induced LABD, who developed bullous rash five days after the initiation of vancomycin and improved with withdrawal of systemic vancomycin. Unique to this case is complete resolution of rash despite the antibiotic spacer that was left in place due to the risk of compromising the patient's ability to ambulate outweighing the benefit of spacer removal. There are no reported cases of linear IgA bullous dermatosis associated with vancomycin contained spacer placement.

Our primary hypothesis as to how resolution was achieved in this context is the following: The patient's rash initially manifested around the joint space where the vancomycin impregnated joint spacer was located suggesting that there was a higher concentration of vancomycin (systemic vancomycin plus spacer vancomycin) relative to elsewhere within the patient, both of which were sufficient to create an immune response. With the discontinuation of systemic vancomycin as well as initiation of colchicine, the patient's immune response was blunted due to decreased immune stimulatory vancomycin as well as treatment-mediated immunosuppression. The concentration of vancomycin within the spacer that continues to leach from the sediment is insufficient to cause an immune response leading to the physical manifestations observed with systemic vancomycin in other reported cases or the combination of parenteral and local vancomycin in our case.

While the precise mechanism remains unclear as to how resolution was achieved, the result is powerful as resolution was achieved with medical therapy without potentially compromising ambulation in an 84-year-old patient who continues to live independently after the hospitalization.

4. Conclusion

In conclusion, linear IgA bullous dermatosis secondary to vancomycin is an uncommon skin disease that may resemble other blistering diseases. Early recognition and management of linear IgA bullous dermatosis is important to avert potential serious morbidity associated with this disorder. Future research is needed to better understand the pathophysiology of linear IgA bullous dermatosis to create novel therapies. We hope this case adds to the literature given the fascinating resolution despite the presence of inciting drug in the patient throughout the course of treatment.

Competing Interests

The authors declare that they have no competing interests.

References

[1] B. D. Wilson, E. H. Beutner, V. Kumar, T. P. Chorzelski, and S. Jablonska, "Linear IgA bullous dermatosis: an immunologically defined disease," *International Journal of Dermatology*, vol. 24, no. 9, pp. 569–574, 1985.

[2] L. A. Baden, C. Apovian, M. J. Imber, and J. S. Dover, "Vancomycin-induced linear IgA bullous dermatosis," *Archives of Dermatology*, vol. 124, no. 8, pp. 1186–1188, 1988.

[3] J. M. Whitworth, I. Thomas, S. A. Peltz, B. C. Sullivan, A. H. Wolf, and A. S. Cytryn, "Vancomycin-induced linear IgA bullous dermatosis (LABD)," *Journal of the American Academy of Dermatology*, vol. 34, no. 5, pp. 890–891, 1996.

[4] P. A. Klein and J. P. Callen, "Drug-induced linear IgA bullous dermatosis after vancomycin discontinuance in a patient with renal insufficiency," *Journal of the American Academy of Dermatology*, vol. 42, no. 2, pp. 316–323, 2000.

[5] A. Gameiro, C. Gouveia, O. Tellechea, and M. Goncalo, "Vancomycininduced linear IgA bullous dermatosis: associations," *Dermatology Online Journal*, vol. 22, no. 4, 2016.

[6] S. S. Richards, S. Hall, B. Yokel, and S. E. Whitmore, "A bullous eruption in an elderly woman," *Archives of Dermatology*, vol. 131, no. 12, pp. 1447–1452, 1995.

[7] E. Antiga, M. Caproni, and P. Fabbri, "Linear immunoglobulin a bullous dermatosis: need for an agreement on diagnostic criteria," *Dermatology*, vol. 226, no. 4, pp. 329–332, 2013.

[8] C. Piketty, F. Meeus, D. Nochy, J. M. Poux, C. Jacquot, and J. Bariety, "Linear IgA dermatosis related to vancomycin," *British Journal of Dermatology*, vol. 130, no. 1, pp. 130–131, 1994.

[9] M. J. Kang, H. O. Kim, and Y. M. Park, "Vancomycin-induced Linear IgA bullous dermatosis: a case report and review of the literature," *Annals of Dermatology*, vol. 20, no. 2, pp. 102–106, 2008.

[10] N. Ramesh, A. Magno, D. Lingutla, and A. Khan, "Vancomycin and linear iga bullous dermatosis," *Journal of Hospital Medicine*, vol. 8, supplement 2, 2013.

[11] R. A. Palmer, G. Ogg, J. Allen et al., "Vancomycin-induced linear IgA disease with autoantibodies to BP180 and LAD285," *British Journal of Dermatology*, vol. 145, no. 5, pp. 816–820, 2001.

[12] D. H. Jones, M. Todd, and T. J. Craig, "Early diagnosis is key in vancomycin-induced linear IgA bullous dermatosis and Stevens-Johnson syndrome," *Journal of the American Osteopathic Association*, vol. 104, no. 4, pp. 157–163, 2004.

14

Successful Treatment of Facial Acne Fulminans: Antimicrobial Agents and Oral Prednisolone as Promising Regimes

Amir Hossein Siadat,[1] Anis Bostakian,[1] Bahareh Abtahi-Naeini,[2,3] and Masoom Shahbazi[1]

[1]*Skin Diseases and Leishmaniasis Research Center, School of Medicine, Isfahan University of Medical Sciences, Isfahan, Iran*
[2]*Cancer Research Center, Semnan University of Medical Sciences, Semnan, Iran*
[3]*Skin Diseases and Leishmaniasis Research Center, Department of Dermatology, Isfahan University of Medical Sciences, Isfahan, Iran*

Correspondence should be addressed to Masoom Shahbazi; masoom_sh1982@yahoo.com

Academic Editor: Ichiro Kurokawa

Acne fulminans (AF), also known as acne maligna, is a rare painful ulcerative form of acne with an abrupt onset and systemic symptoms. Its incidence appears to be decreasing, possibly because of earlier and better treatment of acne. This report highlights a case on a necrotizing facial wound due to AF that was successfully treated with oral prednisolone and antimicrobial medication.

1. Introduction

Acne fulminans (AF), also known as acne maligna, acute febrile ulcerative acne, and acute febrile ulcerative conglobate acne with polyarthralgia [1], is a serious variant of acne characterized by an abrupt onset of painful, inflammatory, ulcerative lesions covered with hemorrhagic crusts, which is accompanied by severe acne scarring. The lesions often appear on the upper chest and back [2, 3].

Systemic constitutional symptoms of AF include fluctuating fever, painful joints, malaise, loss of appetite, and laboratory abnormalities [4, 5]. The face is usually less severely involved than the trunk [5].

AF is a rare medical condition, with reports describing only approximately 150 cases. It needs to be treated immediately to avoid severe medical problems, such as permanent disfiguring scars [3]. Nowadays, fewer cases with this condition occur, possibly due to earlier and better acne treatment [3, 4].

Here we report a case with the abovementioned symptoms to highlight the need for early diagnosis and treatment of AF.

2. Case Presentation

A 15-year-old boy presented with a necrotizing bilateral facial wound on the jaw. He had been diagnosed with cystic acne on the face and upper back 3 months ago. He suddenly developed severe worsening of the acne lesions on the face and upper back, and nodular and ulcerated lesions appeared. Associated with the appearance of cutaneous lesions, he also reported fever, chills, arthralgia, and myalgia. On physical examination, he presented with pustules, nodules, and crusts on the face. Hemorrhagic ulcerations with purulent adherent crust were also present on both lateral jaws, as shown in Figure 1.

Also he presented papules, pustules, and small hemorrhagic crusts which were scattered on the upper back and shoulders, as shown in Figure 2.

Physical examination of musculoskeletal system by an expert rheumatologist demonstrated no bony and joint involvement. There were not any palmoplantar pustulosis or psoriasis skin lesions.

Laboratory tests revealed abnormal white blood cell counts (16,000/mm3; segments 72.7%), hemoglobin (13.6 g/dL), erythrocyte sedimentation rate (75), serum ferritin level (178.8 ng/mL), and raised C-reactive protein levels.

Radiologic evaluation of axial skeleton and also sternoclavicular region revealed no sclerosis and osteolysis and periosteal reaction formation.

Magnetic resonance imaging (MRI) was also performed for detection of any occult bony involvement and the result was negative.

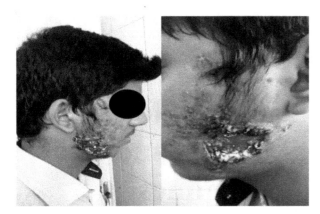

FIGURE 1: Acne fulminans. Hemorrhagic ulcerations with purulent crust scattered on both sides of the face.

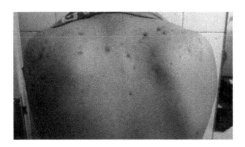

FIGURE 2: Some papules, pustules, small hemorrhagic crusts, and scar formation were scattered on the upper back of patient with acne fulminant.

A biopsy specimen from the facial ulcer showed hyperkeratosis, acanthosis associated with follicular ostium destruction, and neutrophil infiltrations, which confirmed the diagnosis of AF. Treatment with broad-spectrum systemic antibiotics included 300 mg clindamycin thrice daily and 750 mg levofloxacin daily (according to the result of microbial colonization) in conjunction with 1 mg/kg/day oral prednisolone.

Primary control of the lesions was obtained over the course of 4 weeks with this therapeutic regimen, with noticeable decrease in the ulcerative lesions after treatment (Figure 3). Prednisolone was gradually reduced over a 2-month period, and a low dose of oral isotretinoin was initiated. The patient's acne fulminans gradually cleared within 3 months and healed, leaving a cicatricial scar on both lateral jaws.

3. Discussion

The etiology of AF is uncertain, but relationships with circulating androgens, infection, and explosive hypersensitivity reaction to surface bacteria have been postulated. Genetic and hereditary factors may also play an important role in the pathogenesis of AF in some patients [6, 7]. The term fulminans describes the sudden onset of the lesion and the course of this disease [3].

Patients with AF should immediately consult a dermatologist. The management of AF can be difficult; in addition to general supportive care, systemic corticosteroids, such as prednisone (20–60 mg/day), are the mainstay of therapy [8].

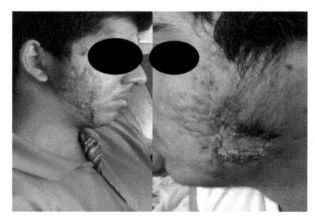

FIGURE 3: Acne fulminans after 28 days of oral prednisone and systemic antimicrobial regimen.

Other medications may be useful but usually require longer treatment periods. These medications include aspirin, dapsone [8], cyclosporine [2], antibiotic treatment probably due to their anti-inflammatory effect, and low-dose isotretinoin (after control of the acute phase of the disease) [4]. The data demonstrate that the treatment protocols that use a combination of prednisolone and isotretinoin lead to a faster control of systemic features as well as a faster clearance of the acne [9].

The use of antibiotics alone is ineffective but antibiotics can be effective if the microbial colonization or anti-inflammatory effects have been considered [8].

In our patient administration of antibiotic was based on the result of culture and microbial colonization.

Recurrences may be prevented by gradually reducing corticosteroids and possibly by the continuation or addition of systemic isotretinoin [10]. Although AF is usually identified because of its unique clinical features, the differential diagnosis should be considered especially at uncommon sites, including the face. Other potential diagnoses include rosacea fulminans [11], pyoderma gangrenosum, acne conglobate [8], and synovitis-acne-pustulosis-hyperostosis-osteitis (SAPHO) syndrome [12–14].

Although the clinical feature of severe rosacea fulminans can be similar to the acne fulminant, usually it is seen in women with higher age [11, 15]. Thus it is less probable for our patient.

Pyoderma gangrenosum characterized by painful progressive necrosis of the wound margins and the border of lesions typically is undermined and violaceous [16].

Acne conglobata rarely can affect the face but it has a more chronic course without a sudden onset [8].

SAPHO syndrome is suspected when a patient presents with a pustular skin disease in association with rheumatic pain but our patient had not any bony involvement and internal organs like the hematopoietic system [17].

Thus, clinicians should consider AF as a differential diagnosis for facial wounds as early diagnosis and treatment can reduce the associated morbidity.

4. Conclusion

AF should be suspected in patients presenting with an abrupt onset of a painful necrotizing facial wound of unknown etiology. In these settings antimicrobial agents combined with oral prednisone are an effective treatment for stabilizing clinical and laboratory parameters and preventing diseases progression.

Conflicts of Interest

The authors declare that there are no conflicts of interest regarding the publication of this paper.

References

[1] D. C. Seukeran and W. J. Cunliffe, "The treatment of acne fulminans: a review of 25 cases," *British Journal of Dermatology*, vol. 141, no. 2, pp. 307–309, 1999.

[2] P. Giavedoni, J. M. Mascaró-Galy, P. Aguilera, and T. Estrach-Panella, "Acne fulminans successfully treated with cyclosporine and isotretinoin," *Journal of the American Academy of Dermatology*, vol. 70, no. 2, pp. e38–e39, 2014.

[3] R. Zaba, R. A. Schwartz, S. Jarmuda, M. Czarnecka-Operacz, and W. Silny, "Acne fulminans: explosive systemic form of acne," *Journal of the European Academy of Dermatology and Venereology*, vol. 25, no. 5, pp. 501–507, 2011.

[4] E. Rodríguez-Lomba, I. Molina-López, I. Monteagudo-Sáez, R. Suárez-Fernández, and M. Campos-Domínguez, "A case of acne fulminans with sacroiliitis successfully treated with methotrexate and isotretinoin," *Dermatologic Therapy*, vol. 29, no. 6, pp. 476–478, 2016.

[5] L. R. Grando, O. G. Leite, and T. F. Cestari, "Pseudo-acne fulminans associated with oral isotretinoin," *Anais Brasileiros de Dermatologia*, vol. 89, no. 4, pp. 657–659, 2014.

[6] M. Saint-Jean, C. Frenard, M. Le Bras, G. G. Aubin, S. Corvec, and B. Dréno, "Testosterone-induced acne fulminans in twins with Kallmann's syndrome," *JAAD Case Reports*, vol. 1, no. 1, pp. 27–29, 2015.

[7] S. L. Karvonen, L. Räsänen, W. J. Cunliffe, K. T. Holland, J. Karvonen, and T. Reunala, "Delayed hypersensitivity to propionibacterium acnes in patients with severe nodular acne and acne fulminans," *Dermatology*, vol. 189, no. 4, pp. 344–349, 1994.

[8] R. B. Lages, S. H. Bona, F. V. M. E. Silva, A. K. L. Gomes, and V. Campelo, "Acne fulminans successfully treated with prednisone and dapsone," *Anais Brasileiros de Dermatologia*, vol. 87, no. 4, pp. 612–614, 2012.

[9] D. Blanc, M. Zultak, D. Wendling, and F. Lonchampt, "Eruptive pyogenic granulomas and acne fulminans in two siblings treated with isotretinoin. A possible common pathogenesis," *Dermatologica*, vol. 177, no. 1, pp. 16–18, 1988.

[10] S.-L. Karvonen, "Acne fulminans: report of clinical findings and treatment of twenty-four patients," *Journal of the American Academy of Dermatology*, vol. 28, no. 4, pp. 572–579, 1993.

[11] L. A. Smith, S. A. Meehan, and D. E. Cohen, "Rosacea fulminans with extrafacial lesions in an elderly man: successful treatment with subantimicrobial-dose doxycycline," *Journal of Drugs in Dermatology*, vol. 13, no. 6, pp. 763–765, 2014.

[12] L. Mantovani, S. Zauli, A. Virgili, and V. Bettoli, "Rosacea fulminans or acute rosacea? Report of 5 cases and review of the literature," *Giornale Italiano di Dermatologia e Venereologia*, vol. 1, no. 5, pp. 53–57, 2016.

[13] B. Abtahi-Naeini, F. Bagheri, M. Pourazizi, M. Forozeshfard, and A. Saffaei, "Unusual cause of breast wound: postoperative pyoderma gangrenosum," *International Wound Journal*, vol. 14, no. 1, pp. 285–287, 2017.

[14] Z. Shahmoradi, F. Mokhtari, M. Pourazizi, B. Abtahi-Naeini, and A. Saffaei, "Extensive abdominal wall and genital pyoderma gangrenosum: combination therapy in unusual presentations," *Journal of Cutaneous and Aesthetic Surgery*, vol. 7, no. 4, pp. 238–240, 2014.

[15] L. B. P. Ribeiro and M. Ramos-e-Silva, "Rosacea fulminans," *Cutis*, vol. 92, no. 1, pp. 29–32, 2013.

[16] G. Faghihi, B. Abtahi-Naeini, Z. Nikyar, K. Jamshidi, and A. Bahrami, "Postoperative pyoderma gangrenosum: a rare complication after appendectomy," *Journal of Postgraduate Medicine*, vol. 61, no. 1, pp. 42–43, 2015.

[17] B. L. Divya and P. N. Rao, "SAPHO syndrome with acne fulminans and severe polyosteitis involving axial skeleton," *Indian Dermatology Online Journal*, vol. 7, no. 5, pp. 414–417, 2016.

15

Nevus Lipomatosus Superficialis on the Left Proximal Arm

Alexander K. C. Leung[1,2] and Benjamin Barankin[3]

[1]*Department of Pediatrics, The University of Calgary, Calgary, AB, Canada T2M 0H5*
[2]*The Alberta Children's Hospital, Calgary, AB, Canada T2M 0H5*
[3]*Toronto Dermatology Centre, Toronto, ON, Canada M3H 5Y8*

Correspondence should be addressed to Alexander K. C. Leung; aleung@ucalgary.ca

Academic Editor: Jacek Cezary Szepietowski

We report a 58-year-old woman with a solitary type of nevus lipomatosus superficialis on the left proximal arm. To our knowledge, the occurrence of a solitary type of nevus lipomatosus superficialis on the arm has very rarely been reported. A perusal of the literature revealed but one case, to which we are going to add another one. Recognition of this clinical manifestation is important so that a proper diagnosis can be made.

1. Introduction

Nevus lipomatosus superficialis is a hamartoma characterized by ectopic mature adipose tissue in the papillary dermis. The condition was first described by Hoffman and Zurhelle in 1921 [1]. Two types of nevus lipomatosus cutaneous superficialis are recognized, namely, the classical multiple type (also known as the Hoffman-Zurhelle type) and the solitary type [2, 3]. We describe a 58-year-old woman with a solitary type of nevus lipomatosus superficialis on the left proximal arm. To our knowledge, the occurrence of a solitary type of nevus lipomatosus superficialis on the arm has very rarely been reported.

2. Case Report

A 58-year-old woman presented with a slow-growing multilobulated plaque on the left proximal arm of approximately 2 years' duration. The lesion was asymptomatic with no history of ulceration or discharge. There was no history of preceding trauma. The patient was otherwise in good health. Family history was noncontributory.

Physical examination revealed a soft, skin-colored, multilobulated, nontender, well-defined, discrete, dome-shaped plaque on the left lateral proximal arm adjacent to the axilla (Figure 1). There was no axillary lymphadenopathy.

There was no comedo-like lesions, café au lait macules, or hypertrichosis on the surface of the lesion. The rest of the physical examination was normal.

Excisional biopsy of the lesion showed islands of mature adipocytes in the papillary dermis, confirming the clinical diagnosis of nevus lipomatosus superficialis (Figure 2).

3. Discussion

Nevus lipomatosus superficialis is an uncommon condition. In a retrospective study, 8 cases were seen in an 11-year-period from 2001 to 2011 at the Department of Dermatology, Venerology and Leprology, Postgraduate Institute of Medical Education and Research in Chandigarh, India [4]. In another retrospective study, 8 cases were seen in a 14-year-period from 1997 to 2010 at the Department of Dermatology, Charles Nicole Hospital in Tunis, Tunisia [5]. There is no familial or sex predilection [3].

The condition is usually idiopathic and the exact pathogenesis is not known [2]. Theories such as mesenchymal perivascular differentiation of lipoblasts, focal heterotopic development of adipose tissue, and adipose metaplasia in the course of degenerative changes of dermal collagen bundles and elastic tissue have been proposed to account for the heterotopic occurrence of adipose tissues but not substantiated [4, 5].

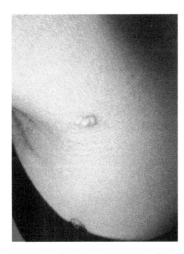

FIGURE 1: A soft, skin-colored, multilobulated, well-defined, discrete, dome-shaped plaque on the left lateral proximal arm adjacent to the axilla.

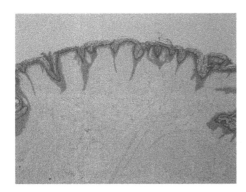

FIGURE 2: Histopathology showing islands of mature adipocytes in the papillary dermis.

Deletion of 2p24 has been described, suggesting that genes may have a role to play [6].

The classical type is usually present at birth or appears within the first two decades of life [3]. Typically, the classical type presents as asymptomatic, multiple, soft, yellowish or skin-colored, sessile or pedunculated, papules or nodules, often coalescing into plaques whose surface may be smooth, wrinkled, or cerebriform or have a peau d'orange appearance that are present in a linear, zosteriform, or segmental pattern [3, 7]. Sites of predilection include the pelvic girdle, gluteal region, lower trunk, and upper thigh [3, 7].

The solitary type, on the other hand, often appears between the third and sixth decade of life and typically presents as an asymptomatic, solitary, yellowish to skin-colored, dome-shaped or sessile papule or nodule, as is illustrated in the present case [7]. The lesion has no predilection for any particular site and can develop anywhere on the body, including the scalp, neck, face, eyelid, nose, knee, axilla, arm, scrotum, vulva, and clitoris [3, 7–11]. The occurrence on the arm has been rarely reported and a perusal of the literature revealed only one case. In 1975, Jones et al. reported a male

patient with a solitary nevus lipomatosus superficialis on the arm [11]. The authors, however, did not specify the age of the patient and the laterality of the lesion. The occurrence of the lesion on the arm may be more common than is presently appreciated. Recognition of this clinical manifestation is important so that a proper diagnosis can be made.

4. Conclusion

Although the solitary type of nevus can develop anywhere on the body, the occurrence on the arm has rarely been reported; a perusal of the literature revealed only one case. The occurrence of the lesion on the arm may be more common than is presently appreciated. Recognition of this clinical manifestation is important so that a proper diagnosis can be made.

Conflicts of Interest

Professor Leung and Dr. Barankin have disclosed no relevant financial relationship. They have received no external funding for the preparation of this manuscript.

References

[1] E. Hoffman and E. Zurhelle, "Ubereinen nevus lipomatodes cutaneus superficialis der linkenglutaalgegend," *Arch dermatol Syph*, vol. 130, pp. 327–333, 1921.

[2] R. Chopra, Y. M. Al Marzooq, F. A. Siddiqui, S. Aldawsari, and A. A. Ameer, "Nevus lipomatosus cutaneous superficialis with focal lipocytic pagetoid epidermal spread and secondary calcinosis cutis: A case report," *American Journal of Dermatopathology*, vol. 37, no. 4, pp. 326–328, 2015.

[3] M. Goyal, V. H. Wankhade, J. I. Mukhi, and R. P. Singh, "Nevus lipomatosus cutaneous superficialis - A rare hamartoma: Report of two cases," *Journal of Clinical and Diagnostic Research*, vol. 10, no. 10, pp. WD01–WD02, 2016.

[4] M. S. Kumaran, T. Narang, S. Dogra, U. N. Saikia, and A. J. Kanwar, "Nevus lipomatosus superficialis unseen or unrecognized: A report of eight cases," *Journal of Cutaneous Medicine and Surgery*, vol. 17, no. 5, pp. 335–339, 2013.

[5] S. Goucha, A. Khaled, F. Zéglaoui, B. Fazaa, S. Rammeh, and R. Zermani, "Nevus lipomatosus cutaneous superfcialis: Report of eight cases," *Dermatology and Therapy*, vol. 1, no. 2, pp. 25–30, 2011.

[6] N. Cardot-Leccia, A. Italiano, M. C. Monteil, E. Basc, C. Perrin, and F. Pedeutour, "Naevus lipomatosus superficialis: a case report with a 2p24 deletion," *British Journal of Dermatology*, vol. 156, no. 2, pp. 380-381, 2007.

[7] P. Bhushan, S. Thatte, and A. Singh, "Nevus lipomatosus cutaneous superficialis: A report of two cases," *Indian Journal of Dermatology*, vol. 61, no. 1, p. 123, 2016.

[8] S. Weitzner, "Solitary Nevus Lipomatosus Cutaneus Superficialis of Scalp," *Archives of Dermatology*, vol. 97, no. 5, pp. 540–542, 1968.

[9] V. Sathyanarayana and S. Weitzner, "Solitary Nevus Lipomatosus Cutaneus Superficialis of the Knee," *Archives of Dermatology*, vol. 114, no. 8, pp. 1226-1227, 1978.

[10] S.-L. Karvonen, "Acne fulminans: report of clinical findings and treatment of twenty-four patients," *Journal of the American Academy of Dermatology*, vol. 28, no. 4, pp. 572–579, 1993.

[11] L. A. Smith, S. A. Meehan, and D. E. Cohen, "Rosacea fulminans with extrafacial lesions in an elderly man: successful treatment with subantimicrobial-dose doxycycline," *Journal of Drugs in Dermatology*, vol. 13, no. 6, pp. 763–765, 2014.

[12] L. Mantovani, S. Zauli, A. Virgili, and V. Bettoli, "Rosacea fulminans or acute rosacea? Report of 5 cases and review of the literature," *Giornale Italiano di Dermatologia e Venereologia*, vol. 1, no. 5, pp. 53–57, 2016.

[13] B. Abtahi-Naeini, F. Bagheri, M. Pourazizi, M. Forozeshfard, and A. Saffaei, "Unusual cause of breast wound: postoperative pyoderma gangrenosum," *International Wound Journal*, vol. 14, no. 1, pp. 285–287, 2017.

[14] Z. Shahmoradi, F. Mokhtari, M. Pourazizi, B. Abtahi-Naeini, and A. Saffaei, "Extensive abdominal wall and genital pyoderma gangrenosum: combination therapy in unusual presentations," *Journal of Cutaneous and Aesthetic Surgery*, vol. 7, no. 4, pp. 238–240, 2014.

[15] L. B. P. Ribeiro and M. Ramos-e-Silva, "Rosacea fulminans," *Cutis*, vol. 92, no. 1, pp. 29–32, 2013.

[16] G. Faghihi, B. Abtahi-Naeini, Z. Nikyar, K. Jamshidi, and A. Bahrami, "Postoperative pyoderma gangrenosum: a rare complication after appendectomy," *Journal of Postgraduate Medicine*, vol. 61, no. 1, pp. 42–43, 2015.

[17] B. L. Divya and P. N. Rao, "SAPHO syndrome with acne fulminans and severe polyosteitis involving axial skeleton," *Indian Dermatology Online Journal*, vol. 7, no. 5, pp. 414–417, 2016.

[18] G. Gaitanis and I. D. Bassukas, "Immunocryosurgery for non-superficial basal cell carcinomas ≤ 20 mm in maximal diameter: Five-year follow-up," *Journal of Geriatric Oncology*, 2018.

[19] P. W. Hashim, J. K. Nia, S. Singer, and G. Goldenberg, "An investigator-initiated study to assess the safety and efficacy of ingenol mebutate 0.05% gel when used after cryosurgery in the treatment of hypertrophic actinic keratosis on dorsal hands," *Journal of Clinical and Aesthetic Dermatology*, vol. 9, no. 7, pp. 16–22, 2016.

[20] G. Penna and L. Adorini, "1α,25-Dihydroxyvitamin D3 inhibits differentiation, maturation, activation, and survival of dendritic cells leading to impaired alloreactive T cell activation," *The Journal of Immunology*, vol. 164, no. 5, pp. 2405–2411, 2000.

[21] M. D. Griffin, W. Lutz, V. A. Phan, L. A. Bachman, D. J. McKean, and R. Kumar, "Dendritic cell modulation by 1α,25 dihydroxyvitamin D3 and its analogs: a vitamin D receptor-dependent pathway that promotes a persistent state of immaturity in vitro and in vivo," *Proceedings of the National Academy of Sciences of the United States of America*, vol. 98, no. 12, pp. 6800–6805, 2001.

[22] M. Hewison, "An update on vitamin D and human immunity," *Clinical Endocrinology*, vol. 76, no. 3, pp. 315–325, 2012.

16

A Supernumerary Nipple-Like Clinical Presentation of Lymphangioma Circumscriptum

Dustin Taylor [ID],[1] **Natalie Kash** [ID],[2] **and Sirunya Silapunt** [ID][2]

[1]University of Texas McGovern Medical School, Houston, TX, USA
[2]Department of Dermatology, University of Texas McGovern Medical School, Houston, TX, USA

Correspondence should be addressed to Sirunya Silapunt; sirunya.silapunt@uth.tmc.edu

Academic Editor: Ichiro Kurokawa

Lymphangioma circumscriptum is a superficially localized variant of lymphangioma. The characteristic clinical presentation is a "frogspawn" grouping of vesicles or papulovesicles on the proximal limb or limb girdle areas. Though most lymphangiomas develop congenitally, the lymphangioma circumscriptum subtype is known to present in adults. We report a case of lymphangioma circumscriptum on the left inframammary area of an African American female with an unusual supernumerary nipple-like clinical presentation. Our patient presented with a firm, smooth, hypopigmented papule, and the clinical diagnosis of keloid was made initially. However, she returned reporting growth of the lesion and was noted to have a firm, exophytic, lobulated, pink to skin-colored nodule. Histopathological examination demonstrated dilated lymphatic vessels, consistent with the diagnosis of lymphangioma. The presentation as a firm, hypopigmented papule and later exophytic, lobulated, skin-colored nodule in our case represents a clinical presentation of lymphangioma circumscriptum not previously described in the literature. Correct diagnosis in lymphangioma circumscriptum is vital, as recurrence following surgical resection and secondary development of lymphangiosarcoma and squamous cell carcinoma following treatment with radiation have been reported. Thus, it is important to consider lymphangioma circumscriptum in the differential of similar lesions in the future to allow appropriate diagnosis, treatment, and monitoring.

1. Introduction

Lymphangiomas are malformations of lymphatic tissue characterized by distended channels. They are most frequently seen in children, with up to 90% of cases occurring within the first 2 years of life [1]. One theory for the pathophysiology of lymphangiomas is that erratic lymph vessels fail to connect with the general lymphatic system during development [2]. A similar hypothesis attests that lymphangiomas develop from a failure of the lymphatic system to communicate with the venous system [2, 3]. Both hypothesized mechanisms are congruent with the fact that lymphangiomas most commonly present as a congenital problem. However, a superficially localized variant, lymphangioma circumscriptum (LC), is known to present in adulthood and is the most common adult-onset form [2, 4]. Lymphangioma circumscriptum most commonly occurs on the proximal limbs or limb girdle areas [2, 4]. It is histopathologically characterized by dilated lymphatic vessels in the papillary dermis that elevate the epidermis above that of the surrounding skin, leading to the characteristic "frogspawn" grouped vesicles or papulovesicles seen clinically [2, 3].

2. Case Presentation

A 42-year-old African American female initially presented with a several month history of an asymptomatic lesion on the left inframammary area. She denied any antecedent trauma to the area or any other predisposing factors. The patient had a history of breast cancer that was being treated with tamoxifen at that time; however, she had not received radiation to the area as part of her treatment regimen. Physical exam revealed a 3-mm, firm, smooth, hypopigmented papule on the left inframammary area. The lesion was diagnosed as a keloid, and the patient was reassured and asked to return to the clinic for treatment if the area became irritated.

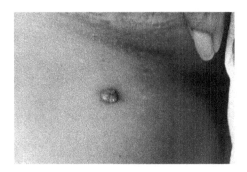

FIGURE 1: Left inframammary area with a 1.5-cm, exophytic, lobulated, pink to skin-colored nodule surrounded by a hyperpigmented patch.

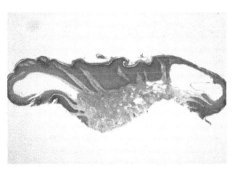

(a) Dilated vessels are present in the papillary dermis. There is elongation of the rete ridges, epidermal atrophy, and some degree of acanthosis and hyperkeratosis in the center (H&E, 40x)

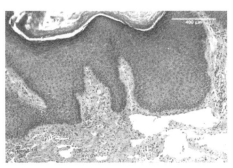

(b) Higher power magnification demonstrates epidermal hyperplasia in the center (H&E, 200x)

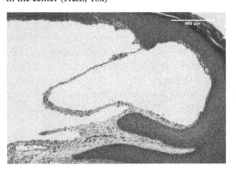

(c) Dilated lymphatic vessels characterized by thin walls lined by endothelial cells and a lack of red blood cells (H&E, 200x)

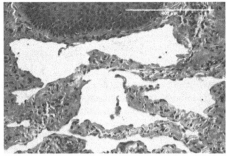

(d) Valves are present within the lymphatic vessels (H&E, 400x)

FIGURE 2

The patient presented 1.5 years later because the lesion had been growing and rubbing on clothing. She denied any associated bleeding, pruritus, or pain. On exam, the left inframammary area was noted to have a 1.5-cm, firm, exophytic, lobulated, pink to skin-colored nodule with a surrounding hyperpigmented patch (Figure 1). The clinical differential diagnosis included supernumerary nipple, eccrine poroma, clear cell acanthoma, papillary eccrine adenoma, tubular apocrine adenoma, keloid, melanoma, and nonmelanoma skin cancer. The lesion was entirely removed, and histopathology demonstrated dilated lymphatic vessels with thin walls lined by endothelial cells and no associated red blood cells in the papillary dermis, overlying epidermal atrophy, some degree of acanthosis and hyperkeratosis, and elongation of the rete ridges, consistent with a diagnosis of lymphangioma (Figure 2). The patient has since done well with no evidence of recurrence at one-year follow-up.

3. Discussion

Literature search reveals several cases of LC arising on the abdomen, breast, and inframammary region; however, these cases manifested clinically with papulovesicular lesions [5, 6]. The firm, exophytic, lobulated, pink to skin-colored nodule with a surrounding hyperpigmented patch detailed in our case clinically mimicked a supernumerary nipple given its location along the milk line in the inframammary area and represents a clinical presentation of LC not previously described in the literature.

Additionally, adult-onset or acquired cases of LC in the literature usually report some history of antecedent trauma, particularly in areas that are subject to friction or previous radiation therapy or in the setting of chronic lymphedema [5, 7, 8]. Those near the breast are associated with previous breast conservation therapy or radiation to the area [5]. Our patient had no history of previous surgery, radiation therapy, or lymphedema. While our patient could not attest to any trauma to the area, its distribution near the bra could likely have subjected it to frequent friction, suggesting a possible inciting event.

Histologically, lymphangiomas are characterized by dilated lymphatic vessels present in the papillary dermis, positivity of the lymphatic channels to the lymphatic endothelial marker D2-40, atrophy of the overlying epidermis, and elongation of the rete ridges [3, 9]. The verrucous variety demonstrates epidermal hyperplasia, papillomatosis, and hyperparakeratosis [10]. The histologic findings in our case are consistent with the diagnosis of lymphangioma. Our case did show epidermal atrophy with some degree of epidermal hyperplasia. However, given that the epidermal hyperplasia and hyperkeratosis were minimal and that clinically there was clearly no verrucous component, our case is not consistent with the verrucous variety.

The importance of the correct diagnosis in cases of LC is multifold; risks associated with this diagnosis include recurrence and the secondary development of malignancy. One study reports that the risk of recurrence in surgically resected cases of LC is 11% [11]. Further, cases of secondary development of lymphangiosarcoma and squamous cell carcinoma within these lesions following radiation have been reported [12, 13]. The complete removal of the lesion in our patient appears to have minimized her risk for future complications, and appropriate monitoring revealed no evidence of recurrence in her case. This case warrants consideration and inclusion of LC in the clinical differential diagnosis of a firm, skin-colored nodule to enable appropriate diagnosis and management.

Conflicts of Interest

The authors declare that there are no conflicts of interest regarding the publication of this article.

References

[1] A. Alqahtani, L. T. Nguyen, H. Flageole, K. Shaw, and J.-M. Laberge, "25 years' experience with lymphangiomas in children," *Journal of Pediatric Surgery*, vol. 34, no. 7, pp. 1164–1168, 1999.

[2] J. Patterson, "Vascular Tumors," in *In: Weedon's Skin Pathology*, pp. 1069–1115, Elsevier Inc., 4th edition, 2016.

[3] I. W. Whimster, "The pathology of lymphangioma circumscriptum," *British Journal of Dermatology*, vol. 94, no. 5, pp. 473–486, 1976.

[4] R. D. G. Peachey, C. C. Lim, and I. W. Whimster, "Lymphangioma of skin: a review of 65 cases," *British Journal of Dermatology*, vol. 83, no. 5, pp. 519–527, 1970.

[5] I. Tasdalen, S. Gokgoz, E. Paksoy et al., "Acquired lymphangiectasis after breast conservation treatment for breast cancer: Report of a case," *Dermatol Online Journal*, vol. 10, no. 1, p. 9, 2004.

[6] H. M. Omprakash and S. C. Rajendran, "Lymphangioma circumscriptum (microcystic lymphatic malformation): palliative coagulation using radiofrequency current," *Journal of Cutaneous and Aesthetic Surgery*, vol. 1, no. 2, pp. 85–88, 2008.

[7] Y. Hamada, K. Yagi, A. Tanano et al., "Cystic lymphangioma of the scrotum," *Pediatric Surgery International*, vol. 13, no. 5-6, pp. 442–444, 1998.

[8] X. C. Mu, T.-A. N. Tran, M. Dupree, and J. A. Carlson, "Acquired vulvar lymphangioma mimicking genital warts. A case report and review of the literature," *Journal of Cutaneous Pathology*, vol. 26, no. 3, pp. 150–154, 1999.

[9] A. Sultan, S. S. Dadras, J. M. Bay, and N. N. H. Teng, "Prox-1, Podoplanin and HPV staining assists in identification of lymphangioma circumscriptum of the vulva and discrimination from vulvar warts," *Histopathology*, vol. 59, no. 6, pp. 1274–1277, 2011.

[10] C. F. Poh and R. W. Priddy, "Acquired oral lymphangioma circumscriptum mimicking verrucous carcinoma," *Oral Oncology Extra*, vol. 41, no. 10, pp. 277–280, 2005.

[11] K. Niitsuma, M. Hatoko, H. Tada, A. Tanaka, S. Yurugi, and H. Iioka, "Recurrence of cutaneous lymphangioma after surgical resection: Its features and manner," *European Journal of Plastic Surgery*, vol. 27, no. 8, pp. 367–370, 2005.

[12] D. T. King, D. M. Duffy, F. M. Hirose, and A. W. Gurevitch, "Lymphangiosarcoma Arising From Lymphangioma Circumscriptum," *JAMA Dermatology*, vol. 115, no. 8, pp. 969–972, 1979.

[13] G. R. Wilson, N. H. Cox, N. R. McLean, and D. Scott, "Squamous cell carcinoma arising within congenital lymphangioma circumscriptum," *British Journal of Dermatology*, vol. 129, no. 3, pp. 337–339, 1993.

17

Asymmetric Bilateral Lichen Striatus: A Rare Presentation following Multiple Blaschko's Lines

Jeffrey S. Dickman (ID),[1] **McKay D. Frandsen,**[1] **and Andrew J. Racette**[2]

[1]*Midwestern University, Arizona College of Osteopathic Medicine, 19555 N 59th Ave, Glendale, AZ 85308, USA*
[2]*Omni Dermatology, Inc., KCU-GMEC Phoenix Dermatology Residency Program, 4840 E Indian School Rd, Suite 102, Phoenix, AZ 85018, USA*

Correspondence should be addressed to Jeffrey S. Dickman; jdickman26@midwestern.edu

Academic Editor: Soner Uzun

Lichen striatus (LS) is an uncommon, acquired, self-limited, and benign linear dermatosis of unknown etiology that most often occurs unilaterally and is confined to the lines of Blaschko. A healthy 7-year-old girl presented to our clinic with bilateral asymmetric LS occurring on the right arm and left leg of 1-year duration. Very few cases of bilateral LS have been previously reported in the literature, with none from clinics within the United States. The etiology of LS is currently unknown; however its confinement to Blaschko's lines, which represent embryologic migration of skin cell clones, does provide insight into a possible pathogenesis. It seems most likely that an individual's development of LS is linked to their genetic predisposition and a subsequent triggering event. Our case serves as a strong example of a rare presentation of LS and facilitates discussion of the clinical diagnostic process and possible pathogenesis of this dermatosis.

1. Introduction

Lichen striatus (LS) is an uncommon linear dermatosis that most commonly affects children aged 4 months to 15 years and is distributed along the lines of Blaschko. Diagnosis is made based on clinical appearance of 2 to 4 mm, flat-topped, lichenoid papules ranging from red color to flesh color that are distributed linearly and may be discrete or confluent [1, 2]. A variant presentation may more commonly present with hypochromic macules that are singular or coalesce into a patch [2]. Classically, LS occurs unilaterally and along a singular Blaschko line (BL) typically on the extremities, but a few rare cases have been found occurring bilaterally. To the best of our knowledge less than ten bilateral presentations have been previously reported in the literature, making our patient very unique [3–7]. The etiology of LS remains unclear, though the lesions are benign and the condition is self-limited. Some have hypothesized that the LS may develop in a genetically predisposed individual who encounters an immunologic trigger [1, 8].

In this article we present a patient with bilateral asymmetric LS who reported gradual onset one year prior to presentation. Very few cases of bilateral LS have been previously reported in the literature; and to the best of our knowledge none was from clinics within the United States of America [3–7].

2. Case Presentation

A healthy 7-year-old girl of Indian descent presented with one-year duration of hypochromic linear bands in two regions. The lesions were present on the right forearm and left leg and buttocks. Neither the patient nor her parents were able to recall any inciting illness, allergy, or environmental or social exposure that may have preceded the onset, which was gradual. There was no associated pruritus, pain, hair loss, or nail involvement. No recent growth had been noted. The patient had not received any previous topical or systemic treatment for the lesions. The patient's past medical history

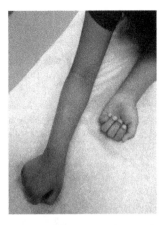

FIGURE 1: Hypopigmented linear eruption on the right forearm.

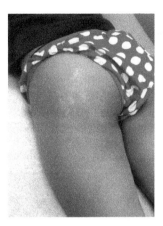

FIGURE 3: Hypopigmented macules and patch following the lines of Blaschko.

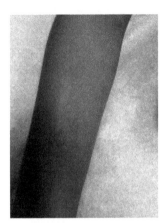

FIGURE 2: Hypopigmented macules coalescing into patch along BL.

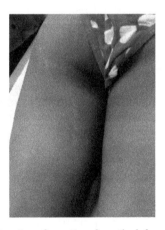

FIGURE 4: Extension of eruption along the left posterior thigh.

was negative for atopy and otherwise unremarkable, as was her family history.

On examination 2 mm hypopigmented lichenoid macules were noted coalescing into a linear patch on the dorsal aspect of the patient's right forearm (Figures 1 and 2). The eruption ended at the distal forearm, sparing the right hand, fingers, and nails. The distribution was consistent with BL. Similar lesions were also noted on the left buttock, though somewhat more diffuse, but also progressing distally along a BL to the left posterior thigh (Figures 3 and 4). The lesions in both locations were nonscaling, nonpainful, nonpruritic, and stable in appearance according to the patient's parents.

No biopsies were taken at the request of the patient's parents. A diagnosis of LS was made clinically, and observation was recommended with explanation of the disease course. A follow-up visit was scheduled but the patient did not return to the clinic.

3. Discussion

Lichen striatus is an acquired, self-limited, benign dermatosis of unknown etiology that most commonly occurs unilaterally

TABLE 1: LS differential diagnosis [1, 8–10].

Inflammatory linear verrucous epidermal nevus
Linear epidermal nevus
Linear psoriasis
Linear lichen planus
Linear verruca plana
Linear porokeratosis
Linear Darier's disease
Blaschkitis

and is confined to the lines of Blaschko. Its diagnosis can be made based on clinical presentation alone, but careful consideration of other linear eruptions must be given (Table 1) [1, 8–10]. Biopsy and histopathological analysis, when tolerable to the patient, may help to distinguish LS from other lesions but are somewhat nonspecific. Typical histological findings include spongiotic and lichenoid interface dermatitis with superficial and deep perivascular infiltrate and epidermal changes including hyperkeratosis, parakeratosis, focal spongiosis, and lymphocytic exocytosis. The deep lymphohistiocytic infiltrates are also seen surrounding adnexal structures such as hair follicles and eccrine glands [11–13].

Three morphological variants of LS have been described [2]. Typical lichen striatus is most common, presenting as 2 to 4 mm, flat-topped, lichenoid papules ranging in color from red to flesh-colored. This accounts for approximately 80% of patients. Lichen striatus albus presents with hypopigmented macules and/or papules that coalesce into a patch as seen in our patient. The final variant is nail lichen striatus, which in addition to cutaneous lesions affects the nail matrix of usually a single digit. LS in all its forms is more common in females with a ratio of 2:1 [1, 2]. Of note, four of the six comparable cases (including ours) of bilateral LS have occurred in patients of Indian descent [3–5]. A recent analysis performed in an outpatient dermatology department in South India showed that LS made up 1.77% of presenting hypopigmentary disorders [14]. Because the pathogenesis of LS is poorly understood more research is necessary to determine if this association is incidental.

The etiology of LS remains unclear. Its confinement to BL, representing embryologic migration of skin cell clones, does however provide insight into a possible pathogenesis. It has been suggested that a postzygotic somatic mutation followed by an immunologic response directed at these clonal cells may be the cause [11, 15]. Happle later proposed the theory that transposable elements or retrotransposons within the human genome, which affect the activation or silencing of genes, could cause linear skin lesions following BL. This model had been demonstrated in the variegated coat patterns resembling BL in animals [16]. It seems most likely that an individual's development of LS is linked to their genetic predisposition and a subsequent triggering event. It remains unclear however if that event is the activation or suppression of a gene, an immunological response against previously mutated cells, or the result of some external agent.

Our patient is especially interesting because the dermatosis was bilateral. Very few cases with bilateral distribution have been reported in the literature [3–7]. While the disease itself is benign and self-limited, it may present a diagnostic challenge and its pathogenesis is complex. Exploration of additional cases like ours will help us to better diagnose and understand this disease.

Conflicts of Interest

The authors declare that they have no conflicts of interest.

References

[1] T. Shiohara and Y. Kano, "Lichen Planus and lichenoid dermatoses," in *Dermatology*, J. Bolognia, J. Jorizzo, and J. Schaffer, Eds., pp. 183–202, Elsevier/Saunders, Philadelphia, PA, USA, 3rd edition, 2012.

[2] A. Patrizi, I. Neri, C. Fiorentini, A. Bonci, and G. Ricci, "Lichen striatus: Clinical and laboratory features of 115 children," *Pediatric Dermatology*, vol. 21, no. 3, pp. 197–204, 2004.

[3] F. Aloi, C. Solaroli, and M. Pippione, "Diffuse and bilateral lichen striatus," *Pediatric Dermatology*, vol. 14, no. 1, pp. 36–38, 1997.

[4] A. Gupta, R. Gautam, and M. Bhardwaj, "Bilateral lichen striatus: A case report with review of literature," *Indian Dermatology Online Journal (IDOJ)*, vol. 8, no. 4, pp. 264–266, 2017.

[5] R. Mittal, B. K. Khaitan, M. Ramam, K. K. Verma, and M. Manchanda, "Multiple lichen striatus-An unusual presentation," *Indian Journal of Dermatology, Venereology and Leprology*, vol. 67, pp. 204-204, 2001.

[6] M. Kurokawa, H. Kikuchi, K. Ogata, and M. Setoyama, "Bilateral Lichen Striatus," *The Journal of Dermatology*, vol. 31, no. 2, pp. 129–132, 2004.

[7] P. Patri, "Lichen striatus bilaterale," *Giornale Italiano di Dermatologia e Venereologia*, vol. 118, no. 2, pp. 101–103, 1983.

[8] A. J. Racette, A. D. Adams, and S. E. Kessler, "Simultaneous lichen striatus in siblings along the same Blaschko line," *Pediatric Dermatology*, vol. 26, no. 1, pp. 50–54, 2009.

[9] K. Denk and K. Flux, "Blaschkitis in children - A new entity?" *Journal of the German Society of Dermatology*, vol. 9, no. 1, pp. 48-49, 2011.

[10] L. L. Kruse, "Differential diagnosis of linear eruptions in children," *Pediatric Annals*, vol. 44, no. 8, pp. e194–e198, 2015.

[11] Y. Zhang and N. S. McNutt, "Lichen striatus: Histological, immunohistochemical, and ultrastructural study of 37 cases," *Journal of Cutaneous Pathology*, vol. 28, no. 2, pp. 65–71, 2001.

[12] J. N. Graham and E. W. Hossler, "Lichen striatus," *Cutis; Cutaneous Medicine for the Practitioner*, vol. 97, no. 2, pp. 86–122, 2016.

[13] M. Johnson, D. Walker, W. Galloway, J. M. Gardner, and S. C. Shalin, "Interface dermatitis along Blaschko's lines," *Journal of Cutaneous Pathology*, vol. 41, no. 12, pp. 950–954, 2014.

[14] T. Sori, A. Nath, D. Thappa, and T. Jaisankar, "Hypopigmentary disorders in children in South India," *Indian Journal of Dermatology*, vol. 56, no. 5, pp. 546–549, 2011.

[15] A. Taieb, A. El Youbi, E. Grosshans, and J. Maleville, "Lichen striatus: A Blaschko linear acquired inflammatory skin eruption," *Journal of the American Academy of Dermatology*, vol. 25, no. 4, pp. 637–642, 1991.

[16] R. Happle, "Transposable elements and the lines of blaschko: A new perspective," *Dermatology*, vol. 204, no. 1, pp. 4–7, 2002.

18

PUVA Induced Bullous Pemphigoid in a Patient with Mycosis Fungoides

Birgül Özkesici,[1] **Saliha Koç,**[2] **Ayşe Akman-Karakaş,**[3] **Ertan Yılmaz,**[3] **İbrahim Cumhur Başsorgun,**[4] **and Soner Uzun**[3]

[1]*Clinic of Dermatology, Adıyaman University Training and Research Hospital, Adıyaman, Turkey*
[2]*Clinic of Dermatology, Kepez State Hospital, Antalya, Turkey*
[3]*Department of Dermatology and Venereology, Akdeniz University School of Medicine, Antalya, Turkey*
[4]*Department of Pathology, Akdeniz University School of Medicine, Antalya, Turkey*

..

Correspondence should be addressed to Birgül Ozkesici; birgulozkesici@gmail.com

Academic Editor: Thomas Berger

Background. Bullous pemphigoid is an autoimmune subepidermal blistering skin disease in which autoantibodies are directed against components of the basement membrane. The disease primarily affects the elderly people and in most of the patients inducing factors cannot be identified. Herein, we report a case of BP that occurred in a patient who was receiving PUVA therapy for the treatment of mycosis fungoides. *Main Observation.* A 26-year-old woman with mycosis fungoides developed blisters while receiving PUVA therapy. On physical examination tense bullae on the normal skin, remnants of blisters, and erosions were observed on her breasts, the chest wall, and the upper abdomen. Histopathological investigations revealed subepidermal blisters with eosinophilic infiltration and in direct immunofluorescence examination linear deposition of IgG along the basement membrane zone was observed. The diagnosis of bullous pemphigoid was also confirmed by ELISA and BIOCHIP mosaic-based indirect immunofluorescence test. *Conclusions.* PUVA therapy is an extremely rare physical factor capable of inducing bullous pemphigoid. So the development of blistering lesions during PUVA therapy may be suggestive sign of a bullous disease such as bullous pemphigoid and it should be excluded with proper clinical and laboratory approaches immediately after withdrawal of PUVA therapy.

1. Introduction

Bullous pemphigoid (BP) is an autoimmune subepidermal blistering skin disease, characterized by autoantibodies against structural proteins of the dermal-epidermal junction and clinically presented with cutaneous and/or mucosal blisters or erosions. It usually affects the elderly people. In the most cases, BP occurs sporadically without any obvious precipitation factors. However, the limited BP cases have been reported that are precipitated by UV radiation, medications, vaccination, radiation therapy, thermal burn, amputation stump, incisional hernia scar, and injection [1, 2]. Herein, we report a case of BP that occurred in a patient who was receiving PUVA therapy for the treatment of mycosis fungoides.

2. Case Report

A 26-year-old woman with mycosis fungoides developed blisters while receiving 8-methoxypsoralen and ultraviolet A (PUVA) therapy, at session 17 when the dose of UVA was 7.01 J/cm^2 (cumulative dose was 70.66 J/cm^2) (Figure 1). The patient had no history of any other drug use. On physical examination tense bullae on the normal skin, remnants of blisters, and erosions were observed on her breasts, the chest wall, and the upper abdomen. The patch lesions of mycosis fungoides were also present on buttocks and lower abdomen of the patient (stage 1A). PUVA therapy had been stopped and skin biopsies have been taken from a newly formed blister for histopathology and perilesional uninvolved skin for direct immunofluorescence (IF) examination for

TABLE 1: Cases of BP due to PUVA therapy.

Cases	Sex	Age (year-old)	Why the treatment of PUVA was given	Type of UVA
1 (2)	Female	45	Vitiligo	Topical PUVASOL
2 (3)	Male	50	Psoriasis	Oral PUVA (methoxsalen)
3 (4)	Male	80	Psoriasis	Oral PUVA (5-MOP)
4 (5)	Female	57	Mycosis fungoides	Oral PUVA (8-MOP)
5 (6)	Female	65	Psoriasis	Oral PUVA (8-MOP)
6 (7)	Female	67	Psoriasis	UVA
7 (8)	Male	58	Psoriasis	PUVA (unspecified)
8 (9)	Male	61	Psoriasis	Oral PUVA (oxsoralen)
9 (present case)	Female	26	Mycosis fungoides	Oral PUVA (8-MOP)

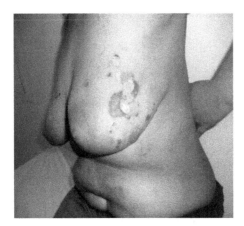

FIGURE 1: Clinical presentation of the patient; blisters, erosions, and remnants of blisters on her breasts and abdomen.

diagnosis. Histopathological examination showed subepidermal blisters with eosinophilic infiltration (Figure 2(a)) and in direct IF examination linear deposition of IgG along the basement membrane zone was observed. ELISA was positive for anti-BP180 antibody (47 U/mL). Also, BIOCHIP mosaic-based indirect IF test demonstrated a linear deposition of IgG along the basement membrane zone on the primate monkey esophagus, epidermal deposition on the salt-split skin substrate (Figure 2(b)), and anti-BP180 and anti-BP230 positivity on transfected EU90 cells.

Topical 0,05% clobetasol propionate cream treatment with a dose of 25 gr/day was started after cessation of the PUVA therapy. Disease was gotten under control after 1 week and complete remission was achieved at 3rd week (Figure 3). Then the dose of clobetasol propionate was tapered monthly as 25 mg on alternate days, twice a week, and once a week till it was discontinued after 4 months. Recurrence was not observed during follow-up period for 3 years. After 3 months of the treatment of BP, although patient had narrow band UVB therapy (25 sessions at the cumulative dose of 25.75 joule/cm^2) for her primary disease, mycosis fungoides, any recurrence of BP was not observed.

3. Discussion

The pathogenesis of BP is characterized by tissue-bound and circulating IgG autoantibodies against two components of the hemidesmosome, BP230 and BP180 [1]. The typical clinical presentation is tense blisters frequently concomitant with urticarial plaques. Most cases of BP occur sporadically without any obvious precipitation factors. Local irritation and damage to the skin have all been implicated in the induction of BP. There are limited numbers of reports suggesting that psoralen plus UVA (PUVA) therapy may trigger the development of BP (Table 1) [3–9]. In the majority of these patients PUVA was administered to treat psoriasis. But BP has also been reported previously in a patient with mycosis fungoides [5]. The role of PUVA in the pathogenesis of BP is poorly understood; however, there are some hypotheses that have been proposed. Danno et al. have demonstrated the alterations of keratinocyte surface and basement membrane markers by PUVA therapy [10]. So such changes may induce the production of BP autoantibodies by polyclonal activation of B cells [1]. On the other hand, PUVA may also alter the immunologic reactivity of T-helper and T-suppressor cells that may result in the development of the autoantibodies against native proteins [6]. Inversely, the protective effect of UVB irradiation has been showed by reducing the expression of pemphigoid antigens in organ-cultured normal human skin in a study [11]. In fact, after healing her PUVA induced BP, our patient was treated by UVB for her mycosis fungoides without recurrence of BP.

Although it is difficult to generalize about the prognosis of PUVA induced BP because of the limited numbers of cases [5], it seems that its prognosis is better with mild and transient behavior than idiopathic ones [6].

4. Conclusion

Our case indicates that the development of blistering lesions during PUVA therapy may be suggestive sign of a bullous disease such as BP and it should be excluded with proper clinical and laboratory approaches immediately after withdrawal of PUVA therapy.

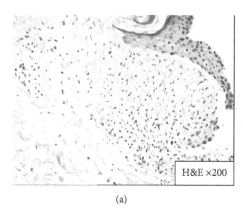

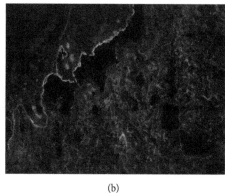

(a)   (b)

FIGURE 2: (a) Subepidermal blisters with eosinophilic infiltration (H&E ×200). (b) BIOCHIP demonstrated epidermal deposition on the salt-split skin substrate.

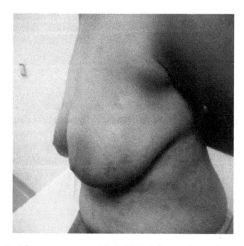

FIGURE 3: After treatment with 0,05% clobetasol propionate cream. Note the complete healing.

Disclosure

This has been presented at the 22nd EADV Congress, İstanbul-TURKEY, 2–6 October 2013.

Conflicts of Interest

The authors declare that they have no conflicts of interest.

References

[1] A. Lo Schiavo, E. Ruocco, G. Brancaccio, S. Caccavale, V. Ruocco, and R. Wolf, "Bullous pemphigoid: etiology, pathogenesis, and inducing factors: Facts and controversies," *Clinics in Dermatology*, vol. 31, no. 4, pp. 391–399, 2013.

[2] N. Riyaz, N. Nasir, V. Bindu, and S. Sasidharanpillai, "Bullous pemphigoid induced by topical PUVASOL," *Indian Journal of Dermatology, Venereology and Leprology*, vol. 80, no. 4, pp. 363–364, 2014.

[3] E. A. Abel and A. Bennett, "Bullous pemphigoid: occurrence in psoriasis treated with psoralens plus long-wave ultraviolet radiation," *Archives of Dermatology*, vol. 115, no. 8, pp. 988–989, 1979.

[4] S. Perl, K. Rappersberger, D. Födinger, B. Anegg, H. Hönigsmann, and B. Ortel, "Bullous pemphigoid induced by PUVA therapy," *Dermatology*, vol. 193, no. 3, pp. 245–247, 1996.

[5] J. W. Patterson, M. Ali, J. C. Murray, and T. A. Hazra, "Bullous pemphigoid: occurrence in a patient with mycosis fungoides receiving puva and topical nitrogen mustard therapy," *International Journal of Dermatology*, vol. 24, no. 3, pp. 173–176, 1985.

[6] M. A. Barnadas, M. Gilaberte, R. Pujol, M. Agustí, C. Gelpí, and A. Alomar, "Bullous pemphigoid in a patient with psoriasis during the course of PUVA therapy: study by ELISA test," *International Journal of Dermatology*, vol. 45, no. 9, pp. 1089–1092, 2006.

[7] H. Washio, H. Hara, H. Suzuki, M. Yoshida, and T. Hashimoto, "Bullous pemphigoid on psoriasis lesions after UVA radiation," *Acta Dermato-Venereologica*, vol. 85, no. 6, pp. 561–563, 2005.

[8] N. Caca-Biljanovska, I. Arsovska-Bezhoska, and M. V'lckova-Laskoska, "PUVA-induced bullous pemphigoid in psoriasis," *Acta Dermatovenerologica Croatica*, vol. 24, no. 3, pp. 214–217, 2016.

[9] P. M. George, "Bullous pemphigoid possibly induced by psoralen plus ultraviolet A therapy," *Photodermatology, Photoimmunology & Photomedicine*, vol. 11, no. 5-6, pp. 185–187, 1995.

[10] K. Danno, M. Tagikawa, and T. Horio, "The alterations of keratinocyte surface and basement membrane markers by treatment with 8-methoxypsoralen plus long-wave ultraviolet light," *Journal of Investigative Dermatology*, vol. 80, no. 3, pp. 172–174, 1983.

[11] T. Muramatsu, Y. Yamashina, T. Shirai, and T. Ohnishi, "UVB irradiation reduces the expression of pemphigoid antigens in organ-cultured normal human skin," *Archives of Dermatological Research*, vol. 286, no. 3-4, pp. 142–144, 1994.

19

A Case of Nonuremic Calciphylaxis in a Caucasian Woman

Bonnie Fergie,[1] Nishant Valecha,[2] and Andrew Miller[1]

[1]Canberra Hospital, ACT Health, Canberra, ACT, Australia
[2]Woden Dermatology, Phillip, ACT, Australia

Correspondence should be addressed to Bonnie Fergie; bonniefergie@gmail.com

Academic Editor: Jacek Cezary Szepietowski

We report a case of nonuremic calcific arteriolopathy (NUCA) in an 82-year-old Caucasian woman from rural Australia. The patient had no history of kidney disease or dialysis. NUCA is rare disease suspected on cutaneous and clinical features and diagnosed by characteristic findings on skin biopsy and vasculature imaging. Calcification induced microvascular occlusion in the absence of renal failure may not be immediately apparent. Clinical suspicion and appropriate investigations are essential for making a diagnosis. A diagnosis of NUCA may be missed given the rarity of the disease, and dermatologists and patients alike would benefit from a greater awareness of this disease.

1. Introduction

Calcific uremic arteriolopathy (CUA), otherwise termed calciphylaxis, characteristically arises in the setting of end stage renal failure and hyperparathyroidism. Calcific arteriolopathy in the setting of normal renal function is a rare entity termed nonuremic calcific arteriolopathy (NUCA). Both NUCA and CUA are caused by microvascular occlusion secondary to calcium deposition in the vessels of the skin and subcutaneous fat. Given the high morbidity and mortality associated with NUCA, recognition and timely diagnosis are essential for patient management.

2. Case

An 82-year-old woman from rural Australia admitted to hospital for an exacerbation of congestive cardiac failure (CCF) developed intensely painful, flesh colored, subcutaneous nodules on both lower legs and left thigh on a background of livedo racemosa. The nodules coincided with a creatinine rise from 96 μmol/L to 120 μmol/L (Table 1) following aggressive diuresis with frusemide for CCF management. Frusemide was subsequently reduced and renal function normalized. Over the subsequent weeks the nodules ulcerated and took on a serpiginous form.

The patient's comorbidities were rheumatoid arthritis, atrial fibrillation, chronic obstructive pulmonary disease, mitral valve replacement (bovine), hypertension, and hypercholesterolemia. Her medications were frusemide, methotrexate 5 mg/week, prednisolone 2.5 mg/day, spironolactone, oxycodone, rabeprazole, potassium, warfarin, salbutamol, budesonide, and formoterol. She had been on the same dose of warfarin for many years and had never smoked cigarettes.

Physical examination showed an afebrile, haemodynamically stable, elderly woman in severe pain from the leg ulcerations. Multiple deep serpiginous ulcerations with overlying necrotic eschars and surrounding macular erythema were present on both lower legs (Figure 1). A new subcutaneous flesh colored nodule with surrounding erythema was present on her left lateral thigh. Livedo racemosa was present on her upper and lower legs bilaterally.

Deep wedge incisional biopsies taken from the left thigh nodule and calf showed panlobular infarction of subcutaneous fat with extensive mural calcification of small and medium sized vessels within the pannus, with luminal occlusion (Figure 2). The left calf showed epidermal and dermal necrosis and ulceration. No features of vasculitis were seen. Direct immunofluorescence was negative. Laboratory investigations (Table 1) showed an elevated intact parathyroid hormone (PTH) 17.7 pmol/L, low urine calcium 0.9 mmol/24 hr, and the aforementioned creatinine elevation. Serum calcium, phosphate, vitamin D, and urea were normal. Plain X-rays of the legs showed extensive vascular

TABLE 1: Blood results.

Test	02.08.2015	21.09.2015	Normal range
Haemoglobin	138	129	115–160 g/L
White cell count	7.0	7.4	4–11 × 10⁹
Platelets	251	220	150–400 × 10⁹
Neutrophils	5.26	6.02	1.8–7.5 × 10⁹
Urea	6.7	12.6	2.5–7.5 mmol/L
Creatinine	96	120	45–90 μmol/L
GFR est	48	36	>90 Mls/min
Glucose	5.0	6.6	3.5–5.5 mmol/L
Osm-calc	291	290	280–300 mOsm/kg
Bilirubin total	25	23	2–20 μmol/L
ALT	14	29	9–33 U/L
Alkaline phosphatase	101	140	30–110 U/L
New GGT	295	502	9–56 g/L
Protein	69	67	69–80 g/L
Albumin	41	43	33–50 g/L
ESR	32	43	1–40 mm/hr
CRP	7.3		<6 Mg/L
ACE level (Buhlmann)	49.8		20–70 U/L
Calcium		2.36	2.1–2.6 mmol/L
Corrected calcium		2.42	2.1–2.6 mmol/L
Phosphate		1.39	0.75–1.50 mmol/L
Intact serum PTH		17.7	1.6–7.2 pmol/L
25-OH vitamin D		82	<60 nmol/L
Urinary Creatinine		5.7	5.3–15.9 mmol/24 h
Urinary calcium		0.9	2.5–7.5 mmol/24 h
Cold agglutinin		Negative	
Cryoglobulin		Negative	
C3		1.58	0.75–1.61 g/L
C4		0.44 H	0.13–0.40 g/L
IgG		5.3	6.5–15.2 g/L
IgA		1.06	0.76–3.89 g/L
IgM		0.6	0.3–2.3 g/L
ANA speckled		1 : 80	Negative
ENA		Negative	<30 AU/mL
dsDNA		5	<40 IU/mL
ANCA		Atypical	Negative
MPO ANCA		Negative	Negative
PR3 ANCA		Negative	Negative
Globulins		Normal	Normal

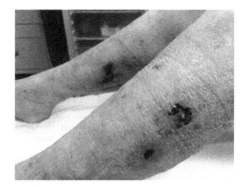

FIGURE 1: Necrotic ulceration on lower legs.

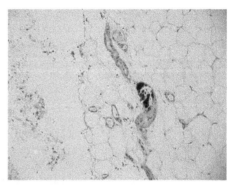

FIGURE 2: Biopsy left calf, illustrating arteriolar calcification in subcutis.

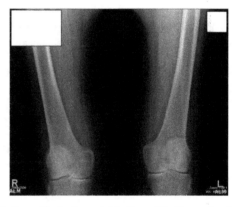

FIGURE 3: X-ray illustrating calcification of the femoral and popliteal vessels.

calcification bilaterally throughout the whole legs including the iliac, femoral, popliteal, and tibial vessels (Figure 3). Abdominal ultrasound showed areas of bilateral medullary nephrocalcinosis. Thyroid ultrasound showed a colloid cyst; the parathyroid glands were not visualized. Nuclear imaging of the parathyroid glands showed no abnormality. These clinical, radiological, and histopathological findings were consistent with a diagnosis of NUCA.

The patient was commenced on doxycycline 50 mg/day and was given an infusion of Zoledronic acid 5 mg. Warfarin was ceased and the patient was commenced on rivaroxaban.

There were no new nodules 6 months after the initial episode and the established erosions were healing slowly.

3. Discussion

NUCA is a rare obstructive vasculopathy caused by calcium deposition within the lumen of small and medium sized blood vessels. In the absence of renal failure, identified risk factors are hypercoagulable states, malignancy, hyperparathyroidism, connective tissue disease, corticosteroids, vitamin D deficiency, calcium based phosphate binders, warfarin, obesity, and diabetes [1–5]. This patient's risk factors were gender, hyperparathyroidism, connective tissue disease, corticosteroid, and warfarin use. Although risk factors for NUCA have been identified the pathogenesis remains poorly understood.

In CUA chronic renal failure causes excess phosphate, which binds with calcium in the blood resulting in blood vessel damage. Reduced vitamin D levels result in increased PTH production. As bones become resistant to PTH the parathyroid glands enlarge to produce more PTH and calcium levels in the blood increase. Although the initial mechanism resulting in calcium deposition in NUCA is not as well characterised as CUA a final common pathway for both CUA and NUCA has been proposed. This pathway involves elevated nuclear factor kB, leading to vascular calcification and thrombosis [4]. Via this pathway, chronic inflammation, impaired liver function, estrogens, parathyroid hormone abnormalities, warfarin, and glucocorticoids may all contribute to the disease.

In this case, given the normal renal function, calcium, phosphate, and vitamin D levels, the elevated PTH represents tertiary hyperparathyroidism. The initial creatinine rise was attributed to hypovolemia caused by aggressive CCF management. Satellite purpuric ulcerations with central overlying necrosis crusts, present in this case, typify the clinical lesions of NUCA. Livedo reticularis or racemosa is usually present on the legs and may precede ulcerations. Clinicopathological correlation is essential for a diagnosis of NUCA.

The characteristic histological features of NUCA, as evident in this case, are calcification of small-medium sized cutaneous vessels, intimal fibrosis, intravascular thrombi, and diffuse calcification of small capillaries in the fat. There may be calcification of adipocytes. Epidermal and dermal ulceration give rise to the typical clinical features of NUCA. Investigations such as plain film X-rays or bone scintigraphy can show arteriolar calcification which may aid diagnosis or monitoring of treatment effects [6].

The management of NUCA involves elimination of identifiable precipitants, adequate analgesia, and early treatment. Meticulous wound management decreases infection risk, and surgical debridement may be warranted. Recent research has suggested that changing warfarin to low molecular weight heparin may be beneficial [5]. Rivaroxaban rather than low molecular weight heparin replaced warfarin in this case due to atrial fibrillation. Other reported treatments are calcimimetic agents, bisphosphonates, hyperbaric oxygen, low dose tissue plasminogen activator, and doxycycline [7]. There is limited evidence for intravenous sodium thiosulfate for its antioxidative properties and ability to increase calcium solubility in NUCA [8].

4. Conclusion

This rare case of NUCA in an 82-year-old Caucasian woman coincided with her hospitalization for the management of her CCF. Her risk factors were gender, connective tissue disease, hyperparathyroid level, glucocorticoid use, and warfarin use. Clinical, histological, and radiological evidence were consistent with a diagnosis of NUCA with no sinister precipitating factors found. The patient improved with meticulous wound care, analgesia, doxycycline 50 mg/day, Zoledronic acid 5 mg, and warfarin cessation. Given the rarity of the disease dermatologists and patients alike would benefit from a greater awareness of NUCA.

Abbreviation List

CUA: Calcific uremic arteriolopathy
CCF: Congestive cardiac failure
NUCA: Nonuremic calcific arteriolopathy
PTH: Parathyroid hormone.

Competing Interests

The authors have no conflict of interests to declare.

Authors' Contributions

All authors are significant contributors and have approved the final copy of this article.

References

[1] S. U. Nigwekar, M. Wolf, R. H. Sterns, and J. K. Hix, "Calciphylaxis from nonuremic causes: a systematic review," *Clinical Journal of the American Society of Nephrology*, vol. 3, no. 4, pp. 1139–1143, 2008.

[2] J. Panuncialman and V. Falanga, "Unusual causes of cutaneous ulceration," *The Surgical Clinics of North America*, vol. 90, no. 6, pp. 1161–1180, 2010.

[3] R. H. Weenig, L. D. Sewell, M. D. P. Davis, J. T. McCarthy, and M. R. Pittelkow, "Calciphylaxis: natural history, risk factor analysis, and outcome," *Journal of the American Academy of Dermatology*, vol. 56, no. 4, pp. 569–579, 2007.

[4] R. H. Weenig, "Pathogenesis of calciphylaxis: hans Selye to nuclear factor κ-B," *Journal of the American Academy of Dermatology*, vol. 58, no. 3, pp. 458–471, 2008.

[5] R. J. Harris and T. G. Cropley, "Possible role of hypercoagulability in calciphylaxis: review of the literature," *Journal of the American Academy of Dermatology*, vol. 64, no. 2, pp. 405–412, 2011.

[6] S. Paul, C. A. Rabito, P. Vedak, S. U. Nigwekar, and D. Kroshinsky, "The role of bone scintigraphy in the diagnosis of calciphylaxis," *JAMA Dermatology*, 2015.

[7] C. Vedvyas, L. S. Winterfield, and R. A. Vleugels, "Calciphylaxis: a systematic review of existing and emerging therapies," *Journal of the American Academy of Dermatology*, vol. 67, no. 6, pp. e253–e260, 2012.

[8] V. M. Smith, T. Oliphant, M. Shareef, W. Merchant, and S. M. Wilkinson, "Calciphylaxis with normal renal function: treated with intravenous sodium thiosulfate," *Clinical and Experimental Dermatology*, vol. 37, no. 8, pp. 874–878, 2012.

20

A Case of Granuloma Annulare Associated with Secukinumab Use

Lauren Bonomo,[1] Sara Ghoneim,[2] and Jacob Levitt[1]

[1]Department of Dermatology, Icahn School of Medicine at Mount Sinai, 5 East 98th Street, 5th Floor, New York, NY 10029, USA
[2]Saba University School of Medicine, The Bottom, Saba, Netherlands

Correspondence should be addressed to Lauren Bonomo; lauren.bonomo@icahn.mssm.edu
and Jacob Levitt; jacoblevittmd@gmail.com

Academic Editor: Ioannis D. Bassukas

Granuloma annulare (GA) is a benign inflammatory dermatosis characterized clinically by dermal papules and annular plaques. The pathogenesis of GA is not well understood, although it is thought to result from a delayed-type hypersensitivity reaction in which inflammatory cells elicit connective tissue degradation. This condition has been seen following the use of several drugs, including tumor necrosis factor-alpha (TNF-α) inhibitors, which paradoxically have also been reported to treat GA. We report the case of a patient who developed GA in association with secukinumab, an interleukin-17A antagonist, and discuss its implications for our understanding of the pathogenesis of GA.

1. Introduction

Granuloma annulare (GA) is a benign inflammatory dermatosis characterized clinically by dermal papules and annular plaques. The characteristic histopathological finding is a lymphohistiocytic granuloma associated with varying degrees of connective tissue degeneration and mucin deposition. The pathogenesis of GA is not well understood, although it is thought to result from a delayed-type hypersensitivity reaction in which inflammatory cells elicit connective tissue degradation [1].

A number of events predisposing to GA have been reported, including mild trauma, various infections, diabetes mellitus, thyroid disease, and malignancy. Additionally, GA has occurred in patients treated with certain drugs, particularly tumor necrosis factor-alpha (TNF-α) inhibitors [2]. We report the case of a patient who developed GA in association with the IL-17A antagonist secukinumab and discuss the implications of this case for our understanding of the pathogenesis of GA.

2. Case Report

A 60-year-old Hispanic woman with a medical history of fibromyalgia, hypothyroidism, and Ménière's disease has been treated in our clinic for psoriasis and psoriatic arthritis since 2006. Over the past ten years, the patient has failed topical therapies, etanercept, infliximab, adalimumab, golimumab, and, most recently, apremilast. Upon failure of apremilast in February 2016, the decision was made to attempt therapy with secukinumab. Her other medications at the time included methotrexate, levothyroxine, omeprazole, and duloxetine. Of note, the patient has a self-reported history of hives after treatment with hydrocodone and ibuprofen.

The patient received her first dose of secukinumab in April 2016, and improvement was noted in both her psoriatic and arthritic symptoms. However, the patient presented in June with concerns that her psoriasis was beginning to return due to "new" spots on the shoulder, face, and neck. She first noticed the spots approximately two weeks after beginning secukinumab. On examination, the patient was found to have scattered tan papules of the neck, back, and shoulders bilaterally (Figure 1).

A three-millimeter punch biopsy was taken from a lesion on her right back for histopathological examination. The specimen showed a superficial dermal scar and underlying dermis containing prominent histiocytes with polygonal and cuboidal cytoplasm, in addition to collagen bundles of the superficial and mid dermis (Figure 2). Colloidal iron stain

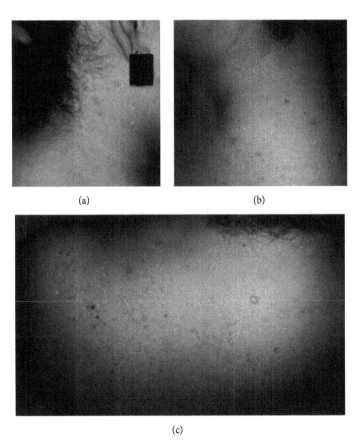

(a)

(b)

(c)

FIGURE 1: The patient on initial presentation. Tan papules were noted on (a) the right neck, (b) the left neck, and (c) the superior back and shoulders.

revealed increased dermal mucin. This pattern of inflammation with interstitial histiocytes, focal collagen degeneration, and mucin deposition is consistent with a diagnosis of GA.

The patient was treated with topical clobetasol propionate (0.05%) with mild improvement in lesion size after two weeks. She continued to use secukinumab with no additional adverse events. However, when she returned to our clinic in August, there was no further clinical improvement noted and secukinumab was discontinued. Over the past eight months, the patient did not receive any monoclonal antibody therapy and has reported marked improvement in the GA lesions present on her face and neck.

3. Discussion

GA has been associated with a variety of predisposing factors. These include chronic conditions (e.g., diabetes mellitus and thyroid disease), infectious diseases (e.g., human immunodeficiency virus (HIV), Epstein-Barr virus (EBV), varicella zoster virus (VZV), and tuberculosis), minor traumas (e.g., bee stings and sun burn), and various malignancies. Our patient was diagnosed with chronic lymphocytic thyroiditis in 2014; however, she has been euthyroid on levothyroxine since that time. Previous case reports of GA associated with hypothyroidism have shown resolution of the lesions upon treatment with synthetic thyroid hormone [3, 4]. Our

patient's chronic medical conditions also included fibromyalgia and psoriatic arthritis. Fibromyalgia is a disorder of pain regulation with no obvious abnormalities on physical examination, while GA is an inflammatory dermatosis. A thorough review of the relevant literature shows no evidence to support the association between fibromyalgia and GA. Likewise, the patient was prescribed duloxetine in 2014 to manage her fibromyalgia symptoms. We believe it is unlikely for duloxetine to be an inciting factor for GA given the well-established safety and adverse profile of the drug. Cutaneous adverse events reported with duloxetine use are rare and include urticaria, contact dermatitis, and Stevens-Johnson syndrome [5]. Psoriatic arthritis (PsA) is an inflammatory arthritis seen in up to 30% of patients diagnosed with psoriasis [6]. While GA and PsA are both inflammatory processes characterized by increased expression of TNF-alpha and matrix metalloproteinases by activated macrophages [7–9], there are no reports to date supporting the role of PsA in the pathogenesis of GA. Further studies are warranted to determine whether the aberrant immunologic signaling observed in psoriasis or PsA plays a direct role in the pathogenesis of GA. Moreover, the patient's psoriasis and PsA symptoms were managed in our clinic since 2006 but the lesions were only observed by the patient two weeks after the administration of secukinumab. Additionally, prior to initiating secukinumab, she was prescribed methotrexate

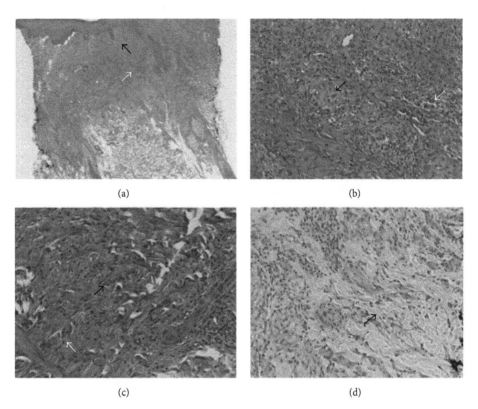

FIGURE 2: Histopathological slides. At 2x magnification (a), there are superficial periadnexal and interstitial granulomatous infiltrates (black arrow). The epidermis is slightly attenuated with subjacent papillary dermal fibrosis (white arrow). At 20x magnification, the superficial dermis (b) contains well-formed granulomas (black arrow) and individual histiocytes that are scaffolded in between collagen bundles; scattered eosinophils are present (white arrow). In the mid dermis (c), there are numerous interstitial histiocytes in small clusters (black arrow) and solitary units (white arrow). Colloidal iron stain (d) reveals interstitial deposition of dermal mucin (black arrow).

for eight years. A previous case report demonstrated the successful treatment of disseminated GA with methotrexate in part due to the medication's anti-inflammatory properties [10]. Therefore, the GA lesions observed are less likely associated with the above-mentioned chronic conditions and medications and more likely associated with the use of secukinumab.

GA has also been seen following the use of multiple drugs, such as gold therapy, allopurinol, diclofenac, quinidine, intranasal calcitonin, and amlodipine. In 2008, Voulgari et al. demonstrated an association between GA and the use of novel biologic agents. This occurred in nine out of 199 patients receiving infliximab, adalimumab, or etanercept for rheumatoid arthritis. Whereas infliximab, adalimumab, and etanercept target TNF-alpha, secukinumab is a high-affinity, human immunoglobulin G1 monoclonal antibody that selectively binds to and neutralizes interleukin-17A (IL-17A). To our knowledge, this is the first published report of a patient developing GA after treatment with secukinumab. The IL-17A inhibitor was initially approved in 2015 for the treatment of plaque psoriasis but has since been approved for use in psoriatic arthritis and ankylosing spondylitis [11, 12]. The most common adverse events reported with secukinumab are nasopharyngitis, diarrhea, and upper respiratory infection. The only previously reported dermatologic side effects of secukinumab are urticaria and infection.

The pathogenetic mechanisms of GA are poorly understood. One proposed mechanism is that expression of TNF-alpha and certain matrix metalloproteinases by activated macrophages results in matrix degradation [7]. This seems to be supported by evidence that recalcitrant disseminated GA can be successfully treated with the TNF-alpha inhibitor infliximab [13]. However, the work of Voulgari et al. demonstrating a significant association between TNF-alpha antagonist use and development of GA implies that the mechanism may be more complicated or that multiple pathways may be involved. Despite decreasing activity of TNF itself, antagonists may upregulate T-helper 1 lymphocytes, which in turn activate macrophages to produce inflammation and tissue degradation. Our finding that an IL-17A antagonist can also provoke GA formation may provide additional evidence for a T-helper 1 cell-mediated process. Further molecular and immunologic studies are needed to determine whether this is the mechanism by which IL-17A blockade produces this effect.

Disclosure

Dr. Jacob Levitt has served on advisory boards for Amgen, Novartis, Janssen Biotech, Promius Pharma, Genentech, Ranbaxy, Pfizer, and Castle Biosciences Incorporated.

Conflicts of Interest

The authors declare that there are no conflicts of interest regarding the publication of this paper.

References

[1] L. A. Thornsberry and J. E. English, "Etiology, diagnosis, and therapeutic management of granuloma annulare: an update," *American Journal of Clinical Dermatology*, vol. 14, no. 4, pp. 279–290, 2013.

[2] P. V. Voulgari, T. E. Markatseli, S. A. Exarchou, A. Zioga, and A. A. Drosos, "Granuloma annulare induced by anti-tumour necrosis factor therapy," *Annals of the Rheumatic Diseases*, vol. 67, no. 4, pp. 567–570, 2008.

[3] F. Vázquez-López, M. A. González-López, C. Raya-Aguado, and N. Pérez-Oliva, "Localized granuloma annulare and autoimmune thyroiditis: a new case report," *Journal of the American Academy of Dermatology*, vol. 43, no. 5, pp. 943–945, 2000.

[4] M. J. Willemsen, A. L. De Coninck, M. H. Jonckheer, and D. I. Roseeuw, "Autoimmune thyroiditis and generalized granuloma annulare: remission of the skin lesions after thyroxine therapy," *Dermatology*, vol. 175, no. 5, pp. 239–243, 1987.

[5] J. R. Strawn, R. Whitsel, J. J. Nandagopal, and M. P. Delbello, "Atypical Stevens-Johnson syndrome in an adolescent treated with duloxetine," *Journal of Child and Adolescent Psychopharmacology*, vol. 21, no. 1, pp. 91-92, 2011.

[6] H. Zachariae, "Prevalence of joint disease in patients with psoriasis: implications for therapy," *American Journal of Clinical Dermatology*, vol. 4, no. 7, pp. 441–447, 2003.

[7] A. Fayyazi, S. Schweyer, B. Eichmeyer et al., "Expression of IFNγ coexpression of TNFα and matrix metalloproteinases and apoptosis of T lymphocytes and macrophages in granuloma annulare," *Archives of Dermatological Research*, vol. 292, no. 8, pp. 384–390, 2000.

[8] D. Tracey, L. Klareskog, E. H. Sasso, J. G. Salfeld, and P. P. Tak, "Tumor necrosis factor antagonist mechanisms of action: a comprehensive review: a comprehensive review," *Pharmacology & Therapeutics*, vol. 117, no. 2, pp. 244–279, 2008.

[9] C. A. Hitchon, C. L. Danning, G. G. Illei, H. S. El-Gabalawy, and D. T. Boumpas, "Gelatinase expression and activity in the synovium and skin of patients with erosive psoriatic arthritis," *Journal of Rheumatology*, vol. 29, no. 1, pp. 107–117, 2002.

[10] A. N. Plotner and D. F. Mutasim, "Successful treatment of disseminated granuloma annulare with methotrexate," *British Journal of Dermatology*, vol. 163, no. 5, pp. 1123-1124, 2010.

[11] P. J. Mease, I. B. McInnes, B. Kirkham et al., "Secukinumab inhibition of interleukin-17A in patients with psoriatic arthritis," *The New England Journal of Medicine*, vol. 373, no. 14, pp. 1329–1339, 2015.

[12] R. G. Langley, B. E. Elewski, M. Lebwohl et al., "Secukinumab in plaque psoriasis—results of two phase 3 trials," *The New England Journal of Medicine*, vol. 371, no. 4, pp. 326–338, 2014.

[13] M. S. Hertl, I. Haendle, G. Schuler, and M. Hertl, "Rapid improvement of recalcitrant disseminated granuloma annulare upon treatment with the tumour necrosis factor-α inhibitor, infliximab," *British Journal of Dermatology*, vol. 152, no. 3, pp. 552–555, 2005.

21

Extensive Cutaneous T-Cell Lymphoma of the Feet Treated with High-Dose-Rate Brachytherapy and External Beam Radiation

Joy Tao ⓘ,[1] **Courtney Hentz,**[2] **Michael L. Mysz,**[2] **Issra Rashed,**[2] **David Eilers,**[3] **James Swan,**[4] **Rebecca Tung,**[4] **and Bahman Emami**[2]

[1]*Stritch School of Medicine, Loyola University Chicago, Chicago, IL, USA*
[2]*Department of Radiation Oncology, Stritch School of Medicine, Loyola University Chicago, Chicago, IL, USA*
[3]*Section of Dermatology, Hines Veterans Affairs Hospital, Hines, IL, USA*
[4]*Division of Dermatology, Department of Medicine, Stritch School of Medicine, Loyola University Chicago, Chicago, IL, USA*

Correspondence should be addressed to Joy Tao; joytao16@gmail.com

Academic Editor: Michela Curzio

Cutaneous T-cell lymphoma (CTCL) is a chronic, debilitating disease that has a severe impact on quality of life. We present a patient with multiple CTCL lesions on the bilateral feet, which impaired his ability to ambulate. His lesions on both feet were successfully treated with a total of 8 Gy in two fractions via high-dose-rate surface brachytherapy using the Freiburg Flap applicator. The deeper aspects of the bulkier lesions on the left foot were boosted with electron beam therapy. The radiation therapy was well tolerated, and the patient was able to regain his mobility after completing radiation therapy. To our knowledge, there are few reports utilizing brachytherapy in treating CTCL. Our case describes treatment of larger, more extensive CTCL lesions than previously reported.

1. Introduction

Cutaneous T-cell lymphoma (CTCL) is a chronic, debilitating condition that accounts for approximately 4% of all non-Hodgkin lymphomas, with mycosis fungoides being the most common type [1]. Current strategies and goals of CTCL treatments include alleviation of symptoms, control of local disease, and improvement in quality of life [2]. We report on a patient with multiple CTCL lesions refractory to standard therapies who received a combination of external beam radiation therapy (EBRT) and high-dose-rate (HDR) brachytherapy for organ preservation and to control his painful disease.

2. Case

A 69-year-old male presented to dermatology clinic with stage T2b mycosis fungoides, diagnosed two years prior, which manifested as a persistent, chronic rash involving both feet, and, to a lesser extent, other sites of his body. The lesions on his feet were painful and pruritic, limiting his ability to wear shoes and ambulate for the past two years. His disease showed little to no response to numerous topical agents including topical nitrogen mustard, imiquimod, clobetasol, vinegar soaks, PUVA soaks, amoxicillin, and doxycycline. Per the patient, consideration was made for amputation of the left foot below the ankle, which he refused. Subsequently, he was referred to radiation oncology.

Physical exam revealed tender, confluent, erythematous, and desquamated patches on the skin extending from the dorsal and ventral surfaces of his left foot to the ankle (Figures 1(a) and 1(b)). His right foot had smaller, erythematous patches proximal to the 4th and 5th digits extending between the digits (Figure 1(e)). He was recommended surface HDR brachytherapy to his symptomatic lesions. The patient agreed to begin radiation therapy first to his most prominent and painful lesions on his left foot and undergo subsequent treatments for his other lesions if results warranted. A preliminary scan of the left foot showed diffuse involvement with some dorsal lesions > 5 mm in thickness. The

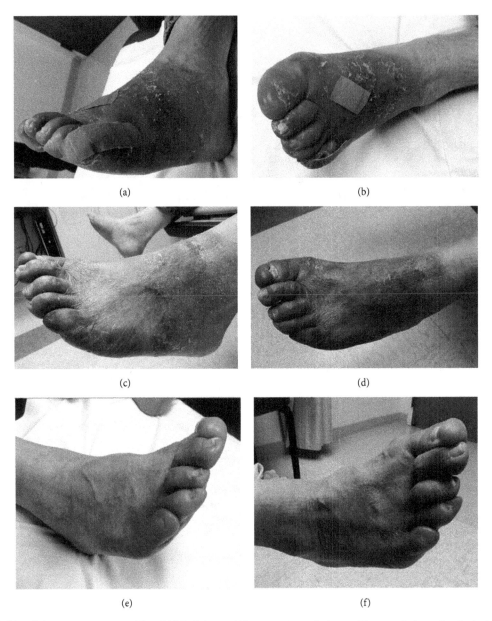

FIGURE 1: (a) and (b) Left foot at presentation. (c) and (d) Left foot at follow-up 11 months later with a new 3-4 cm circular lesion that developed just proximal to the irradiated area. (e) Right foot at presentation. (f) Right foot at follow-up 11 months later.

patient was recommended 8 Gy in 2 fractions of superficial HDR brachytherapy to the entire affected area of his left foot using the Freiburg Flap (FF) applicator (Elekta AB, Stockholm, Sweden) followed by 20 Gy in 10 fractions of 6 MeV external beam electron treatments to the bulky dorsal lesions.

The FF applicator consists of a planar array of 1 cm diameter silicone spheres with longitudinal channels for insertion of treatment catheters and flexible connections laterally which enable the FF to conform to highly curved and irregular surfaces. The FF is often affixed to a thermoplastic mesh (TM), commonly used in radiation therapy, to maintain a reproducible orientation relative to the patient's anatomy.

In preparation for this patient's left foot HDR treatment, two pieces of TM material (Extremity EMRT-8430, Bionix Inc., Toledo, OH) were heated and formed around the patient's left foot consisting of a dorsal part and corresponding plantar portion. This two-part, clam shell construction allowed the entire foot to be tightly enveloped by TM yet provided ease of ingress and egress (Figure 2(a)). The FF was attached to the TM with dental floss interwoven between the FF beads and through the TM struts. This TM design and position of the FF catheters enabled the Ir-192 HDR source to travel in close proximity to the cutaneous tissue to be treated. A total of 39 catheters were required to encompass the entire treatment area of his left foot (Figures 2(b) and 2(c)).

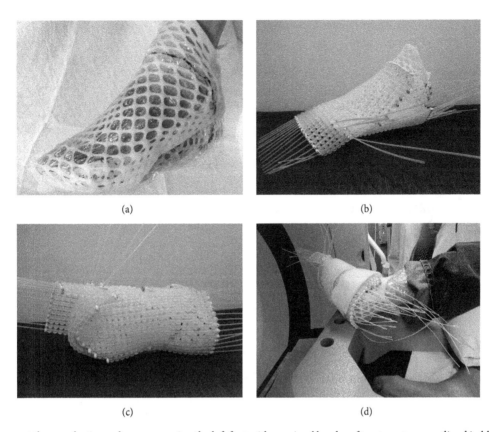

(a)   (b)

(c)   (d)

FIGURE 2: (a) Two-part thermoplastic mesh encompassing the left foot with proximal border of treatment area outlined in black. (b) Complete Freiburg device consisting of a total of 39 catheters. (c) Plantar aspect of the Freiburg device. (d) Positioning of the left foot for CT scan and treatment.

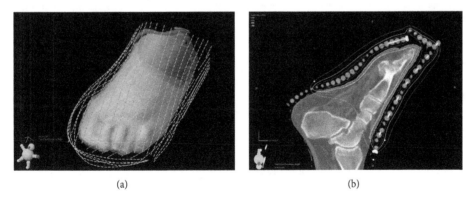

(a)   (b)

FIGURE 3: (a) Left foot treatment plan: 3D view of source dwell positions. (b) Left foot treatment plan: cutaneous planning treatment volume is shown in cyan, and the delivery of a highly conformal 4 Gy of radiation is shown in yellow isodose line.

For treatment planning, a CT scan was performed with the FF device firmly affixed to the patient's foot and a thin metal marker wire attached to the TM to delineate the intended treatment borders (Figure 2(d)). The images were imported into Eclipse (Varian Medical Systems, Palo Alto, Ca). The planning treatment volume (PTV) outlined or 'contoured' on the CT images consisted of a 1 cm proximal margin and all cutaneous surface tissue below the level of the marker wire to a depth of 3 mm. The path of each FF catheter

was identified in three dimensions, and dwell positions for the HDR source were selected in step increments of 5 mm (Figure 3(a)). The dwell times of these source positions were adjusted to provide uniform coverage of 4 Gy to the peripheral margins of the PTV (Figure 3(b)). Overall, the left foot treatment plan involved 1326 active sources across 39 catheters, with a total dwell time of 1407 seconds (for a 10 Ci source). Two fractions of 4 Gy were delivered every other day during one week.

The treatment was well tolerated with some mild radiation-related edema and associated left foot pain that was managed conservatively and resolved within a week of completing treatment. At one-week follow-up, his lesions were regressing with significant improvement in pain, scaling, and erythema. Four months later, the deeper aspect of the gross tumor lesions involving the left foot was boosted with 20 Gy in 10 daily fractions using 6 MeV external beam electrons. Additionally, the same brachytherapy process without EBRT was subsequently followed for the patient's right foot, which responded well to HDR brachytherapy.

At each short-term follow-up (≤ 6 weeks) after completing his HDR brachytherapy, he reported a rewarding response with improvement of disease-related erythema, pain, and swelling in all treated areas, with near resolution of treatment related hyperpigmentation (Figures 1(c), 1(d), and 1(f)). Both feet were still in remission at his most recent follow-up 21 months and 19 months after completing his left and right foot treatments, respectively. Additionally, he was ambulating and wearing shoes, which he was unable to do at presentation due to his painful lesions. He did develop a new 3-4 cm mildly erythematous, circular lesion on the dorsal surface of his left foot just proximal to the irradiated area, which was treated and controlled with topical steroids (Figures 1(c) and 1(d)).

3. Discussion

CTCL lesions are extremely radiosensitive, with some reports suggesting that low-dose radiation therapy can achieve successful results (Table 1) while allowing for fewer clinic visits, decreased costs, less toxicity to the skin, and reirradiation in the future due to symptom relapse [3, 4]. Neelis et al. utilized low-dose external beam radiotherapy to treat mycosis fungoides lesions refractory to PUVA and topical steroids. They reported that 65 lesions in 24 patients treated with 8 Gy in two fractions had a complete response rate of 92% with no skin toxicities noted [3]. Thomas et al. found a complete response rate of approximately 94.4% among 58 patients with CTCL treated with a single fraction of radiation therapy, the majority between 7 and 8 Gy, using either photons or electrons. The mean follow-up time was 41.3 months, and no significant long-term side effects were observed [4]. Low-dose total skin electron beam therapy has also shown satisfactory results with a good side effect profile for patients with more diffuse skin disease [5–8].

Brachytherapy is a technique in which a radioactive source is placed directly into or adjacent to target lesions via implants or surface applicators [9, 10]. One such applicator is the Freiburg Flap, which is designed to allow the HDR Ir-192 source to travel approximately 5 mm from the skin surface. This method is noninvasive and ideal for delivering tumoricidal doses of radiotherapy to superficial lesions while limiting unfavorable delivery of radiation to healthy tissues due to rapid dose fall-off at the periphery of the lesions. This is especially desirable when treating anatomic sites that are near tissues vulnerable to irradiation or that present significant cosmetic challenges to surgical excision such as the scalp, face, and hands [9]. With use of custom molds such as the FF, this technique also permits delivery of a uniform radiation dose to uneven surfaces, which was advantageous in the treatment of our patient's feet, whereas EBRT is often utilized for deeper lesions and on flat surfaces [11]. Some lesions on the dorsal aspect of our patient's left foot were greater than 5 mm in thickness, and the EBRT was added to treat the deeper, bulkier parts of the tumor, whereas only the FF brachytherapy was required for the thinner patches on the right foot. Therefore, treatment with the FF alone is sufficient for superficial lesions contained within 5 mm of the skin surface.

While brachytherapy treatments for nonmelanoma skin cancers have been extensively studied and found to have high local control rates and excellent cosmetic outcomes [9, 10, 12–14], there are few reports utilizing brachytherapy for CTCL. DeSimone et al. reported on 10 patients with facial mycosis fungoides lesions that were successfully treated with HDR brachytherapy doses of 8 Gy in 2 fractions of 4 Gy. There were no recurrences in the median 6-month follow-up period [15]. Goddard et al. presented a case series utilizing HDR brachytherapy for the treatment of acral CTCL skin lesions on six patients with eight lesions also treated with 8 Gy in 2 fractions. They reported an 88% control rate with only one lesion recurring locally within a mean follow-up period of 15.8 months [16]. Our case describes treatment of more extensive CTCL lesions than previously reported.

The symptom burden of CTCL significantly impairs the quality of life for patients. Patients frequently experience intense pruritus, pain, cracking and bleeding skin, and associated insomnia, depression, and decreased self-esteem [17, 18]. Depending on the location of the lesions, patients may have difficulty using their hands or ambulating [16]. Treatment with radiotherapy improved our patient's symptoms and allowed him to regain his mobility and avoid possible amputation of his afflicted left foot. Our case, as well as the previous literature, suggests that HDR brachytherapy is a potentially valuable palliative, organ sparing treatment for CTCL lesions, particularly those refractory to more traditional therapies. Further studies are needed to establish treatment guidelines as well as evaluate long-term control rates and outcomes.

Abbreviations

CTCL: Cutaneous T-cell lymphoma
Gy: Gray
HDR: High-dose-rate
EBRT: External beam radiation therapy
FF: Freiburg Flap
TM: Thermoplastic mesh
PTV: Planning treatment volume.

Conflicts of Interest

The authors report no conflicts of interest.

TABLE 1: Local cutaneous T-cell lymphoma lesions treated with low-dose radiation therapy.

Reference	Number of Patients	Number of Sites	Radiation Technique	Total Doses (Gy)	Local Recurrence Rate	Mean Follow-up
Neelis et al, 2009 [3]	24	65	Electron beam	8.0 Gy in 2 fractions	5/65 (7.7%)	9.6 months
Thomas et al, 2013 [4]	58	270	Photon or electron beam	≥7.0 Gy in 1 fraction	4/270 (1.5%)	41.3 months
DeSimone et al, 2013 [15]	10	23	HDR brachytherapy	8.0 Gy in 2 fractions	0/23 (0%)	6.3 months (median)
Goddard et al, 2015 [16]	6	8	HDR brachytherapy	8.0 Gy in 2 fractions	1/8 (12.5%)	15.8 months

References

[1] S. I. Jawed, P. L. Myskowski, S. Horwitz, A. Moskowitz, and C. Querfeld, "Primary cutaneous T-cell lymphoma (mycosis fungoides and Sézary syndrome): part I. Diagnosis: clinical and histopathologic features and new molecular and biologic markers," *Journal of the American Academy of Dermatology*, vol. 70, no. 2, pp. 205.e1–205.e16, 2014.

[2] S. I. Jawed, P. L. Myskowski, S. Horwitz, A. Moskowitz, and C. Querfeld, "Primary cutaneous T-cell lymphoma (mycosis fungoides and Sézary syndrome): part II. Prognosis, management, and future directions," *Journal of the American Academy of Dermatology*, vol. 70, no. 2, pp. 223.e1–223.e17, 2014.

[3] K. J. Neelis, E. C. Schimmel, M. H. Vermeer et al., "Low-dose palliative radiotherapy for cutatneous B- and T-cell lymphomas," *International Journal of Radiation Oncology, Biology & Physics*, vol. 74, no. 1, pp. 154–158, 2009.

[4] T. O. Thomas, P. Agrawal, J. Guitart et al., "Outcome of patients treated with a single-fraction dose of palliative radiation for cutaneous T-cell lymphoma," *International Journal of Radiation Oncology, Biology & Physics*, vol. 85, no. 3, pp. 747–753, 2013.

[5] M. R. Kamstrup, L. M. Lindahl, R. Gniadecki et al., "Low-dose total skin electron beam therapy as a debulking agent for cutaneous T-cell lymphoma: An open-label prospective phase II study," *British Journal of Dermatology*, vol. 166, no. 2, pp. 399–404, 2012.

[6] M. Chowdhary, A. M. Chhabra, S. Kharod, and G. Marwaha, "Total Skin Electron Beam Therapy in the Treatment of Mycosis Fungoides: A Review of Conventional and Low-Dose Regimens," *Clinical Lymphoma, Myeloma & Leukemia*, vol. 16, no. 12, pp. 662–671, 2016.

[7] K. Elsayad, K. H. Susek, and H. T. Eich, "Total Skin Electron Beam Therapy as Part of Multimodal Treatment Strategies for Primary Cutaneous T-Cell Lymphoma," *Oncology Research and Treatment*, vol. 40, no. 5, pp. 244–252, 2017.

[8] K. Kroeger, K. Elsayad, C. Moustakis, U. Haverkamp, and H. T. Eich, "Low-dose total skin electron beam therapy for cutaneous lymphoma: Minimal risk of acute toxicities," *Strahlentherapie und Onkologie*, vol. 193, no. 12, pp. 1024–1030, 2017.

[9] M. Alam, S. Nanda, B. B. Mittal, N. A. Kim, and S. Yoo, "The use of brachytherapy in the treatment of nonmelanoma skin cancer: a review," *Journal of the American Academy of Dermatology*, vol. 65, no. 2, pp. 377–388, 2011.

[10] A. Bhatnagar, R. Patel, W. P. Werschler, R. I. Ceilley, and R. Strimling, "High-dose Rate Electronic Brachytherapy: A Nonsurgical Treatment Alternative for Nonmelanoma Skin Cancer," *Journal of Clinical and Aesthetic Dermatology*, vol. 9, no. 11, pp. 16–22, 2016.

[11] S. Aldelaijan, H. Bekerat, I. Buzurovic et al., "Dose comparison between TG-43–based calculations and radiochromic film measurements of the Freiburg flap applicator used for high-dose-rate brachytherapy treatments of skin lesions," *Brachytherapy*, vol. 16, no. 5, pp. 1065–1072, 2017.

[12] D. Delishaj, C. Laliscia, B. Manfredi et al., "Non-melanoma skin cancer treated with high-dose-rate brachytherapy and Valencia applicator in elderly patients: a retrospective case series," *Journal of Contemporary Brachytherapy*, vol. 7, no. 6, pp. 437–444, 2015.

[13] D. Delishaj, A. Rembielak, B. Manfredi et al., "Non-melanoma skin cancer treated with high-dose-rate brachytherapy: a review of literature," *Journal of Contemporary Brachytherapy*, vol. 8, no. 6, pp. 533–540, 2016.

[14] Z. Ouhib, M. Kasper, J. Perez Calatayud et al., "Aspects of dosimetry and clinical practice of skin brachytherapy: The American Brachytherapy Society working group report," *Brachytherapy*, vol. 14, no. 6, pp. 840–858, 2015.

[15] J. A. DeSimone, E. Guenova, J. B. Carter et al., "Low-dose high-dose-rate brachytherapy in the treatment of facial lesions of cutaneous T-cell lymphoma," *Journal of the American Academy of Dermatology*, vol. 69, no. 1, pp. 61–65, 2013.

[16] A. L. Goddard, R. A. Vleugels, N. R. LeBoeuf et al., "Palliative Therapy for Recalcitrant Cutaneous T-Cell Lymphoma of the Hands and Feet With Low-Dose, High Dose-Rate Brachytherapy," *JAMA Dermatology*, vol. 151, no. 12, pp. 1354–1357, 2015.

[17] M. F. Demierre, S. Gan, J. Jones, and D. R. Miller, "Significant impact of cutaneous T-cell lymphoma on patients' quality of life: results of a 2005 National Cutaneous Lymphoma Foundation Survey," *Cancer*, vol. 107, no. 10, pp. 2504–2511, 2006.

[18] T. Beynon, L. Selman, E. Radcliffe et al., "We had to change to single beds because I itch in the night: a qualitative study of the experiences, attitudes and approaches to coping of patients with cutaneous T-cell lymphoma," *British Journal of Dermatology*, vol. 173, no. 1, pp. 83–92, 2015.

22

Pravastatin-Induced Eczematous Eruption Mimicking Psoriasis

Michael P. Salna,[1] Hannah M. Singer,[2] and Ali N. Dana[3,4]

[1]Department of Cardiothoracic Surgery, Stanford University School of Medicine, Stanford, CA, USA
[2]Columbia University College of Physicians and Surgeons, New York City, NY, USA
[3]Dermatology Service, James J. Peters VA Medical Center, Bronx, NY, USA
[4]Department of Dermatology, Columbia University College of Physicians and Surgeons, New York City, NY, USA

Correspondence should be addressed to Ali N. Dana; ali.dana@va.gov

Academic Editor: Jacek Cezary Szepietowski

Background. Statins, an example of the most commonly prescribed medications to the elderly, are not without side effects. Dermatologic events are often overlooked as arising from medications, particularly those which are taken chronically. Moreover, elderly patients are prone to pharmacologic interactions due to multiple medications. In this report, we describe a case of a statin-induced eczematous dermatitis with a psoriasis-like clinical presentation and review the skin manifestations that may arise from statin therapy. *Case Presentation.* An 82-year-old man with gout and hypercholesterolemia presented to dermatology clinic with new onset of pruritic, scaly erythematous plaques bilaterally on the extensor surfaces of his arms. He had never had similar lesions before. Despite various topical and systemic treatments over several months, the rash continued to evolve. The patient was then advised to discontinue his long-term statin, which led to gradual resolution of his symptoms. He was subsequently diagnosed with statin-induced eczematous dermatitis. *Conclusions.* This case report describes an adverse cutaneous reaction to statins that is rarely reported in the literature. Medications, including longstanding therapies, should be suspected in cases of refractory dermatologic lesions.

1. Introduction

Statins have become the cornerstone of hypercholesterolemia pharmacotherapy in the elderly [1]. Despite the widespread use of these medications, their role in the development of new skin conditions may be overlooked and their dermatologic side effects misdiagnosed. Statins have been increasingly associated with drug-induced autoimmune reactions, including systemic lupus erythematosus, dermatomyositis, and lichen planus pemphigoides [2]. In this case report, we describe an unusual eczematous rash in an elderly patient on long-term pravastatin therapy that appeared several months after a dose increase.

2. Case Report

An 82-year-old man with a history of gout, hypercholesterolemia, and multiple nonmelanoma skin cancers was referred to our dermatology clinic for evaluation of pruritic lesions affecting the skin of the bilateral posterior arms for several weeks. He had no personal or family history of psoriasis or atopic dermatitis and denied any new contact exposures, new detergents, or starting any new medications or supplements. His daily medications included the following: allopurinol 300 mg, hydrochlorothiazide 25 mg, aspirin 81 mg, pravastatin 20 mg, and colchicine 0.6 mg. The patient had been on pravastatin therapy for hypercholesterolemia for over 5 years. Several months before onset of the rash his pravastatin had been increased from 10 mg to 20 mg daily.

Clinical examination revealed scaly, confluent, well-circumscribed erythematous plaques on the extensor surfaces of the upper arms extending to the forearms with no other lesions noted on skin exam (Figures 1(a) and 1(b)). Evaluation of the nails did not reveal any significant findings. A 4 mm punch biopsy was obtained from the forearm for routine histological evaluation. Given the psoriasis-like appearance, the patient was prescribed triamcinolone ointment 0.025%.

The biopsy (Figure 1(c)) revealed compact orthokeratosis and significant spongiosis with a perivascular lymphocytic

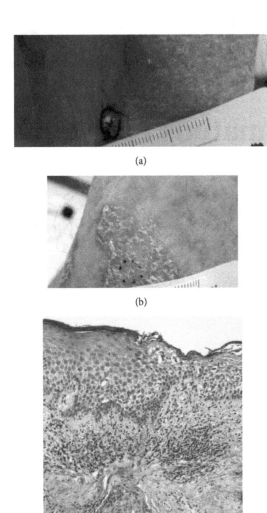

(a)

(b)

(c)

FIGURE 1: (a) Well-demarcated, erythematous patch with scale on the extensor surface of the right arm. (b) Dots indicate site of biopsy within lesion on the right arm. (c) Biopsy revealed spongiosis and perivascular lymphocytic infiltrate (hematoxylin and eosin).

infiltrate, consistent with an eczematous process. There was no evidence of acanthosis or psoriasiform epidermal hyperplasia. At the patient's follow-up appointment two weeks later, the lesions had spread to his anterior thighs and lower back. He was experiencing significant distress due to the pruritus and appearance of the rash and was treated with 40 mg intramuscular triamcinolone acetonide 0.1% solution. One month later, there was no improvement of his symptoms and alternative treatment options including phototherapy and nonsteroidal immunosuppressive therapy were considered. The patient was started on oral methotrexate, 10 mg weekly, as his schedule was unable to accommodate phototherapy. Further studies including complete blood count, metabolic panel, thyroid hormone, prostate specific antigen, serum protein electrophoresis, hepatitis B and hepatitis C, rapid plasma reagin, and autoimmune panel were unrevealing.

Fungal culture and skin scraping for microscopic evaluation for dermatophyte were negative.

Despite an 8-week course of methotrexate, there was no improvement of his lesions. Finally, the patient underwent a trial off his pravastatin to rule out the statin as an etiologic agent. In collaboration with his primary care provider, the patient was switched to cholestyramine for cholesterol management and, after 8 weeks, his cutaneous lesions resolved. The patient was tapered off methotrexate and there was no recurrence of his lesions.

3. Discussion

Statins, an example of the most commonly prescribed medications in adults, lower lipid levels through inhibition of hepatic 3-hydroxy-3-methylglutaryl coenzyme-A reductase. Given the widespread usage of statins, diagnosticians should be aware of cutaneous reactions associated with this class of medications. The most commonly reported adverse dermatological reaction is a widespread, eczematous rash or hypersensitivity reaction. With respect to specific medications, atorvastatin has been reported to cause photosensitivity, edema, cheilitis, urticaria, and skin ulceration; lovastatin has caused pruritus and/or rash in up to 5% of patients; and simvastatin has been associated with lupus-like syndrome, lichenoid drug eruptions, cheilitis, photosensitivity, and vesiculobullous eruptions [3–5]. Any of the aforementioned statin-induced skin reactions can occur soon after initiation of therapy or after many years of stable dosing.

The mechanism of statin-induced cutaneous eruptions is not well understood. Statins have been noted to affect multiple immunological pathways, partially explaining the diversity of adverse cutaneous reactions that have been reported [4]. The anti-inflammatory effects of statins are mediated by inhibiting the expression of intercellular adhesion molecule-I on leukocytes and endothelial cells as well as suppressing antigen presentation and subsequent T-cell activation [6].

Drug interactions that affect the bioavailability and metabolism of statins may also account for variations in adverse cutaneous events. Simvastatin, lovastatin, atorvastatin, and rosuvastatin undergo metabolism in the liver by cytochrome P450 enzymes CYP3A4 and CYP2C9AV; however pravastatin does not undergo metabolism by CYP enzymes [6, 7]. Up to 60% of active pravastatin may undergo renal excretion due to its hydrophilic properties and relatively low binding fraction with plasma proteins. In serum, pravastatin has been found to have a lower rate of binding with plasma proteins of 43–48% compared to lovastatin, simvastatin, and fluvastatin which have plasma protein binding rates of at least 95%. Pravastatin has a lower fraction of hepatic extraction compared to simvastatin and lovastatin, which may result in increased exposure to pravastatin in peripheral tissues. Additionally, several pravastatin metabolites have activity comparable to the native drug. Of note, patients with hepatic failure have increased systemic exposure to all statins [8].

Systemic levels of pravastatin may also be affected by the activity of transport peptides. Permeability glycoprotein

TABLE 1: Cases of pravastatin-induced adverse effects and P-glycoprotein interactions.

Reported case of pravastatin-induced adverse effect	Other medications taken by patient	P-glycoprotein effect	References
Lichenoid drug eruption in 64-year-old woman [12]	Aspirin	Possible inducer	[13]
	Candesartan	—	
	Clopidogrel	Substrate	[9]
	Diltiazem	Substrate, inhibitor, inducer	[9, 14]
	Furosemide	—	
	Hydralazine	—	
	Isosorbide mononitrate	—	
	Insulin	Inducer	[14]
	Metformin	—	
Diffuse, pruritic rash in a 55-year-old woman [15]	Aripiprazole	Substrate	[16]
	Lorazepam	—	
	Sertraline	Substrate and inhibitor	[9, 14, 16]
	Olanzapine	Substrate	[16]
	Quetiapine	Substrate	[16]
	Lithium carbonate	—	
	Levothyroxine	Inducer	[17]
	Magnesium	—	
Acute myopathy in a 65-year-old woman [18]	Aspirin	Possible inducer	[13]
	Colchicine	Substrate, inducer	[14, 18]
	Spironolactone	Inhibitor	[19]
	Furosemide	—	
	Losartan	Substrate, inhibitor	[9, 14]
Pruritic, psoriasis-like eczematous eruption in an 82-year-old man (current case)	Allopurinol	—	
	Aspirin	Possible inducer	[13]
	Colchicine	Substrate, inducer	[14, 18]
	Hydrochlorothiazide	—	

(P-gp) is an ATP-binding cassette transporter found in the small intestine, liver, kidneys, and blood-brain barrier. P-gp is located at luminal apical cells and acts on both endogenous organic compounds and many common medications, including pravastatin [9]. On enterocytes, apical P-gp is an efflux transporter that transports absorbed substrates back into the gut lumen for excretion. In hepatic biliary canaliculi, P-gp excretes substrates back into bile for elimination, and in renal tubules P-gp transports substances into urine [9, 10]. If the P-gp transporters become saturated with substrate then less medication will be eliminated and more will be absorbed systemically. Another transporter, the organic anion-transporting peptide 1B1 (OATP1B1), solute carriers also play a role in the movement of organic compounds and medications, including statins, into hepatocytes [7, 11]. OATP1B1 is located on both apical and basolateral ends of enterocytes and can translocate a variety of organic compounds and drugs. The specific role OATP1B1 and P-gp transporters play in absorption and metabolism of drug compounds is an area of active investigation with many clinical implications [10].

Case reports suggest that drug-drug interactions and genetic predispositions may precipitate adverse reactions for patients taking pravastatin; statins are very well tolerated overall. From searching the literature, three cases identified pravastatin as the cause of an adverse reaction [12, 15, 18]. All of the patients described were taking other medications, which may have influenced systemic exposure to pravastatin. Pravastatin is a substrate for the P-gp efflux transporter, and we outline in Table 1 the medications that are also reported to interface with P-gp. Drugs that are P-gp substrates, if saturated, would allow for more than expected absorption, as would inhibitors. P-gp inducers would decrease systemic exposure by increasing elimination.

4. Conclusion

This case demonstrates that pravastatin may be associated with psoriasis-like eczematous lesions that are resistant to treatment with steroids and immunosuppressive therapy. In any elderly patient with a new rash, it is worth remembering that both recently introduced and longstanding medications may play a role in skin changes and that the resolution of these changes may take weeks to months once the offending agent has been discontinued. Individual factors, slight differences between the metabolism and activity of statins, and interactions with other medication may all play a role in the etiology of statin-induced dermatitis.

Disclosure

Michael P. Salna and Hannah M. Singer are co-first authors.

Conflicts of Interest

The authors declare that there are no conflicts of interest regarding the publication of this article.

References

[1] N. J. Stone, J. G. Robinson, A. H. Lichtenstein, C. N. B. Merz, C. B. Blum, R. H. Eckel et al., "2013 ACC/AHA guideline on the treatment of blood cholesterol to reduce atherosclerotic cardiovascular risk in adults: a report of the American College of Cardiology/American Heart Association Task Force on Practice Guidelines," *Journal of the American College of Cardiology*, vol. 129, no. 25, pp. 2889–2934, 2014.

[2] B. Noël, "Lupus erythematosus and other autoimmune diseases related to statin therapy: A systematic review," *Journal of the European Academy of Dermatology and Venereology*, vol. 21, no. 1, pp. 17–24, 2007.

[3] W. H. Frishman, B. D. Brosnan, M. Grossman, D. Dasgupta, and D. K. Sun, "Adverse dermatologic effects of cardiovascular drug therapy: Part III," *Cardiology in Review*, vol. 10, no. 6, pp. 337–348, 2002.

[4] A. E. Adams, A. M. Bobrove, and A. C. Gilliam, "Statins and 'chameleon-like' cutaneous eruptions: Simvastatin-induced acral cutaneous vesiculobullous and pustular eruption in a 70-year-old man," *Journal of Cutaneous Medicine and Surgery*, vol. 14, no. 5, pp. 207–211, 2010.

[5] B. Noël and R. G. Panizzon, "Lupus-like syndrome associated with statin therapy," *Dermatology*, vol. 208, no. 3, pp. 276-277, 2004.

[6] F. Jowkar and M. R. Namazi, "Statins in dermatology," *International Journal of Dermatology*, vol. 49, no. 11, pp. 1235–1243, 2010.

[7] L. Becquemont, M. Neuvonen, C. Verstuyft et al., "Amiodarone interacts with simvastatin but not with pravastatin disposition kinetics," *Clinical Pharmacology and Therapeutics*, vol. 81, no. 5, pp. 679–684, 2007.

[8] C. B. Blum, "Comparison of properties of four inhibitors of 3-hydroxy-3-methylglutaryl-coenzyme a reductase," *The American Journal of Cardiology*, vol. 73, no. 14, pp. D3–D11, 1994.

[9] J. D. Wessler, L. T. Grip, J. Mendell, and R. P. Giugliano, "The P-glycoprotein transport system and cardiovascular drugs," *Journal of the American College of Cardiology*, vol. 61, no. 25, pp. 2495–2502, 2013.

[10] D. Coyle, E. D. Wittwer, and J. Sprung, "P-glycoprotein and Organic Anion-transporting Polypeptide (OATP) Transporters," in *A Case Approach to Perioperative Drug-Drug Interactions*, C. Marcucci et al., Ed., pp. 67–72, Springer, New York, NY, USA, 2015.

[11] J. Noé, R. Portmann, M.-E. Brun, and C. Funk, "Substrate-dependent drug-drug interactions between gemfibrozil, fluvastatin and other organic anion-transporting peptide (OATP) substrates on OATP1B1, OATP2B1, and OATP1B3," *Drug Metabolism & Disposition*, vol. 35, no. 8, pp. 1308–1314, 2007.

[12] V. S. C. Pua, R. A. Scolyer, and R. S. C. Barnetson, "Pravastatin-induced lichenoid drug eruption," *Australasian Journal of Dermatology*, vol. 47, no. 1, pp. 57–59, 2006.

[13] J. Oh, D. Shin, K. S. Lim et al., "Aspirin decreases systemic exposure to clopidogrel through modulation of P-glycoprotein but does not alter its antithrombotic activity," *Clinical Pharmacology and Therapeutics*, vol. 95, no. 6, pp. 608–616, 2014.

[14] S.-F. Zhou, "Structure, function and regulation of P-glycoprotein and its clinical relevance in drug disposition," *Xenobiotica*, vol. 38, no. 7-8, pp. 802–832, 2008.

[15] A. Walder and P. Baumann, "Mood stabilizer therapy and pravastatin: higher risk for adverse skin reactions?" *Acta Medica (Hradec Kralove)*, vol. 52, no. 1, pp. 15–18, 2009.

[16] Y. Akamine, N. Yasui-Furukori, I. Ieiri, and T. Uno, "Psychotropic drug-drug interactions involving P-glycoprotein," *CNS Drugs*, vol. 26, no. 11, pp. 959–973, 2012.

[17] W. Siegmund, S. Altmannsberger, A. Paneitz et al., "Effect of levothyroxine administration on intestinal P-glycoprotein expression: Consequences for drug disposition," *Clinical Pharmacology and Therapeutics*, vol. 72, no. 3, pp. 256–264, 2002.

[18] G. Alayli, K. Cengiz, F. Cantürk, D. Durmuş, Y. Akyol, and E. B. Menekşe, "Acute myopathy in a patient with concomitant use of pravastatin and colchicine," *Annals of Pharmacotherapy*, vol. 39, no. 7-8, pp. 1358–1361, 2005.

[19] K. M. Barnes, B. Dickstein, G. B. Cutler Jr., T. Fojo, and S. E. Bates, "Steroid transport, accumulation, and antagonism of P-glycoprotein in multidrug-resistant cells," *Biochemistry*, vol. 35, no. 15, pp. 4820–4827, 1996.

23

The Successful Treatment of a Case of Linear Psoriasis with Ixekizumab

Sara Ghoneim,[1] **Alvaro J. Ramos-Rodriguez,**[2]
Fernando Vazquez de Lara,[2] **and Lauren Bonomo**[3]

[1]*Saba University School of Medicine, The Bottom, Netherlands*
[2]*Icahn School of Medicine at Mount Sinai West, New York, NY, USA*
[3]*Icahn School of Medicine at Mount Sinai, New York, NY, USA*

Correspondence should be addressed to Sara Ghoneim; s.ghoneim@saba.edu

Academic Editor: Ravi Krishnan

Linear psoriasis is an unusual clinical variation of psoriasis that manifests segmentally along the lines of Blaschko. A major differential diagnosis is inflammatory linear verrucous epidermal nevus (ILVEN). The treatment of linear psoriasis is often challenging, with inadequate response to biological agents reported in the literature. We report a case of a 25-year-old African-American female who presented with asymptomatic hyperkeratotic papules along the lines of Blaschko and was subsequently diagnosed with linear psoriasis. After failing conventional treatment regimens, the patient received a trial of ixekizumab with complete resolution of cutaneous lesions reported after 4 months and only 8 doses of the anti-IL-17 biologic agent.

1. Introduction

Linear psoriasis is a rare clinical variation of psoriasis that manifests segmentally along the lines of Blaschko. The pathogenesis remains unclear, though some have proposed it could be explained by the well-established concept of genetic mosaicism [1]. Happle (1991) suggested that the loss of heterozygosity in somatic cells during early embryogenesis results in somatic recombination with daughter cells. Subsequently, these daughter cells go on to become clonal stem cells proliferating in a linear pattern during the embryonic development of the skin. A major differential diagnosis for linear psoriasis is inflammatory linear verrucous epidermal nevus (ILVEN), which also presents along the lines of Blaschko with similar morphology [2]. Psoriasis presenting in this manner is often mistaken for ILVEN and undertreated. The treatment of linear psoriasis can be challenging, with reports of inadequate clinical response to various biologic agents approved for the treatment of plaque psoriasis [3]. To our knowledge, we report the first case of this atypical psoriasis morphology successfully treated with the biologic agent ixekizumab.

2. Case Report

A 25-year-old African-American female presented to our clinic with asymptomatic lesions linearly arranged over her left upper extremity. The initial lesion first appeared fifteen years ago and new lesions gradually appeared over time. She denied joint pain and/or a history of infections prior to lesion development. Her past medical history was significant only for posttraumatic distress disorder and depression. There was no personal or family history of psoriasis or other dermatologic disease. Prior to presentation in our clinic, she had a skin biopsy of the right forearm which showed chronic spongiotic dermatitis with parakeratotic foci and superficial perivascular mononuclear infiltrates. No deep dermal or periadnexal infiltrates were seen and periodic acid-Schiff staining was negative for fungal organisms. Based on the results, both lichen striatus and linear psoriasis were considered as potential diagnosis, and she was started on high-potency topical steroids. A month later, the patient was referred to our clinic when she failed to respond to treatment.

Physical examination revealed hyperkeratotic and scaly gray papules coalescing into a linear plaque of the right

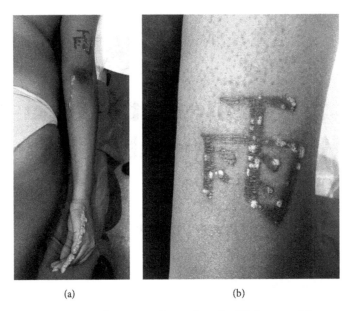

(a)   (b)

FIGURE 1: (a) Linearly arranged hyperkeratotic and scaly gray papules on the right fifth finger and dorsum of the hand extending to the right elbow. (b) Multiple hyperkeratotic papules present within a tattoo on the posterior right arm.

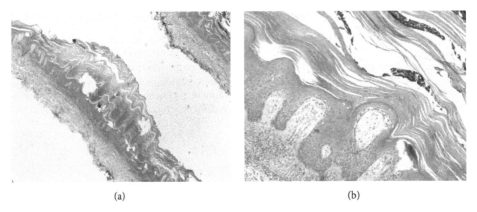

(a)   (b)

FIGURE 2: (a) Histopathological slides. At 2x magnification there is parakeratosis and epidermal acanthosis. (b) Histopathological slides. At 10x magnification a regularly acanthotic epidermis with hyperkeratosis alternating with parakeratosis. Rete ridges show psoriasiform hyperplasia.

dorsal fifth finger extending medially to the right elbow (Figure 1(a)). Of note, scaly papules were also present on a tattoo above the right elbow (Figure 1(b)). There was no nail or palmoplantar involvement. The differential diagnosis included linear psoriasis and ILVEN. The isomorphic reaction seen within the patient's tattoo (Koebner phenomenon) favored a diagnosis of psoriasis. A skin biopsy and electrodessication of one papule on her right dorsal fifth finger were performed. Histological examination of the specimen revealed parakeratosis with uniformly acanthotic epidermis (Figure 2). At a follow-up visit 2 weeks later, the patient developed new papules with similar morphology in the area that was previously electrodessicated (Figure 3(a)). This new episode of Koebnerization and histological findings further supported our diagnosis of linear psoriasis and the decision was made to initiate treatment with ixekizumab, a

monoclonal antibody targeting interleukin- (IL-) 17A. Four months later and after 8 doses of ixekizumab, we observed almost-complete resolution of the cutaneous lesions (Figures 3(b) and 3(c)).

3. Case Discussion

Linear psoriasis is a rare clinical presentation of psoriasis characterized by the linear distribution of psoriatic lesions along the lines of Blaschko. The main differential diagnosis is ILVEN. Gross morphological distinction between these two entities is difficult. Furthermore, the two entities share similar histological findings and the coexistence of ILVEN and psoriasis has also been reported [3, 4]. Histological examination of ILVEN shows areas of hypergranulosis and orthokeratosis alternating with areas of hypogranulosis and

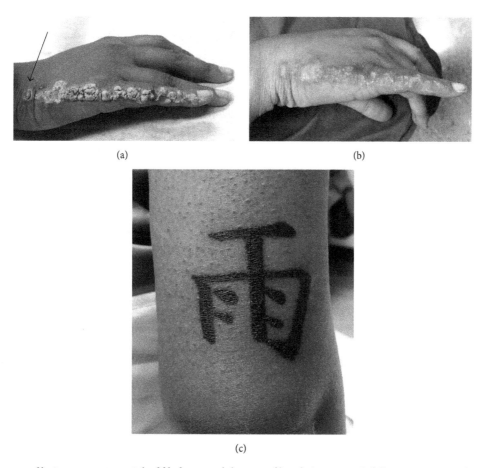

(a)

(b)

(c)

FIGURE 3: (a) Close-up of lesions present on right fifth finger and dorsum of hand. At two-week follow-up, new papules appear in the area that is previously electrodessicated (black arrow). (b) Remarkable clearing of the lesions and postinflammatory hypopigmentary changes can be seen after 8 doses of ixekizumab. (c) Psoriatic lesions are no longer present on the tattoo after treatment with 8 doses of ixekizumab.

parakeratosis [5]. Under these circumstances, immunohistochemical studies are helpful in distinguishing these two cutaneous disorders. For example, involucrin is a marker whose expression is absent in the parakeratotic areas of ILVEN but present in psoriasis [6]. Moreover, the number of Ki-67 positive nuclei is higher in psoriasis compared to ILVEN, while the number of keratin-10 positive cells is higher in ILVEN [7]. In practice, these tests are rarely ordered. It is often more practical to simply initiate therapy for psoriasis if the diagnosis is suspected.

We are now able to conclude that linear psoriasis was the correct diagnosis in this case based on several observations. First, our patient's lesions were nonpruritic, and ILVEN tends to be more pruritic than psoriatic lesions [8]. Additionally, Koebner phenomenon affects 25–30% of patients with psoriasis [9], and our patient developed lesions on her tattoo and on the electrodessicated site of her right dorsal hand. To our knowledge, Koebner phenomenon has not been described in any reported case of ILVEN. Finally, ILVEN responds minimally to antipsoriatic agents, and our patient had a remarkable response to only 8 doses of the biologic agent ixekizumab, a drug approved by the US Food and Drug

Administration in 2016 for the treatment for moderate to severe plaque psoriasis.

It is known from a small number of reports that segmental manifestations of psoriasis respond less favorably to systemic therapies such as methotrexate, acitretin, and, more recently, biologics [3, 10–13]. The chronicity and resistance of linear psoriasis to available antipsoriatic agents were suggested to be in part due to the loss of heterozygosity in cells where the lesions occur [12]. In our literature review, patients treated with either anti-IL-23 or tumor necrosis-alpha inhibitor agents had significant improvements on all of the types of psoriasis except in linear psoriasis (Table 1). Multiple studies have also demonstrated that even though psoriatic lesions might look similar, they differ substantially in the activation status of inflammatory and cytokine pathways and such networks might contribute to the different treatment responses observed with biologic agents [14]. Furthermore, by analyzing psoriasis transcriptosome in nontreated biopsied lesions, one study was able to differentiate between etanercept responders and nonresponders [15]. This heterogeneity in response further underscores the potential role of gene-expression profiling as potential predictors of response to biologics.

TABLE 1: Summary of reported cases of linear psoriasis treated with a biological agent.

Authors (year)	Gender	Age	Distribution of linear psoriasis (LP)	Other features	Biological agent used and outcome
Colombo et al. (2011) [3]	Male	67 years	Middle of ventral trunk and left side of arm, hand, thigh, knee, and tibia	Psoriatic arthritis and diffuse plaque psoriasis. Failed to respond to acitretin, cyclosporine, and methotrexate	Plaque psoriasis responded to *etanercept* but not LP
Rott et al. (2007) [10]	Male	11 years	Left side of the body	Psoriatic arthritis, nail changes. Failed methotrexate, cyclosporine and etanercept	Psoriatic arthritis responded to *infliximab* but not LP
Sfia et al. (2009) [11]	Male	29 years	Left arm and left leg	Additional psoriatic plaques on the body	Psoriatic plaques responded to *infliximab* but not LP
Arnold et al. (2010) [12]	Male	50 years	Left flank	Diffuse plaque psoriasis. Failed to respond to topical steroids, PUVA, UVB, cyclosporine, and etanercept	Plaque psoriasis responded to *adalimumab* but not LP
Weng and Tsai (2017) [13]	Male	27 years	Right upper arm, shoulder, and back	In addition to plaque psoriasis. Failed to respond to methotrexate, acitretin, topical vitamin D3 analogs and steroids	Plaque psoriasis responded to *ustekinumab* but not LP
Ghoneim et al. (2017)	Female	25 years	Dorsum of right hand, forearm and arm, and suprapubic region, left thigh and occiput	Failed topical high-potency steroids	Linear psoriasis responded favorably to 8 doses of *ixekizumab*

There are no current formal guidelines for the treatment of linear psoriasis, and larger studies are needed to determine optimal therapy for this rare variant. In our case, the patient responded favorably to ixekizumab, which opens the possibility of using new biologic agents and individualized therapy in patients with recalcitrant linear psoriasis.

Conflicts of Interest

The authors declare that there are no conflicts of interest regarding the publication of this paper.

References

[1] R. Happle, "Somatic recombination may explain linear psoriasis," *Journal of Medical Genetics*, vol. 28, no. 5, p. 337, 1991.

[2] Y. Oram and et al., "Bilateral inflammatory linear verrucous epidermal nevus associated with psoriasis," *Cutis*, vol. 57, 275, no. 4, p. 278, 1996.

[3] L. Colombo and et al., "Superimposed linear psoriasis: low effectiveness of biologic therapy," *Giornale Italiano di Dermatologia e Venereologia*, vol. 146, no. 4, pp. 311–313, 2011.

[4] T. Hofer, "Does inflammatory linear verrucous epidermal nevus represent a segmental type 1/type 2 mosaic of psoriasis?" *Dermatology*, vol. 212, no. 2, pp. 103–107, 2006.

[5] A. Brinca, F. Santiago, D. Serra, P. Andrade, R. Vieira, and A. Figueiredo, "Linear Psoriasis – A Case Report," *Case Reports in Dermatology*, vol. 3, no. 1, pp. 8–12, 2011.

[6] F. R. Ferreira, N. G. Di Chiacchio, M. L. De Alvarenga, and S. H. Mandelbaum, "Involucrin in the differential diagnosis between linear psoriasis and inflammatory linear verrucous epidermal nevus: A report of one case," *Anais Brasileiros de Dermatologia*, vol. 88, no. 4, pp. 604–607, 2013.

[7] W. H. Vissers and et al., "Immunohistochemical differentiation between inflammatory linear verrucous epidermal nevus (ILVEN) and psoriasis," *European Journal of Dermatology*, vol. 14, no. 4, pp. 216–220, 2004.

[8] J. Altman and A. H. Mehregan, "Inflammatory Linear Verrucose Epidermal Nevus," *JAMA Dermatology*, vol. 104, no. 4, pp. 385–389, 1971.

[9] N. Kluger, E. Estève, S. Fouéré, F. Dupuis-Fourdan, M. Jegou, and C. Lévy-Rameau, "Tattooing and psoriasis: a case series and review of the literature," *International Journal of Dermatology*, vol. 56, no. 8, pp. 822–827, 2017.

[10] S. Rott, R. M. Küster, and U. Mrowietz, "Successful treatment of severe psoriatic arthritis with infliximab in an 11-year-old child suffering from linear psoriasis along lines of Blaschko [5]," *British Journal of Dermatology*, vol. 157, no. 1, pp. 191-192, 2007.

[11] M. Sfia, B. Roth-Mall, M.-C. Tortel, J.-C. Guillaume, and B. Cribier, "Blasch-kolinear psoriasis revealed by infliximab therapy," *Annales de Dermatologie et de Venereologie*, vol. 136, no. 12, pp. 898–903, 2009.

[12] A. W. Arnold, R. Happle, and P. H. Itin, "Superimposed linear psoriasis unmasked by therapy with adalimumab," *European Journal of Dermatology*, vol. 20, no. 5, pp. 573-574, 2010.

[13] H. Weng and T. Tsai, "Response of superimposed linear psoriasis to ustekinumab: A case report," *Indian Journal of*

Dermatology, Venereology and Leprology, vol. 83, no. 3, p. 392, 2017.

[14] J. Karczewski, B. Poniedziałek, P. Rzymski, and Z. Adamski, "Factors affecting response to biologic treatment in psoriasis," *Dermatologic Therapy*, vol. 27, no. 6, pp. 323–330, 2014.

[15] W. R. Swindell, A. Johnston, J. J. Voorhees, J. T. Elder, and J. E. Gudjonsson, "Dissecting the psoriasis transcriptome: inflammatory- and cytokine-driven gene expression in lesions from 163 patients," *BMC Genomics*, vol. 14, no. 1, article 527, 2013.

24

Double Morphology: Tertiary Syphilis and Acquired Immunodeficiency Syndrome

R. M. Ngwanya, B. Kakande, and N. P. Khumalo

Groote Schuur Hospital and The University of Cape Town, Cape Town, South Africa

Correspondence should be addressed to R. M. Ngwanya; laduma.ngwanya@uct.ac.za

Academic Editor: Alireza Firooz

Background. Human immunodeficiency virus (HIV) and *Treponema pallidum* coinfection is relatively common and accounts for about 25% of primary and secondary syphilis. Tertiary syphilis in HIV-uninfected and HIV-infected patients is vanishingly rare. This is most likely due to early treatment of cases of primary and secondary syphilis. There is rapid progression to tertiary syphilis in HIV-infected patients. *Case Presentation.* A 49-year-old woman diagnosed with HIV Type 1 infection and cluster of differentiation 4 (CD4) count of 482 presented with a four-week history of multiple crusted plaques, nodules, and ulcers on her face, arms, and abdomen. Her past history revealed red painful eyes six months prior to this presentation. She had generalized lymphadenopathy, no alopecia, and no palmar-plantar or mucosal lesions. There were no features suggestive of secondary syphilis. Neurological examination was normal. Her rapid plasma reagin test was positive to a titer of 64. She was treated with Penicillin G 20 mu IVI daily for 2 weeks. *Conclusion.* Penicillin remains the treatment of choice in syphilitic infected HIV negative and HIV-infected individuals. In neurosyphilis, the dose of Penicillin GIVI is 18–24 mu daily for 10–14 days. This case report demonstrates the importance of excluding syphilis in any HIV-infected patient.

1. Background

Human immunodeficiency virus and *Treponema pallidum* coinfection is relatively common and accounts for about 25% of primary and secondary syphilis [1]. Tertiary syphilis in the antibiotic era is rare and tertiary syphilis in human immunodeficiency virus- (HIV-) uninfected and HIV-infected patients is vanishingly rare. This is most likely due to the judicious use of antibiotics and early treatment of cases of primary and secondary syphilis. The standard of care for syphilis is penicillin. We present a 49-year-old female patient who had tertiary syphilis characterized by gummas and papillitis on a background of HIV coinfection.

2. Case Presentation

A 49-year-old woman patient diagnosed with HIV Type 1 infection and cluster of differentiation 4 (CD4) count of 482 presented to the Dermatology Department at Groote Schuur Hospital, Cape Town, South Africa, with a four-week history of multiple crusted plaques, nodules, and ulcers on her face, arms, and abdomen (Figures 1 and 2). She was on antiretroviral therapy. Her past medical history revealed red painful eyes six months prior to this presentation. She did not seek medical care for her eye condition. She had generalized lymphadenopathy. no alopecia, no palmar-plantar, and no mucosal lesions or lesions of lues maligna. There were no features suggestive of secondary syphilis such as a papulosquamous nonitchy eruption on her body. Neurological examination was normal. Ophthalmological examination revealed unilateral acute papillitis. The physical examination showed a well looking female patient with crusted plaques and nodules on face and abdomen and an ulcer on her forearm, hence double morphology (Figures 1 and 2).

Our initial evaluation centered around lues maligna but this was excluded on the basis of the fact that lesions of lues maligna are usually multiple, well demarcated rupioid nodules and papules. A black eschar is sometimes observed on the lesions. Infections such as tuberculosis and deep fungal infections were also considered as atypical presentations are common in HIV infections. The patient was referred to an ophthalmologist and a diagnosis of papillitis was made. Rapid

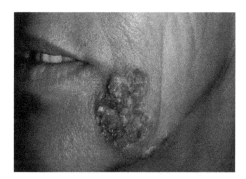

FIGURE 1: Plaque on chin before Penicillin G treatment.

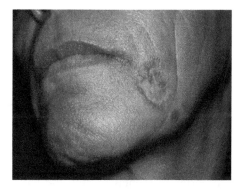

FIGURE 3: Plaque on chin after IVI Penicillin G treatment.

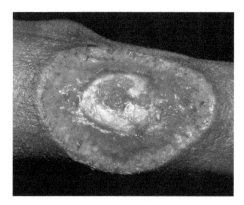

FIGURE 2: Ulcer on forearm before Penicillin G treatment.

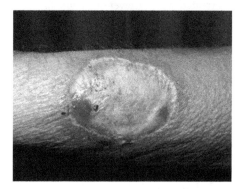

FIGURE 4: Ulcer on forearm after IVI Penicillin G treatment.

plasma reagin (RPR) test was positive (titer = 1 : 256, normal < 1 : 16). A diagnosis of tertiary syphilis with HIV coinfection was made. Tertiary syphilis diagnosis was made on the basis of the skin findings of gummas and papillitis, a manifestation of neurosyphilis. Lumbar puncture and skin biopsy were not done. She was treated with intravenous Penicillin G 5 MU IVI 6 hourly for 2 weeks. Healing occurred with atrophic scaring (Figures 3 and 4).

3. Discussion

Human immunodeficiency virus and *Treponema pallidum* coinfection is relatively common and accounts for about 25% of primary and secondary syphilis [1]. Tertiary syphilis in the antibiotic era is rare and tertiary syphilis in HIV-uninfected and HIV-infected patients is vanishingly rare. This is most likely due to the judicious use of antibiotics and early treatment of cases of primary and secondary syphilis. There is rapid progression to tertiary syphilis in HIV-infected patients, resulting in earlier onset of cardiovascular and neurologic sequelae [2]. Optic neuritis, uveitis, and other ocular manifestations of syphilis are common among HIV-infected patients [3]. Syphilis, a multisystem bacterial infection, is caused by the spirochete *Treponema pallidum*. It is characterized by three stages of active disease primary, secondary, and tertiary with latent periods between the secondary and tertiary stages. Gummatous mucocutaneous lesions of tertiary syphilis snd advanced secondary syphilis can be seen simultaneously [4]. Left untreated patients

with latent syphilis will develop tertiary syphilis. Tertiary syphilis usually is slowly progressive and without treatment will appear after many years characterized by the presence of neurosyphilis, cardiovascular syphilis, and gummas. The gummas occur in any organ but are seen more often in bone, mucous membrane, and the skin. Skin gummas which are by far very common are indurated, nodular, or ulcerative and spirochetes in these lesions are rare. Our patient presented with both the ulcers and nodules with plaques hence the double morphology. Our patient also presented with generalized lymphadenopathy. Lymphadenopathy is a usual finding in patients with both primary and secondary syphilis. It was not a surprising finding in our patient as this is a normal finding in HIV infection. Histopathological findings include a central area of coagulative necrosis, obliterative endarteritis, plasma cells, and epithelioid histiocytes. Papillitis and gummas, which were present in our patient, are manifestations of tertiary syphilis. Syphilis and HIV frequently coexist and this is not surprising [5]. The rate of coinfection has been noted to be on the rise in men having sex with men. Unusual and atypical forms of syphilis are usually observed in the setting of syphilis. In the presence of HIV infection syphilis can appear at any stage. The eye changes of syphilis can involve any structure of the eye with uveitis being the initial manifestation in patients who have acquired immunodeficiency syndrome [6]. Panuveitis is common in patients who are HIV infected [7]. Papillitis, also known as optic neuritis, is characterized by inflammation and deterioration of the optic disc. It is one of the many manifestations of neurosyphilis. Neurosyphilis is a serious complication of syphilis and can occur at any time during the course of syphilis. Syphilitic optic neuropathy has been described in seven patients who had syphilitic optic neuropathy on a background of HIV infection [8]. The presence of neurosyphilis should be looked for as this impacts on management. Diagnosis of syphilis is based on serological tests for both the non-*Treponema* and *Treponema* antibodies. It is important to actively test for syphilis in HIV-infected patients even when the initial test may be negative [9]. In our laboratory a titer of more than 1:16 is considered positive. Penicillin remains the treatment of choice in all forms of syphilis in both the HIV negative and HIV-infected individuals. In neurosyphilis the dose is Penicillin G intravenous (IVI) 18–24 mu daily for 10–14 days

She was treated with intravenous Penicillin G 5 MU IVI 6 hourly for 2 weeks. Healing occurred with atrophic scaring (Figures 3 and 4). That which occurs commonly must always be excluded even for rarer variants of that disease. This case report demonstrates the importance of excluding syphilis in any HIV-infected patient.

Abbreviations

AIDS: Acquired immunodeficiency syndrome
HIV: Human immunodeficiency virus
CD4:   Cluster of differentiation 4
RPR: Rapid plasma reagin
IVI: Intravenous.

Conflicts of Interest

The authors declare that they have no conflicts of interest.

References

[1] H. W. Chesson, J. D. Heffelfinger, R. F. Voigt, and D. Collins, "Estimates of primary and secondary syphilis rates in persons with HIV in the United States, 2002," *Sexually Transmitted Diseases*, vol. 32, no. 5, pp. 265–269, 2005.

[2] N. Gregory, M. Sanchez, and M. R. Buchness, "The spectrum of syphilis in patients with human immunodeficiency virus infection," *Journal of the American Academy of Dermatology*, vol. 22, no. 6 I, pp. 1061–1067, 1990.

[3] C. M. Marra, "Update on neurosyphilis," *Current Infectious Disease Reports*, vol. 11, no. 2, pp. 127–134, 2009.

[4] E. N. Nnoruka and A. C. J. Ezeoke, "Evaluation of syphilis in patients with HIV infection in Nigeria," *Tropical Medicine & International Health*, vol. 10, no. 1, pp. 58–64, 2005.

[5] N. M. Zetola and J. D. Klausner, "Syphilis and HIV infection: an update," *Clinical Infectious Diseases*, vol. 44, no. 9, pp. 1222–1228, 2007.

[6] C. Tsen, S. Chen, Y. Chen, and S. Sheu, "Uveitis as an initial manifestation of acquired immunodeficiency syndrome," *International Journal of STD & AIDS*, vol. 28, no. 12, pp. 1224–1228, 2017.

[7] S. Y. Lee, V. Cheng, D. Rodger, and N. Rao, "Clinical and laboratory characteristics of ocular syphilis: a new face in the era of HIV co-infection," *Journal of Ophthalmic Inflammation and Infection*, vol. 5, no. 1, article 26, 2015.

[8] S. Apinyawasisuk, A. Poonyathalang, P. Preechawat, and K. Vanikieti, "Syphilitic optic neuropathy: re-emerging cases over a 2-year period," *Neuro-Ophthalmology*, vol. 40, no. 2, pp. 69–73, 2016.

[9] G. Smith and R. P. Holman, "The Prozone Phenomenon with Syphilis and HIV-1 Co-infection," *Southern Medical Journal*, vol. 97, no. 4, pp. 379–382, 2004.

25

Photopheresis Provides Significant Long-Lasting Benefit in Nephrogenic Systemic Fibrosis

Ranran Zhang and William Nicholas Rose

Department of Pathology and Laboratory Medicine, University of Wisconsin, Madison, WI, USA

Correspondence should be addressed to William Nicholas Rose; wrose@uwhealth.org

Academic Editor: Alireza Firooz

Nephrogenic systemic fibrosis (NSF), previously known as nephrogenic fibrosing dermopathy, is a rare complication of exposure to gadolinium-based contrast agents in patients who have significantly decreased renal function. Manifestations include fibrosis of the skin and other tissues. Effective therapies are lacking. Photopheresis has been tried with variable rates of improvement, and small numbers of cases (20 as of 2016) have been reported of NSF patients treated with photopheresis. We report a case of patient with nephrogenic systemic fibrosis who was treated with photopheresis and demonstrated significant lasting improvements.

1. Introduction

Nephrogenic systemic fibrosis is a rare but well-recognized severe systemic complication of gadolinium-based contrast agents. It occurs exclusively in patients with renal insufficiency [1, 2]. The pathophysiology is emerging. A process similar to wound healing driven by proinflammatory and profibrotic pathways may be one of the underlying causes [1]. Extracorporeal photopheresis (ECP) is a treatment method that improves several autoimmune or inflammatory conditions. Scattered case reports and case series suggest that ECP improves symptoms in patients with NSF [2].

The 2016 evidence-based guidelines from the American Society for Apheresis state that outcomes have been reported for 20 patients who were treated with ECP for NSF [3]. Thus, due to the very small number of reports, our goal is to contribute another data point, however meager, in an effort to help practitioners manage these patients.

Furthermore, coverage decisions typically depend on published evidence or the lack thereof. Due to the expense of photopheresis, the treatment is often highly scrutinized by Medicare in the United States, and coverage denials are very common. We advocate for a reconsideration of summary coverage denials of ECP for NSF.

2. Case Report

A 60-year-old male presented with progressive fibrotic indurated skin plaques, multiple contractures, severely limited range of motion of all limbs, and joint pain. Symptoms started while he was recovering from an episode of severe sepsis four years prior to presentation.

His sepsis at that time (four years prior to presentation) was complicated by acute renal injury requiring temporary hemodialysis and cervical spine epidural abscess causing paraplegia.

At that time (four years prior to presentation), multiple MRI studies with gadolinium-based contrast agents were performed, while he was on hemodialysis. The combination of gadolinium exposures in concert with dialysis dependence was most likely the cause of his NSF.

At the time of presentation, the diagnosis of NSF was based on clinical suspicion (i.e., the aforementioned plaques, indurations, and joint contractures in the setting of gadolinium exposure while being dialysis-dependent). Skin punch biopsy performed at presentation was noteworthy for increased cellularity, thick and thin collagen fibers, and elastic preservation (Figures 1(a) and 1(b)).

After a one-month trial of sodium thiosulfate without improvement, he was started on ECP using the Therakos

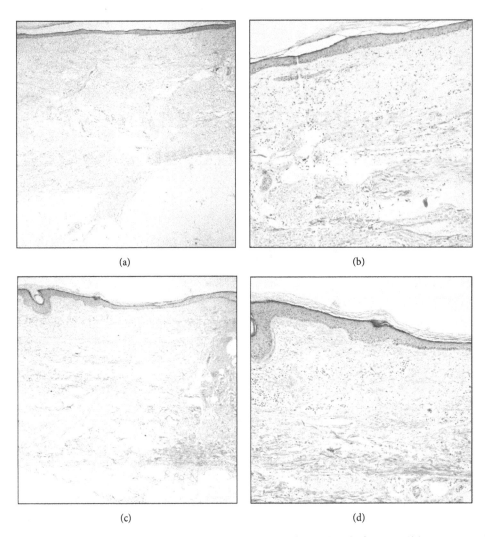

FIGURE 1: Skin punch biopsies before ((a) at 4x magnification; (b) at 10x magnification) and after ECP ((c) at 4x magnification; (d) at 10x magnification). Despite clinical improvement, interval changes in histology were not dramatic. Fibrocollagenous thickening of dermis was seen in both biopsies. In addition, dermal perivascular plasmacytic infiltrates were minimal in both biopsies.

UVAR XTS for two consecutive days (i.e., one cycle) per week for four weeks (i.e., eight total ECP procedures over four weeks). The patient reported and showed improvement as early as one week after the completion of this first batch of four cycles of ECP. Bilateral knee joints contractures and reduced range of motion (ROM) were the main limitations of patient's mobility and their improvement was relatively well-documented.

This initial 4-week course was based on ASFA's guidelines for using ECP in a variety of diseases such as cutaneous T-cell lymphoma, hematopoietic stem cell transplant associated graft-versus-host disease, and cellular rejection of lung transplant [3]. This starting protocol was also what others reported in case reports that described ECP as a treatment for NSF [4, 5].

A very common principle of using ECP is to start with this schedule initially and then taper to every 2 weeks times 4-5 cycles and then every month times 3 cycles (and continue as needed depending on response).

We must emphasize that the precise quantity of cycles beyond the initial 4-week period was relatively arbitrary and guided by clinical judgment and prudence for patient finances since there was no ASFA guideline for ECP in NSF at the time and because there was uncertainty about reimbursement coverage.

After the initial four cycles, a three-month interval passed without ECP. An important reason for pausing ECP at that time was concern about reimbursement coverage. ECP was then restarted with a schedule of one cycle every two weeks for six cycles. This was then tapered to one cycle every month for seven cycles. A summary of ECP treatments is shown in Table 1.

Interestingly, despite significant clinical improvement, biopsies after completion of ECP treatment did not reveal significant changes compared to biopsies prior to ECP (Figures 1(c) and 1(d)). The benefit of ECP appeared to plateau 14 months after the initiation of therapy.

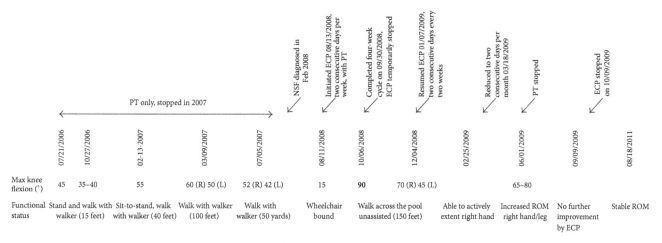

FIGURE 2: Disease and treatment timeline.

TABLE 1: Summary of ECP treatments.

One cycle q week × 4

(three-month interval without ECP)

One cycle q2 weeks × 6

One cycle q month × 7

Note. One "cycle" equals ECP on two consecutive days.

Subsequently, patient was maintained on tacrolimus alone which continued to slowly improve his symptoms. The summary of the disease course is shown in Figure 2.

3. Discussion

Exceptional reviews with visual aids are highly recommended for further reading on the general aspects of NSF [6, 7]. For this case specifically, we were initially impressed with the rapid onset of improvements in this patient. This was largely a result of comparing this patient to our usual experience with photopheresis in the treatment of chronic graft-versus-host disease after hematopoietic progenitor cell transplant in which improvements tend to be relatively slower and require at least a few to several months of ECP to gauge benefit.

Upon further reading, we discovered that the rapidity of improvement is not necessarily unique to this patient nor is it necessarily that rapid compared to other reports. Kafi et al. reported that a patient treated with phototherapy (a similar but not identical modality to ECP) and that "softening of the patient's skin lesions was first noted during the second week of therapy" [4].

More specific to ECP, Gilliet et al. reported 3 NSF patients treated with ECP [5]. They reported that "[a]ll three patients showed a softening of the skin lesions and a marked improvement of the joint motility starting after four cycles of ECP" and that "after two cycles of therapy, [one] patient noted a marked softening of her lesions on the lower leg."

Thus, if a patient improves from ECP, then it would not be unexpected to see such benefits within approximately 2–6 weeks. This is speculated to depend upon many variables including the frequency of ECP, duration of ECP, other additional treatments, heterogeneity of disease, and interpatient biological heterogeneity.

4. Conclusion

We report a case of NSF treated with ECP over a period of 14 months which demonstrated significant movement improvement that was sustained after cessation of ECP. ECP may be useful for NSF patients with longstanding disease. It is important to keep in mind that clinical improvement may not be proportional to histological improvement, and the ideal ECP regimen is highly personalized. For further characterization of the benefit of ECP in NSF patients, standard methods to assess disease improvement are needed.

Disclosure

This case report was presented as an abstract poster at the American Society for Apheresis 2015 Annual Meeting in San Antonio, Texas, USA [8].

Conflicts of Interest

The authors declare that there are no conflicts of interest regarding the publication of this paper.

References

[1] Z. Zou, H. L. Zhang, G. H. Roditi, T. Leiner, W. Kucharczyk, and M. R. Prince, "Nephrogenic systemic fibrosis: Review of 370 biopsy-confirmed cases," *JACC: Cardiovascular Imaging*, vol. 4, no. 11, pp. 1206–1216, 2011.

[2] H. Richmond, J. Zwerner, Y. Kim, and D. Fiorentino, "Nephrogenic systemic fibrosis: relationship to gadolinium and response to photopheresis," *Archives of Dermatology*, vol. 143, no. 8, pp. 1025–1030, 2007.

[3] J. Schwartz, A. Padmanabhan, N. Aqui et al., "Guidelines on the use of therapeutic apheresis in clinical practice—evidence-based approach from the writing committee of the american

society for apheresis: the seventh special issue," *Journal of Clinical Apheresis*, vol. 31, no. 3, pp. 149–162, 2016.

[4] R. Kafi, G. J. Fisher, T. Quan et al., "UV-A1 phototherapy improves nephrogenic fibrosing dermopathy," *Archives of Dermatology*, vol. 140, no. 11, pp. 1322–1324, 2004.

[5] M. Gilliet, A. Cozzio, G. Burg, and F. O. Nestle, "Successful treatment of three cases of nephrogenic fibrosing dermopathy with extracorporeal photopheresis," *British Journal of Dermatology*, vol. 152, no. 3, pp. 531–536, 2005.

[6] T. Chopra, K. Kandukurti, S. Shah, R. Ahmed, and M. Panesar, "Understanding nephrogenic systemic fibrosis," *International Journal of Nephrology*, vol. 2012, Article ID 912189, 14 pages, 2012.

[7] S. Swaminathan and S. V. Shah, "New insights into nephrogenic systemic fibrosis," *Journal of the American Society of Nephrology*, vol. 18, no. 10, pp. 2636–2643, 2007.

[8] R. Zhang and W. N. Rose, "Nephrogenic systemic fibrosis significantly improved by extracorporeal photopheresis," *Journal of Clinical Apheresis*, vol. 30, no. 2, 121 pages, 2015.

Diagnostic Challenge: A Report of Two Adult-Onset Still's Disease Cases

Sakunee Niranvichaiya and Daranporn Triwongwaranat

Department of Dermatology, Faculty of Medicine Siriraj Hospital, Mahidol University, Bangkok, Thailand

Correspondence should be addressed to Daranporn Triwongwaranat; t daranporn@hotmail.com

Academic Editor: Julia Y. Lee

This study reports two adult-onset Still's disease (AOSD) cases that met both Yamaguchi's and Fautrel's criteria and that presented with notable clinical manifestations. One case presented with atypical dermographism-like rash with an extremely high ferritin level. The other case presented with typical salmon-pink maculopapular rash but had atypical positive rheumatoid factor. This suggests that although negative rheumatoid factor is one of the criteria used for the diagnosis of AOSD, a positive rheumatoid factor result does not exclude AOSD. Beside a classic rash, characterized by transient salmon-pink maculopapular rash, we also find atypical dermographism-like rash. These findings remind us that there exist various types of rash from AOSD.

1. Introduction

Adult-onset Still's disease (AOSD) is a rare systemic inflammatory condition with unknown etiology that is characterized by high spiking fever, arthritis, typically salmon-pink maculopapular rash, leukocytosis with neutrophilia, and multiple organs' involvement [1]. The diagnosis can be made by excluding other serious conditions. The cutaneous manifestation of AOSD varies, ranging from typical salmon-pink maculopapular rash to atypical rashes such as persistent purpuric papules and plaques, urticaria, dermographism-like rash, generalized erythema, and vesiculopustules on hands and feet [2–4].

2. Case Reports

2.1. Patient 1. A 36-year-old male with history of chronic symmetrical polyarthritis of hand joints was diagnosed with seronegative rheumatoid arthritis for five years. His current medicines were methotrexate 5 mg/week and chloroquine 250 mg/week. Prior to admission, the patient developed high-grade fever, rash with intense pruritus, interphalangeal joint pain, myalgia, and sore throat for three weeks. Antibiotics were given but no improvement was noted. On examination, his temperature was 39.5°C with mild pharyngeal hyperemia, hepatomegaly, and oligoarthralgia of the interphalangeal joints. Lung, spleen, and lymph node examinations were unremarkable. The persistent hyperpigmented plaques with excoriation and some scale were observed on his trunk, back, shoulders, and both thighs. He also had linear edematous erythematous wheal lesions, similar to dermographism in appearance on his back and shoulders (Figure 1). We observe no evanescent rash in this case. Laboratory findings are shown in Table 1. Chest radiography revealed bilateral perihilar interstitial infiltration. After excluding other conditions, he was diagnosed with AOSD. Prednisolone 60 mg/day was given with continued methotrexate 5 mg/week and increased dose of chloroquine from 250 mg/week to 250 mg/day. At the follow-up, corticosteroids were gradually decreased as symptoms, such as skin rash, fever, and arthralgia, showed improvement. Hepatitis, anemia, and interstitial infiltration of lung were also resolved.

2.2. Patient 2. A previously healthy 27-year-old woman developed high-grade fever, maculopapular rash with mild itching, weight loss, and polyarthralgia for 4 months. Hepatomegaly and bilateral symmetrical polyarthralgia of shoulders, wrists, knees, and phalangeal joints were also observed. The salmon-pink colored maculopapular rash was observed

TABLE 1: Laboratory findings from two patients presenting with adult-onset Still's disease.

Laboratory data	Patient 1	Patient 2
Hemoglobin (12–18 g/dL)	11.7	11.3
MCV/MCH (80–99 fL/27–37 pg)	79.8/26	84.8/27.8
WBC* count ($4-11 \times 10^3/mm^3$)	29,020	25,040
Neutrophils (40–74%)	82.0	93.5
ESR† (0–20 mm/hr)	86	94
CRP‡ (<5 mg/L)	N/A	89
Ferritin (30–400 ng/ml)	>100,000	13,753
AST§ (0–40 U/L)	385	100
ALT‖ (0–41 U/L)	73	39
ALP¶ (40–130 U/L)	179	94
Albumin (3.5–5.2 g/dl)	2.9	3.9
LDH** (240–480 U/L)	6,883	872
Antinuclear antibodies	Homogeneous pattern titer 1 : 320; rim-like pattern; anti-cytoplasmic antibodies	Nucleolar pattern titer 1 : 100; fine-speckled pattern
Anti-double stranded DNA	Negative	Negative
Rheumatoid factor (<4.5 IU/ml = negative; 4.5–≤6.0 U/ml = borderline; >6.0 U/ml = positive)	Negative	23.36 (positive)
Anti-CCP††	Negative	N/A
Cultures	No growth (blood, urine)	No growth (blood)

*White blood cell. †Erythrocyte sedimentation rate. ‡C-reactive protein. §Aspartate transaminase. ‖Alanine transaminase. ¶Alkaline phosphatase. **Lactate dehydrogenase. ††Anti-cyclic citrullinated peptide antibody.

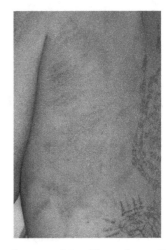

FIGURE 1: Linear, dermographism-like, and vague lichenoid papules.

on her trunk, back, and extremities, with no residual hyperpigmentation observed when the rash subsided (Figure 2(a)). Skin biopsy was revealed as in Figure 2(b). Laboratory findings are shown in Table 1. Chest radiography was unremarkable. High-resolution computer tomography showed enlargement of multiple bilateral lymph nodes at axillary regions, with several subcentimeter lymph nodes noted at prevascular, periaortic, right paratracheal, and left upper paratracheal regions. Naproxen 500 mg/day, chloroquine 250 mg/day, and prednisolone 15 mg/day were prescribed. Fever, salmon-pink rash, and all other symptoms were subsided and completely resolved within a few months.

3. Discussion

Classic rash in AOSD is characterized by transient salmon-pink maculopapular rash, usually coexisting with daily high spiking fever [1]. However, atypical rashes have also been reported, such as persistent purpuric papules and plaques,

urticaria, dermographism or linear pigmentation, generalized erythema, dermatomyositis-like plaques, vesiculopustules on hands and feet, prurigo pigmentosa-like plaques, and lichen amyloidosis-like hyperpigmented plaques [2–7]. Our first case presented with atypical dermographism-like and persistent hyperpigmented plaques. Recent studies have postulated that the pathophysiology of dermographism might be an underreported symptom of the Koebner phenomenon or related to mast cell degranulation [4, 5, 7].

AOSD has no pathognomonic histopathology. However, our review of the literature revealed highly distinctive findings of the biopsy specimens from persistent papules and plaques, including parakeratosis, scattered necrotic keratinocytes mostly in the upper half of the epidermis, and interstitial and perivascular neutrophilic infiltration in the papillary dermis with no evidence of vasculitis [6, 7]. On the other hand, the histopathology from urticarial evanescent rash shows normal epidermis, sparse perivascular, and interstitial neutrophilic infiltration with dermal edema [6, 7]. Patient 2 with maculopapular rash revealed the histopathology as superficial perivascular infiltration with neutrophils predominance, which can be found in, but not specific to, patient with AOSD.

Fever, arthralgia, typical rash, and leukocytosis are major criteria for Yamaguchi whereas sore throat, lymphadenopathy, hepatosplenomegaly, abnormal liver function tests, negative antinuclear antibodies, and negative rheumatoid factor are considered minor ones [1]. For Fautrel's criteria, spiking fever, arthralgia, transient erythema, pharyngitis, polymorphonuclear cells ≥ 80%, and glycosylated ferritin ≤ 20% are major criteria. Maculopapular rash and leukocytosis are minor criteria [1]. Our patients were diagnosed with AOSD according to both criteria, with other conditions such as infection, autoimmune diseases, and hematologic malignancy being excluded. Fever and joint pain are common symptoms; however, sore throat, myalgia, and weight loss can also be found. In addition, lymphadenopathy, splenomegaly, hepatitis, and/or hepatomegaly have

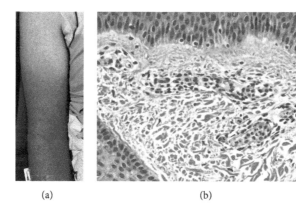

(a)   (b)

FIGURE 2: (a) Salmon-pink rash at forearm. (b) Normal epidermis with no necrotic keratinocytes. Superficial perivascular cells infiltration with neutrophils. No evidence of vasculitis (H&E, ×40).

frequently been reported. Rare interstitial lung infiltration can also develop, as observed in case patient 1 [1].

Some literatures suggested that autoimmunity mechanisms such as macrophage activation and inflammatory cytokines (e.g., IL-1, IL-6, IL-18, IFN-δ, and TNF-α), genetic factors, and infection may play a role of pathogenesis in AOSD [1, 2].

Recent studies have shown that most AOSD patients (93–100%) have negative rheumatoid factor (RF) and usually negative antinuclear antibodies (ANA) [1]. Given the presence of a positive ANA in patient 1, the patient was screened for systemic lupus erythematosus (SLE). Analysis revealed no SLE or specific autoantibodies for SLE in this case. In the second case, although the clinical features of AOSD were present, the patient also had positive RF. This suggests that despite the presence of positive RF and ANA, AOSD should not be dismissed.

Ferritin is usually higher in patients diagnosed with AOSD. If serum ferritin is 5 times above a normal level (normal range 30–400 ng/ml or above 1,000 ng/ml), it is suggested that the patient is having an AOSD, but with only 41–46% specificity [1]. Recent studies found that high serum ferritin level is usually related to disease activity and has been linked to chronic recurrent flares and reactive hemophagocytic lymphohistiocytosis [1, 8, 9]. Zeng et al. found that an elevated serum ferritin level, interstitial pneumonia, pleuritis, and unrecovered fever were still present after prescribing prednisolone 1 mg/kg/day for three days, foretelling poor prognosis [10]. Despite having high ferritin levels, both cases experienced good treatment outcomes. In our view, these positive outcomes might come from patients' good responses to prednisolone, which helped patients to recover from fever. In case 1 with extremely high ferritin level, there was a possibility of chronic recurrent flare in the future. Thus, close observation was needed.

The treatment for AOSD is based on the severity of the disease. Corticosteroids are useful in controlling active disease and inducing remission. NSAIDs are effective in curing mild cases and improving articular symptoms and fever. Steroid-sparing agents, such as methotrexate and hydroxychloroquine, were used and performed well in our cases.

Biologic agents are an alternative treatment for use in the complicated and refractory cases [1, 11].

In conclusion, we report two cases with clinically compelling cutaneous lesions and clinical symptoms of AOSD. Dermographism-like lesions, which have rarely been reported, were found in patient 1. This case also showed a very high ferritin level and interstitial lung infiltration, indicating unfavorable prognosis. Patient 2 presented with typical rash but had positive rheumatoid factor. This suggests that although negative RF is one of the criteria used for the diagnosis of AOSD, a positive RF result does not exclude AOSD. Accordingly, other diagnostic criteria need to be considered and evaluated.

Conflicts of Interest

The authors declare that there are no conflicts of interest regarding the publication of this article.

References

[1] M. Gerfaud-Valentin, Y. Jamilloux, J. Iwaz, and P. Sève, "Adult-onset Still's disease," *Autoimmunity Reviews*, vol. 13, no. 7, pp. 708–722, 2014.

[2] T. Yamamoto, "Cutaneous manifestations associated with adult-onset Still's disease: important diagnostic values," *Rheumatology International*, vol. 32, no. 8, pp. 2233–2237, 2012.

[3] A. Cozzi, A. Papagrigoraki, D. Biasi, C. Colato, and G. Girolomoni, "Cutaneous manifestations of adult-onset Still's disease: a case report and review of literature," *Clinical Rheumatology*, vol. 35, no. 5, pp. 1377–1382, 2016.

[4] P. R. Criado, J. F. De Carvalho, L. A. Ayabe, H. R. C. Brandt, R. Romiti, and C. W. Maruta, "Urticaria and dermographism in patients with adult-onset Still's disease," *Rheumatology International*, vol. 32, no. 8, pp. 2551–2555, 2012.

[5] H.-C. Tseng and C.-H. Lee, "Refractory urticaria in adult-onset Still's disease," *Rheumatology International*, vol. 34, no. 7, pp. 1029-1030, 2014.

[6] J. Y.-Y. Lee, C.-C. Yang, and M. M.-L. Hsu, "Histopathology of persistent papules and plaques in adult-onset Still's disease," *Journal of the American Academy of Dermatology*, vol. 52, no. 6, pp. 1003–1008, 2005.

[7] J. Y.-Y. Lee, C.-K. Hsu, M.-F. Liu, and S.-C. Chao, "Evanescent and persistent pruritic eruptions of adult-onset still disease: a clinical and pathologic study of 36 patients," *Seminars in Arthritis and Rheumatism*, vol. 42, no. 3, pp. 317–326, 2012.

[8] A. Kontzias and P. Efthimiou, "Adult-onset still's disease: pathogenesis, clinical manifestations and therapeutic advances," *Drugs*, vol. 68, no. 3, pp. 319–337, 2008.

[9] X.-D. Kong, D. Xu, W. Zhang, Y. Zhao, X. Zeng, and F. Zhang, "Clinical features and prognosis in adult-onset still's disease: A study of 104 cases," *Clinical Rheumatology*, vol. 29, no. 9, pp. 1015–1019, 2010.

[10] T. Zeng, Y.-Q. Zou, M.-F. Wu, and C.-D. Yang, "Clinical features and prognosis of adult-onset still's disease: 61 Cases from China," *Journal of Rheumatology*, vol. 36, no. 5, pp. 1026–1031, 2009.

[11] N. Mahroum, H. Mahagna, and H. Amital, "Diagnosis and classification of adult Still's disease," *Journal of Autoimmunity*, vol. 48-49, pp. 34–37, 2014.

27

Insight into Natural History of Congenital Vitiligo: A Case Report of a 23-Year-Old with Stable Congenital Vitiligo

Chelsea Casey and Stephen E. Weis

Department of Internal Medicine, University of North Texas Health Science Center, Texas College of Osteopathic Medicine, Fort Worth, TX, USA

Correspondence should be addressed to Chelsea Casey; cdc0308@my.unthsc.edu

Academic Editor: Xing-Hua Gao

Vitiligo is a disorder of skin pigmentation. It affects approximately 1% of the world's population. Vitiligo occurs equally between the sexes with no racial predilections. The majority of cases are acquired and arise between the second and third decades of life. Acquired vitiligo has an unpredictable clinical course. Congenital vitiligo is rare with few reported cases. Due to the rarity of congenital vitiligo, little is known about the clinical course. For patients with acquired or congenital vitiligo, the psychosocial burden can have a profound impact on quality of life. The unknown course of congenital vitiligo can exacerbate the feelings of distress and embarrassment. We report of a case of congenital vitiligo that has been stable for 23 years. The patient had no associated autoimmune disease. The pathogenesis of congenital vitiligo is unknown. This case may be useful to assist clinicians caring for newborns with congenital vitiligo in reassuring parents.

1. Introduction

Vitiligo is a benign disorder of skin pigmentation with a clinical presentation of white macules or patches [1]. It affects approximately 1% of the world's population with most cases appearing in the second and third decades of life. Congenital vitiligo is rare with few reported cases. The etiology of vitiligo is unknown. It is believed to be multifactorial with hypotheses regarding genetics, environment, neurogenic, and autoimmune components. Acquired vitiligo has an unpredictable clinical course with subtypes that include nonsegmental, segmental, or mixed vitiligo. Due to the rarity of congenital vitiligo, little is known about its clinical course. In our research, only 6 cases of congenital vitiligo are reported. However, not all case reports comment on the clinical course of the lesions. Although benign, the psychosocial burden can have a profound impact on quality of life for patients with acquired or congenital vitiligo. The lack of knowledge on the clinical course of congenital vitiligo can intensify the feelings of distress. We present a case of a 23-year-old female patient who was found to have three stable vitiligo patches since birth without any spread of existing lesions or occurrence of new lesions.

2. Case

A 23-year-old Caucasian female presented to the dermatology clinic for multiple dermatologic issues. One of her findings was three depigmented patches. According to her history, and confirmed by her mother, she was born with the three skin lesions. The three lesions had never altered in size or pigmentation, were not painful, and had never blistered. She and her mother denied disease progression since birth. Her prior medical history was only significant for eczema and contact dermatitis. There was no personal or family history of autoimmune diseases, skin malignancies, or trauma.

On physical exam, she had an approximately 3 cm depigmented patch with sharply defined borders on her right inferolateral neck with leukotrichia (Figure 1), a 4 cm depigmented patch with sharply defined borders and leukotrichia on the mons pubis (Figure 2), and a perianal 6 cm depigmented patch with sharply defined borders and leukotrichia

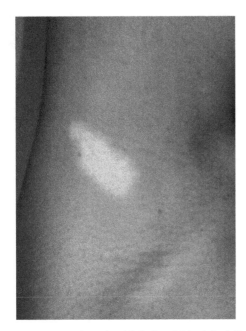

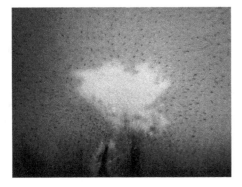

FIGURE 1: Depigmented patch with leukotrichia right inferolateral neck.

FIGURE 2: Depigmented patch with leukotrichia on mons pubis.

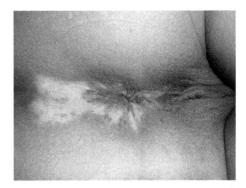

FIGURE 3: Perianal depigmented patch with leukotrichia.

(Figure 3). Considering the clinical history and physical exam findings, the diagnosis of stable congenital vitiligo was given. During the encounter, the patient expressed significant distress, even to the point of being tearful. She was concerned about the inability to obtain a life partner due to her perceived disfigurement. Etiology, clinical course, and treatment were discussed. The patient elected to not seek treatment at the time of presentation as the original three lesions had remained static since birth and she had no new lesions.

3. Discussion

Skin pigmentation occurs by melanocytes that are within the epidermal basal layer. Vitiligo is a skin pigmentation disorder in which the melanocytes are affected. It is traditional in histopathology that vitiligo is characterized by an absence of functioning melanocytes. On developing lesions, an infiltrate of lymphocytes is frequently identified [2]. Clinically, it is manifested by depigmented macules and patches [3].

Although vitiligo has been known for a significant portion of human history, its etiology has remained obscure [4]. Multiple theories have been proposed, which include genetic, environmental, and autoimmune mechanisms. Vitiligo has a 7- to 10-fold increased risk in first-degree relatives. There is high occurrence of comorbid autoimmune diseases such as Hashimoto's disease and Diabetes Mellitus in patients with vitiligo [1]. In 1995, a case of a 31-year-old male with congenital vitiligo who subsequently developed multiple sclerosis is reported [5]. Studies on vitiligo genetics have shown 36 convincing nonsegmental susceptibility loci [4]. Approximately, 10% of genes within or near these loci encode melanocyte proteins. It is theorized that melanocyte proteins might act as autoantigens [6]. Development of vitiligo is believed to be interplay between several factors, including autoantigens and a trigger. Certain triggers, such as oxidative stress or physical trauma, expose antigens and lead to an autoimmune response [7]. It is also postulated that the immune attack may begin in utero in genetically susceptible individuals [6]. There is a single case report of a male child born with congenital vitiligo and his gestation was complicated by his mother acquiring new onset vitiligo [8]. Although a lot has been gleamed from recent advances in vitiligo pathophysiology, the influence of various factors is still poorly understood.

In an attempt to cohesively define nomenclature, clinical progression, outcome, and disease classification, a review was conducted by *Vitiligo Global Issues Consensus Conference [9]*. Vitiligo can be classified as nonsegmental, segmental, or mixed [7]. The subtypes are important for clinical symptoms and etiology [4, 9]. Nonetheless, vitiligo has an unpredictable clinical course. Some lesions remain stable, while others slowly progress, new lesions may appear, or some patients experience flares in between stable periods [10, 11].

Vitiligo can have a significant impact on quality of life due to its psychological aspects [3]. As our patient expressed, individuals often feel a significant burden with low self-esteem due to stigmatization. Our patient with three small, stable lesions that are normally covered with clothing had strong feelings that this would affect her ability to have a normal life. Women and children are often the most impacted by the feelings of embarrassment [12]. Since congenital vitiligo is a rare diagnosis, the inability to provide information on the clinical course further exacerbates the stress of the diagnosis for the patients and their families. Therefore, patients with congenital vitiligo have similar quality of life issues to those with acquired vitiligo.

Of the 6 previously reported cases of congenital vitiligo [6, 11, 13], only one reported the clinical course of vitiligo. The 71-year-old man whose gestation was complicated by his mother acquiring vitiligo had very minimal changes over the course of his life [8]. We report a case of congenital vitiligo that has been stable for 23 years. The patient had no associated autoimmune disease. The pathogenesis of congenital vitiligo is unknown. This case may be useful to assist clinicians caring for newborns with congenital vitiligo in reassuring parents.

Conflicts of Interest

The authors declare that there are no conflicts of interest regarding the publication of this article.

References

[1] T. Kakourou, "Vitiligo in children," *World Journal of Pediatrics*, vol. 5, no. 4, pp. 265–268, 2009.

[2] A. R. Faria, M. T. Mira, R. G. Tarlé, C. C. Silva de Castro, and G. Dellatorre, "Vitiligo—part 2—classification, histopathology and treatment," *Anais Brasileiros de Dermatologia*, vol. 89, no. 5, pp. 784–790, 2014.

[3] P. Manga, N. Elbuluk, and S. J. Orlow, "Recent advances in understanding vitiligo [version 1; referees: 3 approved]," *F1000Research*, vol. 5, article no. 2234, 2016.

[4] R. Czajkowski and K. Męcińska-Jundziłł, "Current aspects of vitiligo genetics," *Dermatology and Allergology*, vol. 31, no. 4, pp. 247–255, 2014.

[5] S. Chandra, A. Kumar, K. K. Singh, and L. Mohan, "Congenital vitiligo," *Indian Journal of Dermatology, Venereology and Leprology*, 1992.

[6] B. N. S. Kambhampati, G. U. Sawatkar, M. S. Kumaran, and D. Parsad, "Congenital vitiligo: a case report," *Journal of Cutaneous Medicine and Surgery*, vol. 20, no. 4, pp. 354-355, 2016.

[7] R. G. Tarlé, L. M. do Nascimento, M. T. Mira, and C. C. S. de Castro, "Vitiligo—Part 1," *Anais Brasileiros de Dermatologia*, vol. 89, no. 3, pp. 461–470, 2014.

[8] A. L. Kedward and D. J. Gawkrodger, "Congenital stable symmetrical type vitiligo in a patient whose mother developed vitiligo during pregnancy," *European Journal of Dermatology*, vol. 18, no. 3, p. 353, 2008.

[9] K. Ezzedine, H. W. Lim, T. Suzuki et al., "Revised classification/nomenclature of vitiligo and related issues: the vitiligo global issues consensus conference," *Pigment Cell and Melanoma Research*, vol. 25, no. 3, pp. E1–E13, 2012.

[10] D. K. Jain, P. Bhargava, K. D. Mathur, U. S. Agarwal, and R. Bhargava, "Congenital familial acral vitiligo," *Indian Journal of Dermatology, Venereology and Leprology*, vol. 63, article 193, 1997.

[11] P. Bhargava, D. K. Mathur, and R. Bhargava, "Congenital leopard vitiligo associated with multiple sclerosis," *Indian Journal of Dermatology, Venereology and Leprology*, vol. 61, no. 6, p. 375, 1995.

[12] D. Parsad, S. Dogra, and A. J. Kanwar, "Quality of life in patients with vitiligo," *Health and Quality of Life Outcomes*, vol. 1, article 58, 2003.

[13] A. B. Lerner and J. J. Nordlund, "Vitiligo: what is it? is it important?" *JAMA: The Journal of the American Medical Association*, vol. 239, no. 12, pp. 1183–1187, 1978.

28

Onychophagia Induced Melanonychia, Splinter Hemorrhages, Leukonychia, and Pterygium Inversum Unguis Concurrently

Sezin Fıçıcıoğlu [iD][1] **and Selma Korkmaz**[2]

[1]*Department of Dermatology, Trakya University Faculty of Medicine, Balkan Yerleskesi, Edirne, Turkey*
[2]*Department of Dermatology, Suleyman Demirel University Faculty of Medicine, Isparta, Turkey*

Correspondence should be addressed to Sezin Fıçıcıoglu; sezinkuru@hotmail.com

Academic Editor: Jacek Cezary Szepietowski

Onychophagia, which refers to compulsive nail-biting behavior, is common among children and young adults. Onychophagia can cause destruction to the cuticle and nail plate, leading to shortening of nails, chronic paronychia, and secondary infections. Relatively uncommon effects include pigmentary changes, such as longitudinal melanonychia and splinter hemorrhages. We report a case of a young adult with longitudinal melanonychia, splinter hemorrhages, punctate leukonychia, and pterygium inversum unguis, concurrently induced by onychophagia. Importantly, patients usually do not report this behavior when asked about nail-related changes. Even upon questioning, they may deny nail-biting behavior. As in many other dermatological disorders, dermoscopy can be helpful in the diagnosis of nail disorders.

1. Introduction

Onychophagia, which refers to compulsive nail-biting behavior, is common among children and young adults. It seems to be related to obsessive-compulsive spectrum disorder and usually cooccurs with psychopathological symptoms [1, 2]. Onychophagia can cause numerous nail changes, including chronic paronychia, longitudinal melanonychia, splinter hemorrhages, nail dystrophy, and partial or total loss of nails [2, 3].

Either melanocytic activation or melanocytic proliferation can be responsible for melanonychia. Melanocytic proliferation is associated with brown-blackish pigmentation, whereas the pigmentation is lighter or even grayish in the presence of melanocytic activation [4]. Melanocytic activation is the most common cause of benign melanonychia in adults. Repeated trauma, periungual tumors, drugs, or systemic diseases can induce melanocytic activation. The activation of melanocytes can also be idiopathic, such as in ethnic-type nail pigmentation, lentigo of the nail apparatus, and Laugier–Hunziker syndrome [3, 5–7].

Splinter hemorrhages are the result of damage to the delicate spiral arteries of the nail bed [8]. The etiology of splinter hemorrhages includes dermatoses (e.g., psoriasis and lichen planus), connective tissue diseases, vasculitis, drugs, particularly kinase inhibitors, infectious diseases, such as acute endocarditis and meningococcemia, and renal failure [4, 8]. In addition, splinter hemorrhages may be idiopathic, as seen in elderly, or they can be caused by various types of trauma, such as playing percussion instruments, housework, sports, and habits/tics.

Leukonychia arising from nail plate abnormalities is called the true form, and it can be longitudinal, transverse, or punctate. In true leukonychia, the discoloration will not disappear when pressure is applied to the nail plate. In contrast, in apparent leukonychia, where the problem is in the nail bed, the discoloration will disappear when pressure is applied [9].

2. Case Report

A 20-year-old male presented with grayish pigmentation on multiple fingernails for a duration of more than two years. He was otherwise healthy, and a physical examination revealed longitudinal hyperpigmented bands of varying widths on the middle parts of his fingernails especially on the right hand.

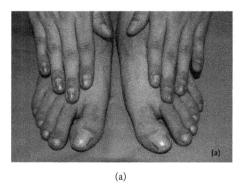
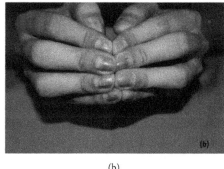

(a)   (b)

FIGURE 1: Whole fingernails and toenails of our patient. Normal toenails except for the second ones which have transverse lamellar splitting (a) and grayish pigmented bands with varying widths and intensities on fingernails, predominantly on right hand; loss of cuticle and erythema of proximal nail folds which can also be seen on both hands (b).

His toenails were normal, except for the second toes of both sides. These showed evidence of transverse lamellar splitting, which was thought to be the result of repeated traumas from ill-fitting footwear. His fingernails also showed punctate leukonychia; small, blackish linear streaks between hyper-pigmented bands; and hyperkeratosis in the hyponychium, which obliterated the distal groove, again predominantly on the right hand (Figure 1, informed consent has been obtained from the patient). In addition, the proximal nail folds of all the fingers were swollen, with erythematous patches, and no cuticles were visible on any of the fingernails. The results of laboratory investigation, including a hemogram (white blood cell count: 7430/μL, normal range: 4230–9070/μL, hemoglobin: 15.7 gr/dl, normal range: 13.7–17.5 gr/dl, and hematocrit: 45.6%, normal range: 40.1–51%), liver, renal, and thyroid function tests, and iron status, were normal. Only vitamin B12 (210 pg/ml, normal range: 211–911 pg/ml) and folic acid (4.29 ng/mL, normal range: 5.38–24 ng/mL) levels were slightly decreased. Immunological studies for antinuclear antibodies were negative. Chest and wrist radiography for the investigation of sarcoidosis were normal. There was no known history of psoriasis or lichen planus and dermatological examination did not reveal any suspicious lesion for them. In addition, a mycological examination with potassium hydroxide smear and a fungal culture was negative. There was no remarkable medical history or contact history of detergents or special chemicals. Family history for similar nail findings or connective tissue diseases was also negative. A dermoscopic examination revealed faintly pigmented longitudinal bands on the middle parts of the patient's fingernails with various intensities, being predominant on the right side. The pigmentation did not extend into the proximal nail fold. The leukonychia did not disappear during the examination when pressure was applied to the nail plates, and they were laid out on the pigmented bands. The blackish linear streaks observed earlier in the physical examination were splinter hemorrhages. In addition, the dermoscopic examination clearly revealed hyperkeratosis in the hyponychium and adherence of the nail bed to the nail plate, raising the suspicion of pterygium inversum unguis (Figure 2). However, it was difficult to identify subungual

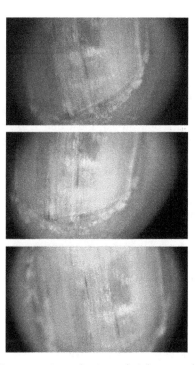

FIGURE 2: Dermoscopic evaluation of right second nail yields longitudinal gray regular lines on a grayish background, splinter hemorrhages as blackish linear streaks, and true leukonychia as it did not disappear with pressure and hyperkeratosis in hyponychium.

extension of the hyponychium because the patient's nails were short. Upon questioning about pain while clipping his nails related to the hyponychium hyperkeratosis, the patient admitted that he had been biting his nails for nearly 4 years, becoming more intense in the last two years.

3. Discussion

The repeated trauma in onychophagia induces melanocytic activation and leads to melanonychia which extends by longitudinal spreading from the nail bed to the distal end of the nail plate. This longitudinal melanonychia is grayish in color, with regular gray parallel lines on a gray background [3, 6]. Onychophagia-induced melanonychia can accompany other trauma-induced nail changes, such as distal nail plate splitting, onychoschizia, and nail plate hypertrophy [3]. Our case had grayish longitudinal parallel lines on nearly all nail plates and they were accompanied with chronic paronychia and onychoschizia.

Splinter hemorrhages in our case were mostly black and located distally so we thought that they were related to onychophagia. This is because when they are traumatic, they are mostly black and located distally, whereas they are red and proximal in the presence of systemic diseases [8].

Multiple punctate leukonychia seen in our case was true leukonychia as it did not disappear upon pressure. True leukonychia can be seen in inherited syndromes, alopecia areata and proximal subungual onychomycosis, or acquired as a result of severe illness or chemotherapeutic exposure [9]. It can also be idiopathic. Trauma can cause true leukonychia [2, 9]. In the present case, we attributed the punctate leukonychia to onychophagia, as they were mostly visible on the pigmented middle parts, where trauma can affect the nail plate.

Pterygium inversum unguis is an infrequent disorder, where an exaggerated stratum corneum in the distal nail bed or hyponychium leads to obliteration of the distal groove. It can be congenital or acquired, and acquired forms have been reported frequently in connective tissue diseases, such as systemic sclerosis [10]. We propose that pterygium inversum unguis may also be associated with reactive hyperkeratosis and an inflammatory reaction to repeated trauma, as described in the present case.

In conclusion, in the present case, all the nail changes were attributed to onychophagia as the shared etiology was trauma. In the literature, we found no case reports of longitudinal melanonychia, splinter hemorrhages, punctate leukonychia, and pterygium inversum unguis appearing concurrently with onychophagia. In the present case, the multiple nail changes may have been due to the severe nature of the trauma and the long duration of onychophagia in a young adult. It is important to question patients specifically about nail-biting or picking behaviors when evaluating nail disorders, as they may not readily admit such behaviors unless questioned. The present case also illustrates the importance of dermoscopes, which are becoming indispensable for dermatologists, in diagnosing diseases in all kinds of patient populations.

Conflicts of Interest

The authors declare that there are no conflicts of interest regarding the publication of this article.

References

[1] P. Pacan, M. Grzesiak, A. Reich, and J. C. Szepietowski, "Onychophagia as a spectrum of obsessive-compulsive disorder," *Acta Dermato-Venereologica*, vol. 89, no. 3, pp. 278–280, 2009.

[2] B. Richert and J. André, "Nail disorders in children: Diagnosis and management," *American Journal of Clinical Dermatology*, vol. 12, no. 2, pp. 101–112, 2011.

[3] H. Jin, J.-M. Kim, G.-W. Kim et al., "Diagnostic criteria for and clinical review of melanonychia in Korean patients," *Journal of the American Academy of Dermatology*, vol. 74, no. 6, pp. 1121–1127, 2016.

[4] A. Lencastre, A. Lamas, D. Sá, and A. Tosti, "Onychoscopy," *Clinics in Dermatology*, vol. 31, no. 5, pp. 587–593, 2013.

[5] H. A. Haenssle, A. Blum, R. Hofmann-Wellenhof et al., "When all you have is a dermatoscope- start looking at the nails," *Dermatology Practical & Conceptual*, vol. 4, no. 4, pp. 11–20, 2014.

[6] R. B. Anolik, K. Shah, and A. I. Rubin, "Onychophagia-induced longitudinal melanonychia," *Pediatric Dermatology*, vol. 29, no. 4, pp. 488-489, 2012.

[7] E. Dowlati, J. Dovico, and B. Unwin, "Skin hyperpigmentation and melanonychia from chronic doxycycline use," *Annals of Pharmacotherapy*, vol. 49, no. 10, pp. 1175-1176, 2015.

[8] R. Haber, R. Khoury, E. Kechichian, and R. Tomb, "Splinter hemorrhages of the nails: a systematic review of clinical features and associated conditions," *International Journal of Dermatology*, vol. 55, no. 12, pp. 1304–1310, 2016.

[9] T. Canavan, A. Tosti, H. Mallory, K. McKay, W. Cantrell, and B. Elewski, "An Idiopathic Leukonychia Totalis and Leukonychia Partialis Case Report and Review of the Literature," *Skin Appendage Disorders*, vol. 1, no. 1, pp. 38–42, 2015.

[10] N. Zaias, S. X. Escovar, M. N. Zaiac et al., "Hyponychium Abnormalities congenital aberrant hyponychium vs. Acquired pterygium inversum unguis vs. Acquired reversible extended hyponychium: A proposed classification based on origin, pathology and outcome," *Journal of the European Academy of Dermatology and Venereology*, vol. 29, no. 7, pp. 1427–1431, 2015.

29

Successful Treatment of Actinic Keratosis with Kanuka Honey

Saras Mane ⓘ,[1] **Joseph Singer,**[1] **Andrew Corin,**[2] and **Alex Semprini** ⓘ[1,3]

[1]*Medical Research Institute of New Zealand, Wellington, New Zealand*
[2]*Clinical Horizons New Zealand, Tauranga, New Zealand*
[3]*Victoria University of Wellington, Wellington, New Zealand*

Correspondence should be addressed to Saras Mane; smane656@gmail.com

Academic Editor: Alireza Firooz

Actinic keratoses form as rough, scaly plaques on sun-exposed areas; they can be an important step in premalignant progression to squamous cell cancer of the skin. Currently, pharmacological treatments consist of topical immunomodulatory agents with poor side effect profiles. Use of honey has been common in both ancient and modern medicine, where it is now a key therapy in the management of wound healing. In vitro studies show the New Zealand native Kanuka honey to have immunomodulatory and antimitotic effects, with recent evidence suggesting efficacy of topical application in a variety of dermatological contexts, including rosacea and psoriasis. Here, we present a case report of a 66-year-old gentleman with an actinic keratosis on his hand, which had been present for years. Regular application of Kanuka honey over three months resulted in remission immediately following the treatment period with no signs of recurrence at nine months.

1. Introduction

Actinic keratoses (AK) are common skin lesions that form as rough, scaly plaques of slow growing epidermal keratinocyte dysplasia. They present largely in the elderly as a result of chronic and cumulative sun exposure. Aside from their unappealing cosmetic appearance and irksome tendency to catch on clothing, they can be an important early step in premalignant progression towards squamous cell carcinoma (SCC). As most SCCs arise from AK, it is important that they be recognised and treated early [1].

AK are principally found in sun-exposed areas such as the shoulders, face, hands, ears, and scalp. Incidence varies globally, with 40–50% of Caucasian Australians developing an AK by the age of 40, and around 10% of Caucasian Europeans are reported to be affected [2].

Current treatments tend to favour surgical removal for single lesions or topical immunomodulatory agents such as 5-fluorouracil or imiquimod for those that are contiguous or diffuse [2]. Efficacy of these topical regimes is good when adhered to; however, there are often unpleasant adverse effects including contact dermatitis, burning, or irritation and even systemic flu-like symptoms, which, combined with long duration of treatment, lead to poor compliance. Furthermore, there is no official consensus with regard to guidelines of management, and most guidelines currently published lack a strong evidence base [3].

Use of Manuka and other honeys in the management of wound healing is well established, and recent literature reveals that honey possesses, in addition to antimicrobial action, complex anti-inflammatory and immunomodulatory properties [4]. Subsequently, honey is emerging as an efficacious treatment of other dermatological conditions.

Here, we present a case of resolution of AK by regular topical application of the New Zealand native Kanuka honey.

2. Case Report

A 66-year-old Caucasian gentleman presented to his GP with a singular, raised, crusted, scaly lesion of 21×20 mm size with marginal erythema on the dorsum of his left hand (Figure 1). He reported that the lesion was present for several years but had noted recent growth.

Medical history included AK, basal cell carcinoma (BCC), and seborrheic keratoses in various distributions over recent years, putting him at a higher risk of keratinocyte

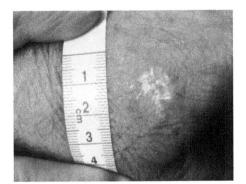

FIGURE 1: Actinic keratosis on the hand prior to honey treatment.

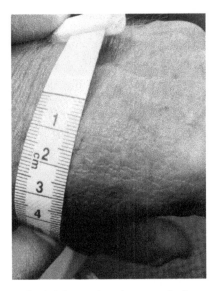

FIGURE 2: Site of actinic keratosis at three months (immediately after honey treatment).

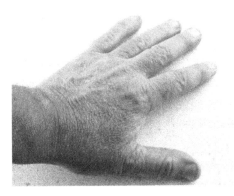

FIGURE 3: Hand at two years after treatment, showing normal skin and no signs of recurrence.

carcinoma [5]. The lesion was diagnosed in the primary care setting as an AK, though possibility of BCC and SCC was considered.

The previous BCC had been managed successfully with six weeks of topical imiquimod treatment. Procedural removal of the AK was offered to the patient, but he expressed interest in trying a different approach. The patient was contemporaneously enrolled in a clinical trial examining the use of Kanuka honey on rosacea [6] and decided to try using the Kanuka honey topically on his AK.

Honevo® medical grade Kanuka honey (90% Kanuka honey, 10% glycerin) was topically applied once daily using a small amount on the fingertip rubbed into the lesion and surrounding 5 mm of normal skin for 10–30 seconds. It was left on for 30–60 minutes and then washed off with water. This was done consecutively for five days, after which the patient took a treatment break of two days due to lesion tenderness. During the break, the lesion was gently picked at, thereby debriding it. This process was repeated for a total of three months; there were no other treatments used prior to or during this regimen and there were no adverse reactions. The lesion gradually reduced in size with an initial rapid reduction in its dry, crusted nature.

After three months, residual appearance of the lesion was a 20 mm by 17 mm area of pink skin with no elements of hypertrophy, crusting, or loss of skin integrity (Figure 2). At six months, there were no signs of recurrence. At nine months, the appearance of the skin had fully returned to normal. A telephone follow-up was conducted at two years after treatment, and the patient reported that his skin in the area was still completely normal and that there were no signs of recurrence. A photograph was taken at this time (Figure 3).

3. Discussion

This case is noteworthy, as, with topical application of Kanuka honey, there was remission of a growing AK within three months and skin returned to normal within nine months. A limitation of our case is that we were not able to obtain biopsies of the lesion. The AK was diagnosed and treated in primary care, where it is not usual for AKs to be biopsied, and the decision to write up the case was made after the course of treatment had finished.

The use of honey to treat AK has not yet been documented; a MEDLINE/PubMed and google scholar search for "honey" AND "actinic keratosis" OR "solar keratosis" (October 2017) did not find any similar cases in the literature. Although spontaneous resolution of AK is seen in its natural history, the mean time for this is 17 months, with a 15% recurrence rate [7]. This suggests that the properties of Kanuka honey may aid and expedite clearance of AK.

The use of honey has been common in both ancient and modern medicine; it is now well established in wound management, where its antimicrobial properties have been shown to inhibit pathogen growth and facilitate healing [8]. In vitro studies show that honeys exert complex anti-inflammatory and immunomodulatory effects, including stimulation and inhibition of various cytokines from granulocytes, as well as the modulation of production of reactive oxygen species from neutrophils [4].

The immunomodulatory properties of Kanuka honey in particular are thought to be more potent than other New Zealand honeys due to the relatively high concentrations of arabinogalactan proteins present [9]. These proteins have been shown to stimulate release of TNF-α from monocytic cell lines in vitro. Immunomodulatory topical agents are already widely used in the treatment of AK as an immune component is evident in its aetiology; immunocompromised patients have 250 times the risk of developing an AK than the general population [2].

In vitro studies are also starting to reveal the significant antimitotic and antiproliferative action of honey on cancer cell lines, including those of breast cancer and colorectal cancer lineages [10]. With relevance to skin cancer, Tualang honey has been shown to decrease proliferation and induce apoptosis of squamous cancer cell lines [11]. Acacia honey has also been shown to pause cell cycle progression of melanoma cell lines in a time- and dose-dependent manner. This is thought to be due to the presence of chrysin, an established antitumour agent, in the honey [12].

Due to its readily topical nature, honey has the potential to be used in a variety of dermatological contexts. A recent pilot randomised control trial demonstrated that topical Kanuka honey decreases objective morbidity of psoriasis lesions compared to traditional aqueous cream, a currently recommended topical agent [13]. Braithwaite et al. conducted a larger, randomised, blinded trial of 138 patients with rosacea (an inflammatory, chronic condition affecting the face), examining the use of topical Kanuka honey. They found that Kanuka was well tolerated and effective in significantly reducing rosacea severity as assessed by a blinded clinical examination [6]. Other reports show success with use of honey in dermatitis and pityriasis [14]. Subsequently, a large trial is now underway, comparing the use of topical aciclovir to Kanuka honey for treatment of active cold sores [15].

In conclusion, when determining treatment of choice for AK, type of lesion, patient preference, price, and availability and tolerance for adverse effects all need to be taken into consideration. Current pharmacological treatments can be effective; however, they often come with undesired side effects including contact dermatitis, burning, or irritation and even systemic flu-like symptoms. The New Zealand native Kanuka honey has been shown to have immunomodulatory and anti-inflammatory effects in vitro and is emerging as a viable and well-tolerated treatment for dermatological lesions. There is, however, a notable paucity of blinded randomised controlled trials regarding honey's use on premalignant dermatological lesions. We hope that case reports such as ours engender further study into this area.

Consent

Full, informed, written consent for publication was obtained from the patient.

Conflicts of Interest

Saras Mane declares no conflicts of interest. Joseph Singer, Andrew Corin, and Alex Semprini declare that they have previously received funding from HoneyLab NZ.

Authors' Contributions

Saras Mane and Joseph Singer contributed equally to the writing of this manuscript. Andrew Corin was the general practitioner who oversaw the care of the patient involved. Alex Semprini reviewed and edited the manuscript.

Acknowledgments

The authors would like to acknowledge the Medical Research Institute of New Zealand for facilitating this work. They would also like to thank Professor Richard Beasley and Dr. Doñah Sabbagh for reviewing the manuscript.

References

[1] E. Stockfleth, K. Peris, C. Guillen et al., "A consensus approach to improving patient adherence and persistence with topical treatment for actinic keratosis," *International Journal of Dermatology*, vol. 54, no. 5, pp. 509–515, 2015.

[2] C. Costa, M. Scalvenzi, F. Ayala, G. Fabbrocini, and G. Monfrecola, "How to treat actinic keratosis? An update," *Journal of Dermatological Case Reports*, vol. 9, no. 2, pp. 29–35, 2015.

[3] J. S. Kirby, T. Scharnitz, E. V. Seiverling, H. Ahrns, and S. Ferguson, "Actinic Keratosis Clinical Practice Guidelines: An Appraisal of Quality," *Dermatology Research and Practice*, vol. 2015, Article ID 456071, 2015.

[4] J. Majtan, "Honey: An immunomodulator in wound healing," *Wound Repair and Regeneration*, vol. 22, no. 2, pp. 187–192, 2014.

[5] J. V. Schmitt and H. A. Miot, "Actinic keratosis: A clinical and epidemiological revision," *Anais Brasileiros de Dermatologia*, vol. 87, no. 3, pp. 425–434, 2012.

[6] I. Braithwaite, A. Hunt, J. Riley et al., "Randomised controlled trial of topical kanuka honey for the treatment of rosacea," *BMJ Open*, vol. 5, no. 6, Article ID e007651, 2015.

[7] R. N. Werner, A. Sammain, R. Erdmann, V. Hartmann, E. Stockfleth, and A. Nast, "The natural history of actinic keratosis: a systematic review," *British Journal of Dermatology*, vol. 169, no. 3, pp. 502–518, 2013.

[8] D. A. Carter, S. E. Blair, N. N. Cokcetin et al., "Therapeutic Manuka Honey: No Longer So Alternative," *Frontiers in Microbiology*, vol. 7, 2016.

[9] S. Gannabathula, M. A. Skinner, D. Rosendale et al., "Arabinogalactan proteins contribute to the immunostimulatory properties of New Zealand honeys," *Immunopharmacology and Immunotoxicology*, vol. 34, no. 4, pp. 598–607, 2012.

[10] O. O. Erejuwa, S. A. Sulaiman, and M. S. Ab Wahab, "Effects of honey and its mechanisms of action on the development and progression of cancer," *Molecules*, vol. 19, no. 2, pp. 2497–2522, 2014.

[11] A. A. Ghashm, N. H. Othman, M. N. Khattak, N. M. Ismail, and R. Saini, "Antiproliferative effect of Tualang honey on oral squamous cell carcinoma and osteosarcoma cell lines," *BMC Complementary and Alternative Medicine*, vol. 10, article 49, 2010.

[12] E. Pichichero, R. Cicconi, M. Mattei, M. G. Muzi, and A. Canini, "Acacia honey and chrysin reduce proliferation of melanoma cells through alterations in cell cycle progression," *International Journal of Oncology*, vol. 37, no. 4, pp. 973–981, 2010.

30

A Severe Case of Lymphomatoid Papulosis Type E Successfully Treated with Interferon-Alfa 2a

Aslı Bilgiç Temel,[1] Betül Unal,[2] Hatice Erdi Şanlı,[3] Şeniz Duygulu,[4] and Soner Uzun[1]

[1]Dermatology and Venereology Department, Akdeniz University Faculty of Medicine, Antalya, Turkey
[2]Pathology Department, Akdeniz University Faculty of Medicine, Antalya, Turkey
[3]Dermatology and Venereology Department, Ankara University Faculty of Medicine, Ankara, Turkey
[4]Dermatology and Venereology Department, Pamukkale University Faculty of Medicine, Denizli, Turkey

Correspondence should be addressed to Soner Uzun; sonuzun@hotmail.com

Academic Editor: Henry Wong

Lymphomatoid papulosis (LyP) is a benign papulonodular skin eruption with histologic features of malignant lymphoma. A new variant of LyP which was termed "type E" was recently described with similar clinical and histological features to angiocentric and angiodestructive T-cell lymphoma. LyP type E is characterized with recurrent papulonodular lesions which rapidly turn into hemorrhagic necrotic ulcers and spontaneous regression by leaving a scar. None of the available treatment modalities affects the natural course of LyP. For therapy various modalities have been used such as topical and systemic steroids, PUVA, methotrexate, bexarotene, and IFN alfa-2b. Here we present a severe and devastating case with a very rare variant of LyP type E, which is, to our knowledge, the first case successfully treated with IFN alfa-2a. Now disease has been maintaining its remission status for six months.

1. Introduction

Lymphomatoid papulosis (LyP) is a benign papulonodular skin eruption with histologic features of malignant lymphoma. It has been listed as a primary, cutaneous, CD30 (+) lymphoproliferative disorder in the current World Health Organization (WHO) and European Organization for Research and Treatment of Cancer (EORTC) classification [1]. Histopathologically, there are well-known 4 LyP types (type A-wedge-shaped infiltrate containing eosinophils and histiocytes, type B-epidermotropism, resembling mycosis fungoides, type C-cohesive sheets of CD30 (+) cells, resembling anaplastic large cell lymphoma, and type D-CD8 (+), resembling primary cutaneous aggressive epidermotropic CD8 (+) cytotoxic T-cell lymphoma) [2]. A new variant of LyP which was termed "type E" by Kempf et al. was recently described with similar clinical and histological features to angiocentric and angiodestructive T-cell lymphoma [3].

Here we present a severe and devastating case with a very rare variant of LyP type E, which is, to our knowledge, the first case successfully treated with IFN alfa-2a.

2. Case Report

A 18-year-old female presented to the outpatient clinic of dermatology with a 15-year history of waxing and waning course of erythematous papules, plaques, hemorrhagic ulcerations, and atrophic scars (Figures 1(a), 1(b), 1(c), and 1(d)). The lesions mostly started as painful erythematous papules and nodules on any site of the body following some constitutional symptoms such as fever and weakness. These lesions then quickly progressed to hemorrhagic deep ulcers resolving with depressed scar tissue either spontaneously or with nonspecific antibiotic therapies between 3 to 4 weeks. For the last 6-month duration, lesions appeared more frequently. She had no family history of similar lesions or other systemic diseases. On physical examination, there were multiple painful ulcers with necrotic base in different sizes scattered all over the body and numerous round atrophic scars (more than one hundred). She has no constitutional symptoms and palpable lymphadenopathy. The skin biopsy revealed regular acanthotic epidermis, a dense dermal infiltrate of pleomorphic atypical lymphoid cells, and

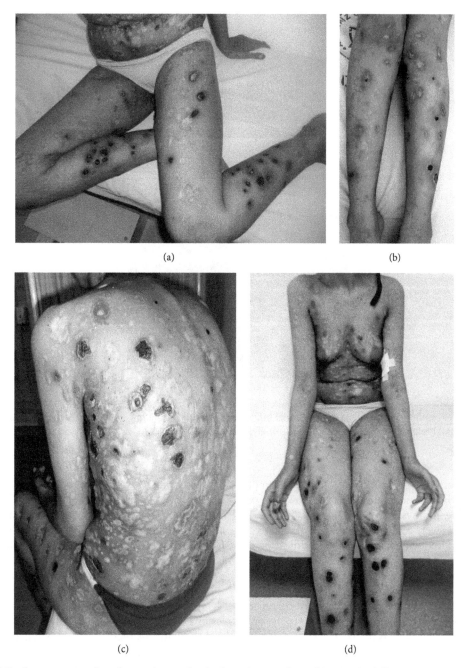

FIGURE 1: (a, b, c, d) Erythematous papules, plaques, hemorrhagic ulcerations, and atrophic scars in different sizes scattered all over the body.

destruction of the blood vessels' walls by abnormal lymphocytes (Figures 2(a) and 2(b)). Biopsy revealed abnormal lymphocytes which were predominantly positive for CD30 (Figure 2(c)) and mostly CD8+ lymphoid cells, especially angiocentric infiltrates. When we closely look at the entire infiltrate, which is both angiocentric and interstitial, an overall predominance of CD8+ cells over CD4+ cells was seen. CD20, CD56, and CD21 were negative. Perforin was negative and granzyme was focal positive. In situ hybridization for Epstein-Barr virus encoded RNA and Latent Membrane Protein 1 (LMP1) was negative. T-cell receptor (TCR) gene rearrangement could not be performed. Based on the clinical history, physical examination, and histological findings, diagnosis of LyP type E was established.

Hematologic laboratory and routine biochemistry workup showed no sign for systemic malignancy nor other systemic diseases. Chest/abdomen/pelvis computed tomography revealed irregular hyperdense areas on skin and subcutaneous tissue and multiple small (<1 cm) lymphadenopathies but neither hepatosplenomegaly nor other abnormalities were seen. On PET examination abdominal, axillary, inguinal, and cervical small hypermetabolic lymph

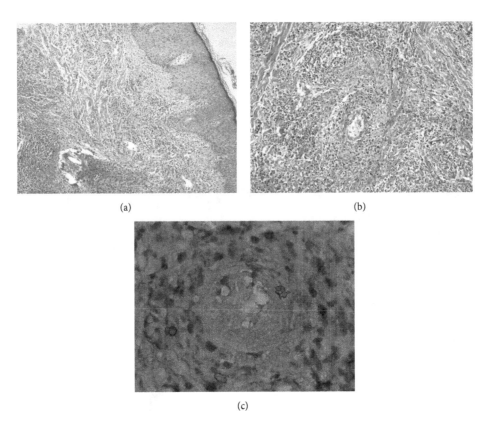

(a)   (b)

(c)

FIGURE 2: (a, b) Regular acanthotic epidermis, a dense dermal infiltrate of pleomorphic atypical lymphoid cells, and destruction of the blood vessels' walls by abnormal lymphocytes. (c) The cells were strongly positive for CD30.

nodes have been detected. Histopathological examination of a posterior cervical lymph node and bone marrow biopsy yielded unremarkable findings.

As the patient has severe course with multiple devastating ulcerative lesions and frequent recurrences, we administered methotrexate with a dose of 15 mg per week. During 3-month follow-up, we observed a relative decrease in the appearance of new lesions. The dose of methotrexate was increased to 20 mg per week. After one month she had a severe recurrence of the disease while on treatment, and the dose was increased to 35 mg per week. However, the liver enzymes were elevated with this approach. The dose of methotrexate had to be discontinued. She was given IFN alfa-2a with a dose of 6 mU three times per week. After two-month treatment with IFN alfa-2a, she was finally feeling well and there were no new lesions and all previous persistent lesions were healed completely (Figures 3(a), 3(b), and 3(c)). A slight leucopenia was observed. Since clinical remission was achieved, the treatment schedule was switched to 6 mU IFN alfa-2a 2 times per week. For the time being the disease has been maintaining its remission status for six months.

3. Discussion

Clinical presentation of LyP is characterized by chronic recurrent, self-healing papulonodules which regress with scar formation. The duration of LyP is variable. It affects especially adults and usually persists with a range from several weeks

to years with an excellent prognosis [4]. However, approximately 10% to 20% of patients with LyP may present with a lymphoproliferative malignancy such as CD30 anaplastic large cell lymphoma (ALCL), mycosis fungoides (MF), or Hodgkin disease [5, 6]. Thus, careful lifelong monitoring is required which allows early detection and treatment of potentially fatal lymphomas especially in children with LyP [7].

LyP type E is characterized with recurrent papulonodular lesions which rapidly turn into hemorrhagic necrotic ulcers and spontaneous regression by leaving a scar [2]. Up to date 18 cases were reported in the literature [3]. All of them had severe clinical features, with a typical progressive course. During follow-up, they all experienced several relapses like current patient [3].

None of the available treatment modalities affects the natural course of LyP. In most cases aggressive treatment is not required because of its favorable prognosis. Treatment can be considered in severe forms of LyP in which the size and number of lesions are extensive or when ulceration, scarring, and pruritus are prominent [4, 8]. For therapy various modalities have been used such as topical and systemic steroids, PUVA, methotrexate, bexarotene, and IFN alfa-2b. Low-dose methotrexate (5 to 25 mg weekly) is the most commonly reported single agent chemotherapy used to treat LyP. According to the results of retrospective analyses, it effectively suppresses the development of new lesions. However, the rapid relapse rate of 63% following methotrexate

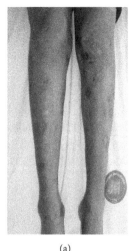
(a)

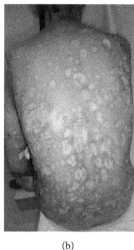
(b)

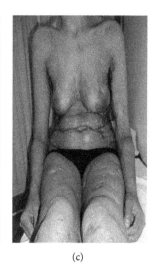
(c)

FIGURE 3: (a, b, c) All previous persistent lesions were healed completely and no new lesions were observed after two-month treatment with IFN alfa-2a.

cessation often necessitates long-term maintenance therapy [4, 9]. Methotrexate was the first-line therapy in our case. However, although it initially suppressed the disease and provided a partial improvement in the clinical picture, it had to be discontinued because of the adverse effects to the liver.

LyP has been observed to progress into anaplastic large cell (CD30+) lymphoma, mycosis fungoides, and Hodgkin or non-Hodgkin lymphoma [8]. IFN alfa has been used successfully in these disorders which is thought to be due to effects on malignant clones [10]. In addition, Yagi et al. have examined the therapeutic efficacy of recombinant IFN-y in two patients with LyP [11]. They suggested that despite being speculative the mechanism of inhibition of CD30+ cell proliferation by IFN-y might involve two actions. First, IFN-y directly downregulates the transcription of cytokine mRNA by CD30+ cells which leads to inhibition of proliferation of these cells. In indirect action, IFN-y enhances mRNA transcription in inflammatory Th1 cells, which might exert antitumor cell activity after activation [11]. In an open trial, researchers compared the clinical, histologic, and immuno-histochemically features from a group of five patients receiving IFN subcutaneously three times per week with the same features from a group of six patients receiving conventional therapy, including photochemotherapy, antibiotics, topical corticosteroids, or surgery [12]. In the IFN group, four patients showed a complete remission, whereas one patient showed a partial remission within 6 weeks. These results indicate that the treatment with IFN of patients with LyP alters the clinical course of the disease with fewer side effects than previous regimens; however, short-term treatment does not induce sustainable remission. Therefore, prolonged treatment appears to be warranted for the long-term remissions in these patients [12]. Because of these reports about the value of interferon in the treatment of cutaneous lymphomas, and in some LyP cases, we decided to use IFN alfa-2a with a dose of 6 mU three times per week subcutaneously [8, 11–13].

In conclusion, we report a very severe case with recently described and rare type E variant of LyP. To our knowledge, this is first case of LyP type E successfully treated with IFN alfa-2a. Even though we think current case may provide some contribution, further knowledge and experiences are needed for morphological features and treatment of this new variant of LyP.

Conflicts of Interest

The authors declare that they have no conflicts of interest.

References

[1] R. Willemze, E. S. Jaffe, G. Burg et al., "WHO-EORTC classification for cutaneous lymphomas," *Blood*, vol. 105, no. 10, pp. 3768–3785, 2005.

[2] W. Kempf, "CD30+ lymphoproliferative disorders: histopathology, differential diagnosis, new variants, and simulators," *Journal of Cutaneous Pathology*, vol. 33, 1, pp. 58–70, 2006.

[3] W. Kempf, D. V. Kazakov, L. Scharer et al., "Angioinvasive lymphomatoid papulosis: a new variant simulating aggressive lymphomas," *The American Journal of Surgical Pathology*, vol. 37, pp. 1–13, 2013.

[4] M. W. Bekkenk, F. A. Geelen, P. C. van Voorst Vader et al., "Primary and secondary cutaneous CD30$^{(+)}$ lymphoproliferative disorders: a report from the Dutch Cutaneous Lymphoma Group on the long-term follow-up data of 219 patients and guidelines for diagnosis and treatment," *Blood*, vol. 95, no. 12, pp. 3653–3661, 2000.

[5] M. E. Kadin, "lymphomatoid papulosis and associated lymphomas: how are they related?" *Archives of Dermatology*, vol. 129, no. 3, pp. 351–353, 1993.

[6] M.-F. Demierre, L. J. Goldberg, M. E. Kadin, and H. K. Koh, "Is it lymphoma or lymphomatoid papulosis?" *Journal of the American Academy of Dermatology*, vol. 36, no. 5 I, pp. 765–772, 1997.

[7] T. Nijsten, C. Curiel-Lewandrowski, and M. E. Kadin, "lymphomatoid papulosis in children: a retrospective cohort study of 35 cases," *Archives of Dermatology*, vol. 140, no. 3, pp. 306–312, 2004.

[8] R. C. Beljaards and R. Willemze, "The prognosis of patients with lymphomatoid papulosis associated with malignant lymphomas," *British Journal of Dermatology*, vol. 126, no. 6, pp. 596–602, 1992.

[9] W. Kempf, K. Pfaltz, M. H. Vermeer et al., "EORTC, ISCL, and USCLC consensus recommendations for the treatment of primary cutaneous CD30-positive lymphoproliferative disorders: lymphomatoid papulosis and primary cutaneous anaplastic large-cell lymphoma," *Blood*, vol. 118, no. 15, pp. 4024–4035, 2011.

[10] M. Duvic, N. A. Lemak, J. R. Redman et al., "Combined modality therapy for cutaneous T-cell lymphoma," *Journal of the American Academy of Dermatology*, vol. 34, no. 6, pp. 1022–1029, 1996.

[11] H. Yagi, Y. Tokura, F. Furukawa, and M. Takigawa, "Th2 cytokine mRNA expression in primary cutaneous CD30-positive lymphoproliferative disorders: successful treatment with recombinant interferon-γ," *Journal of Investigative Dermatology*, vol. 107, no. 6, pp. 827–832, 1996.

[12] M. Schmuth, G. Topar, B. Illersperger, E. Kowald, P. O. Fritsch, and N. T. Sepp, "Therapeutic use of interferon-α for lymphomatoid papulosis," *Cancer*, vol. 89, no. 7, pp. 1603–1610, 2000.

[13] S. J. Proctor, G. H. Jackson, A. L. Lennard, and J. Marks, "Lymphomatoid papulosis: response to treatment with recombinant interferon alfa-2b," *Journal of Clinical Oncology*, vol. 10, no. 1, p. 170, 1992.

31

Two Cases of Delayed Diagnosis of Leprosy in Mauritania

Boushab Mohamed Boushab ⓘ,[1] Fatima-Zahra Fall-Malick,[2] and Leonardo K. Basco[3]

[1]*Department of Internal Medicine and Infectious Diseases, Kiffa Regional Hospital, Assaba, Mauritania*
[2]*National Institute of Hepatitis and Virology, School of Medicine, Nouakchott, Mauritania*
[3]*Aix Marseille Univ, IRD, AP-HM, SSA, VITROME, IHU-Méditerranée Infection, Marseille, France*

Correspondence should be addressed to Boushab Mohamed Boushab; bboushab@gmail.com

Academic Editor: Sergio A. Cuevas-Covarrubias

Leprosy is a chronic infectious disease that mainly affects the skin, mucous membranes, and peripheral nervous system. The clinical manifestations of leprosy are numerous and polymorphic with the most frequent signs involving skin and neurological damage. Some of its manifestations, such as joint pain, are unusual. Its elimination as a public health problem in many countries seems to lead to a lack of practical knowledge among health care personnel and as a consequence a risk of late diagnosis. As in other countries, leprosy has become rare in Mauritania. We report two cases of misdiagnosed leprosy in two male patients aged 17 and 65 years. Clinical manifestations included polyarthritis, bilateral plantar perforation, and severely deformed hands and feet in the first case and lichenoid lesions, hypopigmented papules, and unilateral bronchial rales in the second case. The duration of development and persistence of clinical signs before establishment of correct diagnosis was seven to ten years despite the presence of anesthetic, hypochromic maculopapular skin lesions and neurologic signs suggestive of leprosy in both cases. A multilevel chemotherapeutic regimen recommended by the World Health Organization (WHO) was effective, and the patients' condition evolved satisfactorily. The scarcity of leprosy in our health care facilities often leads to a wrong diagnosis. It is imperative to inform physicians to increase their vigilance for appropriate screening and reporting of these cases. The prognosis depends largely on early diagnosis and appropriate treatment.

1. Introduction

Leprosy, or Hansen's disease, is a chronic infectious disease caused by the bacillus *Mycobacterium leprae*, which mainly affects the skin, mucous membranes, and peripheral nervous system [1]. Transmitted by droplets of buccal or nasal origin during close and frequent contact with an infected and untreated subject [2], this disease may manifest itself as a result of motor sequelae in relation to neurological or mutilating bone damage and visceral dissemination that can be life threatening [3]. Although leprosy still occurs with a relatively high prevalence in some countries in Asia and South America [1], leprosy has become a rare disease in Mauritania. We report here two cases of late diagnosis of leprosy despite the persistence of pathognomonic signs.

2. Case Report 1

A 17-year-old farmer residing in Kankossa (Kankossa/Assaba region), Mauritania, spontaneously presented for consultation at Kiffa Regional Hospital on December 2, 2016, for severe chronic arthralgia affecting joints of the hands associated with bilateral perforating plantar ulcer. The patient's clinical history showed that the cutaneous and neurological signs had evolved for 7 years, which initially presented with hypopigmented maculopapular lesions and paresthesia at the interphalangeal extremities and on the plantar surfaces of the feet. Prior to consultation in our hospital, the patient had seen several dermatologists and traditional healers over the past 7 years. None of these practitioners considered leprosy for differential diagnosis, and the prescribed analgesic, antibiotic,

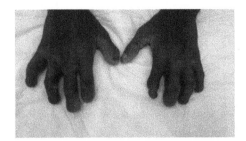

FIGURE 1: Bilateral atrophied hands with hypopigmented and hypoesthesic lesions in interdigital spaces.

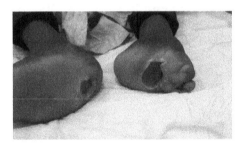

FIGURE 2: Bilateral neuropathic plantar ulcer.

and topical treatments had not improved the patient's condition.

Physical examination revealed anesthetic distal phalangeal atrophy associated with severe deformity of the hands, hypochromic, anesthetic macular lesions (Figure 1), atrophy of the metatarsals and phalanges with severe deformity of the feet, and bilateral plantar perforations (Figure 2). Hypertrophied nerve trunks were palpable at the ulnar and popliteal level. Visual examination was normal. Clinical diagnosis of lepromatous leprosy was established on the basis of 2 of 3 criteria set by the World Health Organization (WHO) [1]: hypochromic anesthetic skin lesions and palpable peripheral nerves. The third criterion, bacteriological examination of skin smears and/or skin biopsy of infiltrated lesions, was not sought to demonstrate the presence of *M. leprae* since these examinations are not available in the country.

Human immunodeficiency virus (HIV) serology was negative. The radiographs of the hands and feet showed osteoporosis (Figure 3). After routine pretherapeutic laboratory examinations that proved to be normal, antileprosy treatment (rifampicin 600 mg/day, dapsone 100 mg/day, and clofazimine 100 mg/day) was prescribed and was generally well tolerated, resulting in good clinical progress. After six months of therapy, the superficial skin lesions regressed and were completely healed. No relapse was noted during the follow-up period.

3. Case Report 2

A 65-year-old farmer residing in Gougui (Kobeni/Hodh El Gharbi region), Mauritania, consulted on December 2, 2016, at the Aïoun Regional Hospital for maculopapular, nodular lesions associated with chest pain and chronic productive

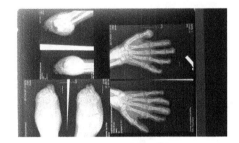

FIGURE 3: Bilateral osteoporosis.

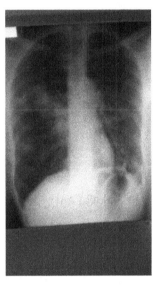

FIGURE 4: Reticulonodular infiltrates at the apex of the right lungs associated with bilateral hilar lymphadenopathy.

cough. On admission to hospital, the skin signs had evolved over the past ten years, at first consisting of lichenoid lesions and multiple hypopigmented papules. A few months before consultation, a productive cough associated with progressive deterioration of the general condition occurred. There was no history of tuberculosis. Various analgesics, antibiotics, and topical treatment, including traditional medicines, had not improved his condition. The physical examination revealed the presence of diffuse hypopigmented lichenoid lesions varying from 2 to 5 cm in diameter at the base of the nose with sensory loss. Visual examination was normal. Auscultation revealed rales over the right bronchus. Sputum examination and Ziehl-Neelsen skin smears were negative. Skin biopsy was not performed due to inadequate medical facilities. HIV serology was negative. Laboratory examinations showed anemia (9 g/dl hemoglobin), normal blood sugar, and normal renal and hepatic functions. The chest X-ray showed reticulonodular infiltrates at the right lung apex and bilateral hilar lymphadenopathy (Figure 4). The diagnosis of lepromatous leprosy with concomitant disseminated tuberculosis was made. Antileprosy and antituberculosis treatment (rifampicin 600 mg/day, dapsone 100 mg/day, and clofazimine 100 mg/day) was initiated and was generally well tolerated, leading to a favorable response.

4. Discussion

In the 1990s, WHO set the goal of eliminating leprosy as a public health problem from 2000 to 2005, with a prevalence of less than 1 for 10,000 inhabitants. WHO also recommended the establishment of a leprosy surveillance system in endemic countries in order to have indicators for the detection, management, and follow-up of patients [4]. The successful programme for control and elimination of this disease as a public health problem in some countries, such as Mauritania, seems to generate ignorance of leprosy among health personnel and, as a consequence, may increase the risk of late diagnosis, as in our cases.

The peculiarities of our observations were the long duration of disease evolution before correct clinical diagnosis due to initial misdiagnosis, and in our first case, severe deformity of hands and feet, including bilateral deeply perforating plantar ulcer. Delays in the duration of diagnosis were also noted in Senegal and France [3, 5, 6]. Indeed, articular pain, atrophy of the fingers, and polymorphic cutaneous manifestations often evoke rheumatoid arthritis or deforming polyarthritis. However, the diagnosis of musculoskeletal injury due to leprosy is difficult, given its multiple manifestations and the fact that many autoimmune disorders are part of differential diagnosis [7]. The confusion between leprosy and rheumatic disease has already been reported in the literature [8]. The appearance of "pudgy" deformed fingers is certainly misleading, but it may constitute an unsuspected inaugural form of leprosy, especially in its lepromatous form [9]. The perforating plantar ulcer in our first patient initially evoked a diabetic foot, but its bilateral character and hypertrophy of the ulnar and popliteal nerve trunks helped orient our diagnosis toward leprosy. Plantar neuropathic ulcer is a common and frequent complication of diabetes, a common pathology recognized as a pandemic by the WHO. Although frequently encountered during medical practice, the pathophysiology of neuropathic ulcer associated with diabetes remains poorly understood [10]. In our first patient, the presence of plantar perforation is an indirect evidence for the long duration of evolution but is also a risk of tetanus, osteitis, and sepsis. The hypochromic macules alone were not suggestive of leprosy, but their anesthetic character associated with nerve hypertrophy indicated leprosy in our first case.

In the second case, a diagnosis of pulmonary tuberculosis was suggested by the presence of persistent cough and radiological signs despite a well-conducted antibiotic therapy. As for the diagnosis of leprosy, lichenoid lesions and diffuse hypopigmented papules alone were not highly suggestive of leprosy but their anesthetic character was decisive to establish the correct diagnosis.

Leprosy and tuberculosis coinfection is very rare. However, the earliest case of coinfection of leprosy and tuberculosis was detected in the deoxyribonucleic acid of a man discovered in a burial site dating from the first century [8]. In our second case, leprosy had actually preceded tuberculosis, in agreement with earlier reports of several authors [8, 11, 12]. To our knowledge, there has been no reported case of concomitant tuberculosis and leprosy in Mauritania. The duration between the development of leprosy and tuberculosis varied from 2 months to 15 years [12]. In our case, it was 10 years. However, in one study, it was reported that two cases of tuberculosis occurred before leprosy, and it was suggested that tuberculosis can occur together with the full spectrum of leprosy [9]. The interaction between leprosy and tuberculosis and their impact on the incidence of the other remain a subject of debate [10, 13]. Some authors have observed that cases of pulmonary tuberculosis developed after taking a corticosteroid used primarily for the treatment of silent neuropathy associated with leprosy [11, 13].

Misdiagnosis was due to the rarity of leprosy cases seen in health care facilities in Mauritania today and the "atypical" nature of the lesions in the two cases reported here. Leprosy may become a global health problem due to the reactivation of latent, previously undiagnosed cases, even in the Western world, due to the use of strong immunosuppressive regimens for various diseases [14]. In cases of doubt, a skin smear and/or biopsy often helps to establish the final diagnosis [1]. At the country level, central laboratory with the capacity to perform microbiological diagnosis of tuberculosis and leprosy is still required. In our cases, skin biopsy was not done due to inadequate health resources, but the clinical manifestations were typical and obvious, fulfilling 2 of 3 criteria established by WHO. Treatment consisted of multidrug therapy as recommended by WHO, leading to favorable outcomes in our patients.

5. Conclusion

The polymorphic character of leprosy and the lack of knowledge about its clinical manifestations among most health care personnel due to the reduction of its prevalence constitute a source of misdiagnosis. Our reported cases illustrate these points. Early detection as recommended by WHO should reduce the occurrence of new active cases in the community. To attain the goal of elimination of leprosy, it is imperative for physicians and nurses to increase their vigilance in screening, treating, and reporting cases.

Conflicts of Interest

The authors have no conflicts of interest to declare.

References

[1] K. Eichelmann, S. E. González González, J. C. Salas-Alanis, and J. Ocampo-Candiani, "Leprosy. An update: Definition, pathogenesis, classification, diagnosis, and treatment," *Actas Dermo-Sifiliográficas*, vol. 104, no. 7, pp. 554–563, 2013.

[2] "Global leprosy situation," *Weekly Epidemiological Record*, vol. 87, no. 34, pp. 317–328, 2012.

[3] S. O. Niang, M. Diallo, M. Ndiaye et al., "Epidemiologic and clinicopathologic aspects of Leprosy in Dakar; evaluation of 73 new cases," *Dermatology Reports*, vol. 3, no. 2, article no. e18, 2011.

[4] World Health Organization, "Global leprosy situation," *Weekly Epidemiological Record*, vol. 33, pp. 333–340, 2009.

[5] H. D. Donoghue, A. Marcsik, C. Matheson et al., "Co-infection of Mycobacterium tuberculosis and Mycobacterium leprae in

human archaeological samples: A possible explanation for the historical decline of leprosy," *Proceedings of the Royal Society B Biological Science*, vol. 272, no. 1561, pp. 389–394, 2005.

[6] R. Prasad, S. K. Verma, R. Singh, and G. Hosmane, "Concomittant pulmonary tuberculosis and borderline leprosy with type-II lepra reaction in single patient," *Lung India*, vol. 27, no. 1, pp. 19–23, 2010.

[7] F. A. Sendrasoa, I. M. Ranaivo, O. Raharolahy, M. Andrianarison, L. S. Ramarozatovo, and F. Rapelanoro Rabenja, "Pulmonary Tuberculosis and Lepromatous Leprosy Coinfection," *Case Reports in Dermatological Medicine*, vol. 2015, Article ID 898410, 4 pages, 2015.

[8] D. K. Agarwal, A. R. Mehta, A. P. Sharma et al., "Coinfection with leprosy and tuberculosis in a renal transplant recipient," *Nephrology Dialysis Transplantation* , vol. 15, no. 10, pp. 1720-1721, 2000.

[9] G. R. Rao, S. Sandhya, M. Sridevi, A. Amareswar, B. L. Narayana, and Shantisri, "Lupus vulgaris and borderline tuberculoid leprosy: an interesting co-occurrence," *Indian Journal of Dermatology, Venereology and Leprology*, vol. 77, no. 1, article 111, 2011.

[10] T. M. I. Rawson, V. Anjum, J. Hodgson et al., "Leprosy and tuberculosis concomitant infection: a poorly understood, age-old relationship," *Leprosy Review*, vol. 85, no. 4, pp. 288–295, 2014.

[11] S. Prasad, R. Misra, A. Aggarwal et al., "Leprosy revealed in a rheumatology clinic: a case series," *International Journal of Rheumatic Diseases*, vol. 16, no. 2, pp. 129–133, 2013.

[12] M. Meyer, S. Ingen-Housz-Oro, O. Ighilahriz et al., "Polyarthritis and papular eruption revealing leprosy," *La Revue de Médecine Interne*, vol. 29, no. 3, pp. 242–245, 2008.

[13] J. L. Kuntz, R. Meyer, P. Vautravers, D. Kieffer, and L. Asch, "Polyarthritis in leprosy," *La Semaine des hôpitaux de Paris*, vol. 55, no. 41-42, pp. 1889–1892, 1979.

[14] B. Vanlerberghe, F. Devemy, A. Duhamel, P. Guerreschi, and D. Torabi, "Conservative surgical treatment for diabetic foot ulcers under the metatarsal heads. A retrospective case-control study," *Annales de Chirurgie Plastique Esthétique*, vol. 59, no. 3, pp. 161–169, 2014.

32

Bathing Suit Variant of Autosomal Recessive Congenital Ichthyosis (ARCI) in Two Indian Patients

Dharshini Sathishkumar,[1] Dincy Peter,[1] Susanne Pulimood,[1] Henning Wiegmann,[2] Frederic Valentin,[2] Meera Thomas,[1] Hans Christian Hennies,[3,4,5,6] and Vinzenz Oji [iD] [2]

[1]*Department of Dermatology Venereology and Leprosy, Christian Medical College, Vellore, India*
[2]*Department of Dermatology, University Hospital Muenster, Muenster, Germany*
[3]*Center for Dermatogenetics, Division of Human Genetics, Medical University of Innsbruck, Innsbruck, Austria*
[4]*Cologne Center for Genomics, Division of Dermatogenetics, University of Cologne, Germany*
[5]*Cologne Excellence Cluster on Cellular Stress Responses in Aging-Associated Diseases (CECAD), University of Cologne, Cologne, Germany*
[6]*Department of Biological and Geographical Sciences, University of Huddersfield, Huddersfield, UK*

Correspondence should be addressed to Vinzenz Oji; vinzenz.oji@ukmuenster.de

Academic Editor: Sergio A. Cuevas-Covarrubias

Bathing suit ichthyosis (BSI) is a rare variant of autosomal recessive congenital ichthyosis (ARCI) due to transglutaminase-1 gene (*TGM1*) mutations leading to a temperature sensitive phenotype. It is characterized by dark-grey or brownish scaling restricted to the "bathing suit" areas. We report two Indian girls with bathing suit ichthyosis and mutations in *TGM1* (patient 1: homozygous for c.1147G>A; patient 2: compound heterozygous for c.832G>A, c.919C>G).

1. Introduction

Bathing suit ichthyosis (BSI) is a rare variant of lamellar ichthyosis due to transglutaminase-1 gene (*TGM1*) mutations leading to a temperature sensitive phenotype [1]. First case was described in 1972 by Scott [2], followed by a case series by Jacyk, both from South Africa [3]. A current study by Marukian et al. expanded the group of reported BSI cases by additional 9 new mutations in patients from different ethnic origins [4]. Altogether, the majority of BSI reports are from Africa, Europe, Turkey, Middle East, and China but no reports from India so far. We report two cases of unrelated Indian girls with bathing suit ichthyosis and confirmatory mutations in *TGM1*.

2. Case Report

Two unrelated girls aged nine (patient 1) and 12 (patient 2) years born from nonconsanguineous parents presented at birth with collodion membranes and generalized scaling.

The collodion resolved and left behind erythroderma in the neonatal period. At the age of three months patient 1 developed ichthyosis confined to the trunk. In patient 2 this phenotypic shift developed at the age of three years. Both had history of summer exacerbation and improvement in winter. Interestingly the first patient had history of erythroderma during episodes of fever. No members of their family or pedigree had similar symptoms. They had no past history of serious diseases other than ichthyosis. On examination, patient 1 had large brownish, lamellar scales involving the bathing suit area of the trunk including the neck, forehead, axillae, external auditory meatus, and thick scales on the scalp (Figures 1(a) and 1(c)). The centrofacial region was spared. In addition, she had focal plantar keratoderma. There was marked reduction of scaling during the cold season. Patient 2 was seen in winter, and she had mild ichthyosis confined to the bathing suit area (Figures 1(b) and 1(d)). Skin biopsy from her ichthyotic area showed hyperkeratosis with follicular plugging, mild hyperplasia of the epidermis with well-preserved granular layer, no parakeratosis, and patchy

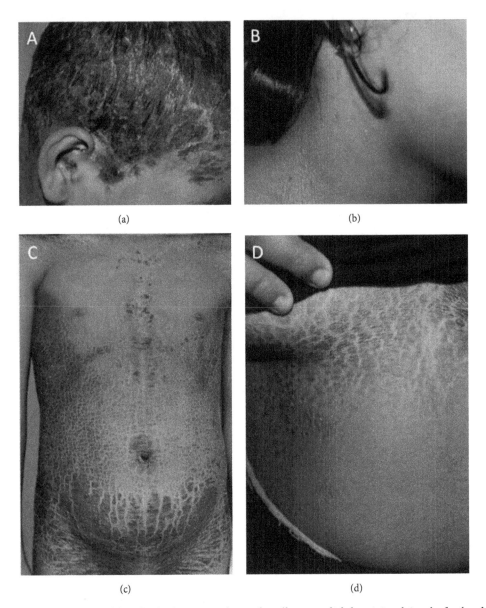

FIGURE 1: **Clinical presentation of patient 1 and 2**. (a, c). Patient 1 shows a lamellar type of ichthyosis involving the forehead, external auditory meatus, and neck, but sparing the centrofacial area by additional involvement of the bathing suit area. (b, d) Patient 2 shows a mild ichthyosis confined to bathing suit area with involvement of the axilla, but sparing of ears and face. The patient has been seen in winter.

perivascular infiltrates of lymphohistiocytes (Figure 2). The diagnosis of bathing suit ichthyosis (BSI) was made in both patients based on the criteria proposed by Jacyk et al. [3]. The patients were treated with bland ointments and mild keratolytics such as urea cream.

3. Results

DNA of each patient has been extracted from full blood and analyzed for mutations in *TGM1* by direct Sanger sequencing of all coding exons and flanking intronic sequences. Patient 1 was homozygous for the mutation c.1147G>A in exon 7, which leads to an exchange of valine by methionine, p.Val383Met. Patient 2 was compound heterozygous for the two *TGM1* mutations c.832G>A in exon 5 and c.919C>G in exon 6. These

DNA changes lead to the missense mutations p.Gly278Arg and p.Arg307Gly, respectively. The aforementioned changes of the amino acids are visualized within a 3-dimensional protein model of TGM1 (Figure 3).

4. Discussion/Conclusion

Bathing suit ichthyosis (BSI) is a rare phenotypic variant of autosomal recessive congenital ichthyosis (ARCI). Patients are born as collodion babies; after shedding of the collodion membrane, large dark grey or black scales develop but are confined to the bathing suit areas. Approximately 50 cases have been reported so far [1, 4–7]. Even though initially thought to be a South African genodermatosis [8] an increasing number of cases have been reported from other parts

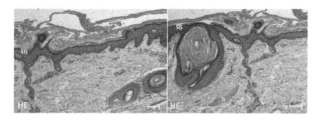

FIGURE 2: Histopathology of the ichthyotic area in patient 2 shows hyperkeratosis with follicular plugging and hyperplasia of the epidermis with well-preserved stratum granulosum. (*HE*: haematoxylin & eosin; *SG*: stratum granulosum; scale bare = 100 μm).

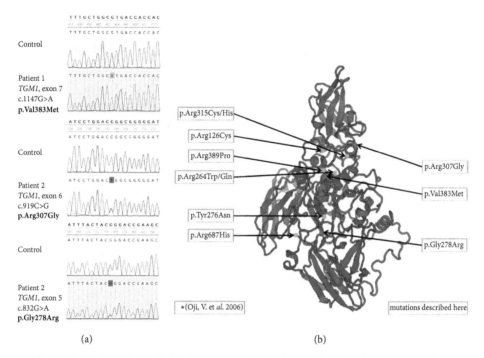

(a)   (b)

FIGURE 3: **Localization of mutations within transglutaminase 1 causing bathing suit ichthyosis.** (a) Results of sanger sequencing of patient 1 and 2 to confirm mutations described here. (b) The localization of the 2006 by Oji et al. published mutations p.Arg315Cys/His, p.Arg126Cys, p.Arg389Pro, p.Arg264Trp/Gln, p.Tyr276Asn, p.Arg687His, p.Arg307Gly (Oji, V. et al. 2006), and the two mutations p.Val383Met and p.Gly278Arg found in two Indian children is depicted within a three-dimensional model of transglutaminase 1. The well-known mutation p.Arg307Gly was also found in the two Indian children. Three-dimensional modeling of transglutaminase 1 isoform 1 was performed by using the online *in-silico* protein structure prediction tool SWISS MODEL (Swiss institute of Bioinformatics, SIB). For structural alignment the structure of transglutaminase 3 was used as template. (b) Results of sanger sequencing of patient 1 and 2 to confirm mutations described here.

of the world [1, 2, 4–6, 8], and this report represents one of the first genetic studies on BSI in Indian patients. Both our patients had characteristic features of BSI. An important diagnostic clinical sign is the involvement of warmer skin areas such as the neck or the excessive desquamation of the external auditory meatus, which required repeated syringing [1, 6].

BSI is caused by transglutaminase-1 deficiency with heat-dependent transglutaminase-1 dysfunction [1, 7]. The enzyme plays a major role in the formation of the cornified cell envelope (CE) by cross-linking of CE precursor proteins and ceramides. Transglutaminase-1 deficiency is supposed to lead to a defective cornified cell envelope formation and a disturbance of the lipid barrier.

Specific mutations of *TGM1* lead to reduced transglutaminase-1 activity at higher temperature [7], which explains the summer exacerbation and fever induced erythroderma seen in patient 2 [6]. Moreover, it is speculated that hypohidrosis following excessive keratinization can result in heat accumulation, which possibly causes additional hyperkeratosis in the summer, and that this vicious circle may contribute to the seasonal variation in BSI [4]. The homozygous missense mutation p.Val383Met, which was identified in patient 1, has been described in other patients with BSI [5] and in one case of lamellar ichthyosis, which would be regarded as a case of BSI retrospectively [6]. The *TGM1* mutation p.Arg307Gly of patient 2 is known from the original BSI series of Oji et al., 2006 [1]. The second mutation p.Gly278Arg found in the compound heterozygous patient 2 was described as a mutation associated with typical lamellar ichthyosis [9]. This observation corroborates the assumption that one temperature responsive mutation in *TGM1* in a compound heterozygous case is sufficient to give rise to the phenotype of BSI [1].

In summary, we confirm that bathing suit ichthyosis can be found in India and is caused by specific mutations in *TGM1*. Clinicians should be aware of the clinical key features of BSI, especially the heat sensitivity of this special ichthyosis variant representing the diagnostic clue. Of note, the refinement of genotype-phenotype correlation within the *TGM1* gene mutation spectrum may improve the counselling situation and management of families with collodion babies.

Conflicts of Interest

The authors have no conflicts of interest to declare.

Authors' Contributions

All listed authors were essentially involved in the generation of the data, the analysis and interpretation of the results, and the preparation of the final manuscript. In the course of manuscript preparation, all authors submitted their intellectual suggestions for improvement and gave their final approval for publication. All authors have agreed to the responsibility for this manuscript.

Acknowledgments

The authors thank the Indian family for their participation and agreement. They would also like to thank all employees and colleagues involved in this study.

References

[1] V. Oji, J. M. Hautier, B. Ahvazi et al., "Bathing suit ichthyosis is caused by transglutaminase-1 deficiency: evidence for a temperature-sensitive phenotype," *Human Molecular Genetics*, vol. 15, no. 21, pp. 3083–3097, 2006.

[2] F. Scott, "The South African "Bathing Suit Ichthyosis" Is a Form of Lamellar Ichthyosis Caused by a Homozygous Missense Mutation, p.R315L, in Transglutaminase 1 Skin diseases in the South African Bantu," in *Essays on Tropical Dermatology*, J. Marshall, Ed., vol. 2, pp. 1–17, Excerpta Medica, Amsterdam, Netherlands, 1972.

[3] V. Oji, G. Tadini, M. Akiyama et al., "Revised nomenclature and classification of inherited ichthyoses: Results of the First Ichthyosis Consensus Conference in Sorèze 2009," *Journal of the American Academy of Dermatology*, vol. 63, no. 4, pp. 607–641, 2010.

[4] N. V. Marukian, R.-H. Hu, B. G. Craiglow et al., "Expanding the genotypic spectrum of bathing suit ichthyosis," *JAMA Dermatology*, vol. 153, no. 6, pp. 537–543, 2017.

[5] E. Bourrat, C. Blanchet-Bardon, C. Derbois, S. Cure, and J. Fischer, "Specific TGM1 mutation profiles in bathing suit and self-improving collodion ichthyoses: Phenotypicand genotypic data from 9 patients with dynamic phenotypes of autosomal recessive congenital ichthyosis," *JAMA Dermatology*, vol. 148, no. 10, pp. 1191–1195, 2012.

[6] B. C. Hackett, D. Fitzgerald, R. M. Watson, F. A. Hol, and A. D. Irvine, "Genotype-phenotype correlations with TGM1: Clustering of mutations in the bathing suit ichthyosis and self-healing collodion baby variants of lamellar ichthyosis," *British Journal of Dermatology*, vol. 162, no. 2, pp. 448–451, 2010.

[7] K. Arita, W. K. Jacyk, V. Wessagowit et al., "The South African "bathing suit ichthyosis" is a form of lamellar ichthyosis caused by a homozygous missense mutation, p.R315L, in t1ransglutaminase 1 [4]," *Journal of Investigative Dermatology*, vol. 127, no. 2, pp. 490–493, 2007.

[8] W. K. Jacyk, "Bathing-suit ichthyosis. A peculiar phenotype of lamellar ichthyosis in South African blacks," *European Journal of Dermatology*, vol. 15, no. 6, pp. 433–436, 2005.

[9] R. Benmously-Mlika, A. Zaouak, R. Mrad et al., "Bathing suit ichthyosis caused by a TGM1 mutation in a Tunisian child," *International Journal of Dermatology*, vol. 53, no. 12, pp. 1478–1480, 2014.

33

Dasatinib-Induced Hypopigmentation in Pediatric Patient with Chronic Myeloid Leukemia

Bader Alharbi ⑩,[1] Samer Alamri,[1] Ahmed Mahdi ⑩,[1] and Siham Marghalani[1,2]

[1]*King Abdullah International Medical Research Center, King Saud bin Abdulaziz University for Health Sciences, P.O. Box 9515, Jeddah 21423, Saudi Arabia*
[2]*Department of Dermatology, King Khaled National Guard Hospital, National Guard Health Affairs, P.O. Box 9515, Jeddah 21423, Saudi Arabia*

Correspondence should be addressed to Bader Alharbi; dr.alharbibader@gmail.com

Academic Editor: Jacek Cezary Szepietowski

Dasatinib is an oral second-generation multitarget tyrosine-kinase inhibitor (TKI) that is efficacious in treating imatinib-resistant chronic myeloid leukemia (CML) or intolerant cases. Noncutaneous adverse effects with dasatinib are well known in the literature, most commonly cytopenias and fluid retention, while pigmentary abnormalities have rarely been reported. We report the case of a 12-year-old male known case of CML, who presented to dermatology clinic approximately 2 years after initiating dasatinib treatment, with new-onset hypopigmentation of his upper limb, upper chest, and both knees of six months' duration.

1. Introduction

Chronic myeloid leukemia (CML) is a hematopoietic stem cell malignancy. It usually occurs in an older population with an age of 60 to 65 years [1]. It is considered to be rare among the young population with an incidence of 2% of all leukemia in an age less than 15 years [2]. CML is a clonal disease that is caused by a gene mutation that consists of a reciprocal translocation between chromosomes 9 and 22, leading to what is known as Philadelphia chromosome (Ph) [3]. Tyrosine kinase inhibitors (TKIs) are currently the mainstay of CML treatment. Dasatinib is an oral multitarget tyrosine-kinase inhibitor. It is efficacious in cases of resistance or intolerance to Imatinib [4]. It works by inhibiting BCR-ABL mutant forms, Src-family tyrosine kinases, c-Kit, ephrin-A2 receptor (EphA2R), and platelet-derived growth factor receptor-B (PDGFR-B). Unlike imatinib, it binds to active and inactive conformations of BCR-ABL [5]. Multiple dermatological side effects such us superficial edema, lichenoid reaction, psoriasis, and Steven-Jonson syndrome have been reported with first generation TKIs like imatinib mesylate [6]. However, depigmentation is reported to be around 41

percent [7]. In contrast, cutaneous side effects of dasatinib have been rarely reported. We report a case of dasatinib-induced hypopigmentation in a young patient with chronic myeloid leukemia and review cases in the literature.

2. Case

A 12-year-old male with a history of chronic myeloid leukemia presented to our dermatology clinic with new-onset hypopigmented patches that are slowly progressive and of varying sizes of six months' duration on his upper limbs, upper chest, and both knees (Figure 1). Also, two depigmented macules were noted on his upper chest and lower abdomen. The patient denied any rashes or other skin changes and also denied any changes in hair, nail, and mucous membranes. Furthermore, Wood's light examination was negative. The patient was switched to dasatinib, at a dose of 70 mg once per day since two years, due to intolerance to imatinib. There was no personal or family history of autoimmune diseases or pigmentary disorders like vitiligo. The patient denied any use of topical medications or bleaching agents. A 3 mm punch biopsy from active hypopigmented lesion on

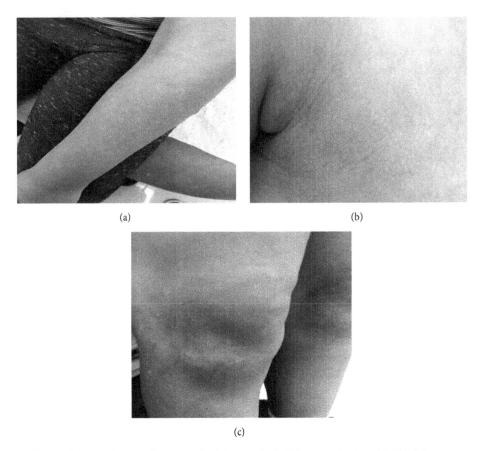

(a)

(b)

(c)

FIGURE 1: Hypopigmented areas on the (a) upper limb, (b) upper chest, and (c) both knees.

the abdomen was performed. Histopathologically, it showed decrease melanocytes and basal layer melanin pigmentation. In immunohistochemistry, Melan A stain revealed decreased melanocyte. All positive and negative controls are examined and show appropriate reactivity. The patient was treated with close observation and reassurance. Through it all, the above clinical clues led to a diagnosis of skin depigmentation during dasatinib treatment.

3. Discussion

Tyrosine Kinase Inhibitors (TKI) are considered the cornerstone in the treatment of chronic myeloid leukemia (CML). Dasatinib, a second generation TKI, is used as a second line therapy in CML cases where patients are resistant or intolerant to first generation TKI, like imatinib [4]. Likewise, our patient was intolerant to imatinib and switched to dasatinib due to severe bone pain before achieving a complete molecular response. In vitro, dasatinib is considered about 300 times more potent than imatinib; this is due to its ability to bind to both active and inactive conformations of BCR-ABL [5].

Multiple well known cutaneous adverse effects were noted with TKI treatment, for example, superficial edema, maculopapular rash, pigmentary changes, lichenoid reaction, and psoriasiform rash [6]. These side effects were reported particularly with first generation TKI, namely, imatinib, while

few cases were reported about the cutaneous side effects with dasatinib. Nevertheless, noncutaneous adverse effects with dasatinib are well known in the literature, most commonly cytopenias and fluid retention [14]. Pigmentary side effects with imatinib were reported in a study done by Arora et al. in which depigmentation and hyperpigmentation were seen in 40.9% and 3.6% of 118 patients, respectively [7].

In addition to BCR-ABL, dasatinib targets multiple tyrosine kinases, such as SCR family kinases, c-Kit, platelet-derived growth factor (PDGFR), and ephrin-A receptor kinases. The protooncogene c-Kit and its ligand stem cell factor (SCF) play a crucial role in the proliferation, migration, and survival of melanocytes. Therefore, inhibiting the c-Kit/SCF signaling pathway is thought to be the reason for pigmentary side effects in a patient receiving TKIs [15]. A clinical example of this signaling pathway is seen in patients with piebaldism, which is an autosomal dominant disorder resulting from a mutation in KIT protooncogene leading to the absence of melanocytes and the appearance of leukoderma on the affected areas [16]. However, dasatinib has a low affinity to c-Kit and PDFGR compared to imatinib, and this is the reason why pigmentary side effects are more pronounced with imatinib compared to dasatinib [6].

The median time for the onset of pigmentary adverse effects is about 2 months after starting TKI therapy (Table 1) [8–13]. Moreover, Webb K et al. reported that a case with dasatinib induced facial depigmentation after almost

TABLE 1

Case number	Age	Gender	Diagnosis	Dasatinib dose	Time to hypopigmentation (Months)	References
Current case	12	Male	chronic myeloid leukemia	70 mg once daily	18	Current case
1	72	Male	chronic myeloid leukemia	100 mg once daily	37	[8]
2	52	Female	Hemangiopericytoma	70 mg twice daily	2	[9]
3	27	Female	chronic myeloid leukemia	100 mg once daily	6	[10]
4	16	Male	Acute lymphoblastic leukemia	100 mg twice daily	1	[11]
5	56	Female	chronic myeloid leukemia	70 once daily	2	[12]
6	29	Female	chronic myeloid leukemia	70 once daily	2	[13]

three years of starting the therapy [8]. In comparison, our patient developed generalized hypopigmentation after about 18 months of switching to dasatinib. The pigmentary changes with TKI appear to be dose-dependent and reversible with a resolution of pigmentary side effects after stopping the treatment [16]. Furthermore, Boudadi et al. reported a case with dasatinib induced hypopigmentation that resolved after stopping the treatment, and then the patient's skin color started to darken beyond her baseline and she experienced diffuse hyperpigmentation. This paradoxical pigmentary changes with TKI were thought to be due to drug-related immune dysregulation in which TKI can act as c-Kit receptor modulator [9].

Regarding the age of patients with dasatinib induced hypopigmentation, our patient is considered the youngest compared to cases reported in the literature (Table 1).

The challenge in the management of pigmentary side effects with TKI is that most patients with hematological malignancies, particularly CML, require the continuation of TKI for long periods even after achieving a complete molecular response. This is because of a high incidence of molecular relapse after withholding the therapy [17]. For this reason, the cessation of dasatinib was not the option in the management for our patient and he was treated with close observation and reassurance.

4. Conclusion

Since TKIs are widely used in the treatment of different hematological and nonhematological malignancies, we encourage physicians to take into account the multiple cutaneous side effects that can be caused by this therapy. Additionally, further studies are needed to explore the role of c-Kit/SCF signaling pathway and the role of other factors in the development of pigmentary changes with different TKI generations.

Conflicts of Interest

The authors declare no conflicts of interest.

References

[1] G. Gugliotta, F. Castagnetti, M. Apolinari et al., "First-line treatment of newly diagnosed elderly patients with chronic myeloid leukemia: Current and emerging strategies," *Drugs*, vol. 74, no. 6, pp. 627–643, 2014.

[2] R. LAG, M. Smith, J. G. Gurney et al., Eds., *Cancer Incidence and Survival among Children and Adolescents: United States SEER Program 1975-1995*, vol. 99, National Cancer Institute, 1999.

[3] Nowell P. C. and D. A. Hungerford, "A minute chromosome in human chronic granulocytic leukemia," *Science*, p. 1497, 132.

[4] A. Hochhaus, S. Saussele, G. Rosti et al., "Chronic myeloid leukaemia: ESMO Clinical Practice Guidelines for diagnosis, treatment and follow-up," *Annals of Oncology*, vol. 28, pp. iv41–iv51, 2017.

[5] M. Lindauer and A. Hochhaus, "Dasatinib," *Recent Results in Cancer Research*, vol. 184, pp. 83–102, 2010.

[6] I. Amitay-Laish, S. M. Stemmer, and M. E. Lacouture, "Adverse cutaneous reactions secondary to tyrosine kinase inhibitors including imatinib mesylate, nilotinib, and dasatinib," *Dermatologic Therapy*, vol. 24, no. 4, pp. 386–395, 2011.

[7] B. Arora, L. Kumar, A. Sharma, J. Wadhwa, and V. Kochupillai, "Pigmentary changes in chronic myeloid leukemia patients treated with imatinib mesylate," *Annals of Oncology*, vol. 15, no. 2, pp. 358-359, 2004.

[8] K. C. Webb, M. Harasimowicz, M. Janeczek, J. Speiser, J. Swan, and R. Tung, "Development of asymmetric facial depigmentation in a patient treated with dasatinib with new-onset hypovitaminosis d: case report and review of the literature," *Case Reports in Dermatological Medicine*, 2017.

[9] K. Boudadi and R. Chugh, "Diffuse hypopigmentation followed by hyperpigmentation in an African American woman with hemangiopericytoma treated with dasatinib," *Journal of Clinical and Diagnostic Research*, vol. 8, no. 11, pp. QD01–QD02, 2014.

[10] S. Samimi, E. Chu, J. Seykora et al., "Dasatinib-induced leukotrichia in a patient with chronic myelogenous leukemia," *JAMA Dermatology*, vol. 149, no. 5, pp. 637–639, 2013.

[11] V. Brazzelli, V. Grasso, V. Barbaccia et al., "Hair depigmentation and vitiligo-like lesions in a leukaemic paediatric patient during chemotherapy with dasatinib," *Acta Dermato-Venereologica*, vol. 92, no. 2, pp. 218-219, 2012.

[12] A. Fujimi, S. Ibata, Y. Kanisawa et al., "Reversible skin and hair depigmentation during chemotherapy with dasatinib for chronic myeloid leukemia," *The Journal of Dermatology*, vol. 43, no. 1, pp. 106-107, 2016.

[13] A. Sun, R. S. Akin, E. Cobos, and J. Smith, "Hair depigmentation during chemotherapy with dasatinib, a dual Bcr-Abl/Src family tyrosine kinase inhibitor," *J Drugs Dermatol*, vol. 8, no. 4, pp. 395–398, 2009.

[14] S. Shayani, "Dasatinib, a multikinase inhibitor: therapy, safety, and appropriate management of adverse events," *Therapeutic Drug Monitoring*, vol. 32, no. 6, pp. 680–687, 2010.

[15] J. M. Grichnik, J. A. Burch, J. Burchette, and C. R. Shea, "The SCF/KIT pathway plays a critical role in the control of normal human melanocyte homeostasis," *Journal of Investigative Dermatology*, vol. 111, no. 2, pp. 233–238, 1998.

[16] N. Oiso, K. Fukai, A. Kawada, and T. Suzuki, "Piebaldism," *The Journal of Dermatology*, vol. 40, no. 5, pp. 330–335, 2013.

[17] I. C. Haznedaroglu, "Current concerns of undertreatment and overtreatment in chronic myeloid leukemia based on European LeukemiaNet 2013 recommendations," *Expert Opinion on Pharmacotherapy*, vol. 14, no. 15, pp. 2005–2010, 2013.

34

Sustained Regression of Hydroxycarbamide Induced Actinic Keratoses after Switching to Anagrelide

Georgios Gaitanis ⓘ,[1] Dora Gougopoulou,[2] Eleni Kapsali,[2] and Ioannis D. Bassukas[1]

[1]*Department of Skin and Venereal Diseases, Faculty of Medicine, School of Health Sciences, University of Ioannina, Ioannina, Greece*
[2]*Hematology Clinic, Department of Internal Medicine, Faculty of Medicine, School of Health Sciences,*
 University of Ioannina, Ioannina, Greece

Correspondence should be addressed to Georgios Gaitanis; ggaitan@cc.uoi.gr

Academic Editor: Kowichi Jimbow

Hydroxycarbamide (HC) is the first-line treatment for certain myeloproliferative neoplasms, such as polycythemia vera and essential thrombocytosis (ET). In a subset of these patients long-term treatment with HC can result in the development of confluent actinic keratoses (AK) followed by invasive keratinocytic carcinomas ("squamous dysplasia"), preferentially on sun-exposed skin. Discontinuation or dose reduction of HC may result in partial improvement. A 59-year-old farmer after 14 years on HC (2 gr/d) and acetylsalicylic acid (100 mg/d) for ET, was referred for numerous, hyperkeratotic AK on face, scalp, and hands that could not be controlled with repeated ($N = 15$) cryosurgery sessions in the previous 3 years. Acitretin (0.32 mg/kg daily) and topical treatments (cryosurgery with ingenol mebutate) were initiated with only marginal improvement after 3 months. Acitretin dose was doubled and HC was switched to anagrelide (0.5 mg twice daily). Within a month the AK load regressed significantly and, at 3 months follow-up, complete clinical remission was achieved and acitretin was discontinued. Twenty months later the patient is clear from AK. In conclusion, the impressive and sustainable AK remission under anagrelide draws attention to a possible role of the phosphodiesterase 3 pathway, the major pharmacological target of anagrelide, as a potential therapeutic target for keratinocytic cancers.

1. Introduction

Hydroxycarbamide (HC) is recommended as the first-line treatment modality for the management of patients within the spectrum of certain myeloproliferative neoplasms, as polycythemia vera and essential thrombocytosis (ET) [1, 2]. HC is a potent inhibitor of the ribonucleotide reductase and slows down the rate of DNA replication decelerating cell cycle progression at the G1/S phase transition point and elongating the S phase both *in vitro* and *in vivo* [3]. However, this exposes cell populations, like epidermal keratinocytes, to the action of carcinogens, as ensuing mutations are established prior to DNA replication and cell division [4]. A subset of patients receiving HC for the above hematologic conditions will develop multiple actinic keratoses (AK) and keratinocytic carcinomas in sun-exposed skin regions ("squamous dysplasia") [5]. This is a serious and therapeutically challenging side-effect [6], which may partly improve after HC discontinuation

or dose reduction [7]. Anagrelide, on the other hand, is a phosphodiesterase 3 (PDE 3) inhibitor that is recommended as a 3rd-line treatment for ET after interferon-α (IFN-α) and busulfan [2].

2. Case Presentation

A 59-year-old farmer on HC for ET was referred due to multiple, hyperkeratotic AK accumulating in chronically sun-exposed skin areas: the hands, ears, almost the entire balding scalp, and large portions of the face, accompanied by severe actinic cheilitis. The majority of the lesions, especially on the scalp, were covered by a hyperkeratotic crust that could be removed relatively easy, revealing an oozing erosion (Figure 1(a)). ET was diagnosed 14 years earlier and was treated since with HC (2 gr/d) and acetylsalicylic acid (100 mg/d). The medical history of the patient

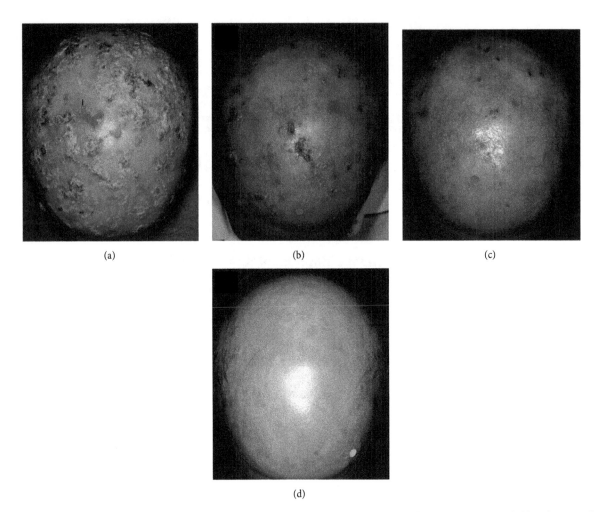

(a)   (b)   (c)

(d)

FIGURE 1: Complete and sustained remission of extensive hydroxycarbamide-associated skin carcinogenesis fields after switching to anagrelide: exemplary presentation of the alterations on the balding scalp skin. (a) At presentation numerous, confluent, hypertrophic actinic keratoses cover almost the entire scalp. Removal of the hyperkeratosis revealed an oozing erosion (arrow). (b) A significant load of actinic keratoses persists 3 months after onset of treatment with cryosurgery plus ingenol mebutate (7 treatment cycles) and daily 0.32 mg/kg b.w. acitretin. At that point acitretin dose was doubled (0.64 mg/kg b.w./d) and the patient was switched from hydroxycarbamide to anagrelide. (c) Impressive improvement after one month in the last treatment scheme (anagrelide and acitretin, no topical treatments). (d) Sustainable "clearance" of the field 20 months after discontinuation of acitretin and still on anagrelide: complete regression of existing and no development of new actinic keratoses.

was also remarkable for hyperlipidemia on simvastatin (20 mg/d) and fenofibrate (145 mg/d), arterial hypertension on atenolol (50 mg/d), and gastroesophageal reflux on rabeprazole (20 mg/d). AK burden had progressively expanded in the past 3 years. During this period, repeated sessions of cryosurgery ($N = 15$) failed to control existing lesions while new ones continued to appear. Biopsies from a hyperkeratotic scalp lesion and from the lower lip confirmed AK and actinic cheilitis, respectively. Due to the hyperlipidemia, the patient was initiated on a moderate acitretin dose (0.32 mg/kg body weight daily). Concurrently, skin segments (25 cm^2 each) with HC induced "squamous dysplasia" [5] were treated topically with the combination of cryosurgery sessions (liquid N$_2$, open spray, 2 cycles of 10 sec each, applied in quarters of the segment) and, starting on the same day, application of ingenol mebutate gel as per manufacturer's recommendations. After 3 months on

this treatment (7 treatment cycles) the AK load had only marginally improved (Figure 1(b)). At this time the dose of acitretin was doubled and HC was switched to anagrelide (0.5 mg twice daily). Already within a month after the latter treatment adaptation an impressive regression of the AK load was evident (Figure 1(c)). At the 3-month follow-up, complete AK remission was recorded and acitretin was discontinued. The temporal regression of lesions was noted concurrently in all affected skin regions and most probably represents sustained remission of the sum of carcinogenesis fields of this occupationally heavily sun-exposed patient. To date, 20 months later, no new AKs have developed (Figure 1(d)) and as we could not identify any clinical signs of AK to sample, a confirmatory biopsy was not performed (Figure 1(d)).

Medline search (January 15, 2018) with conjunction of the terms "'hydroxycarbamide' AND 'skin', 'hydroxycarbamide'

AND ('actinic' OR 'keratosis')" returned 436 and 34 articles, respectively. Extensive search within these articles for comparable cases to the present one located only two relevant reports: the first one [8] describes a 59-year-old man with ET under HC who was switched to anagrelide due to the development of multiple squamous cell carcinomas. The first six months after treatment revision a multitude of skin cancers were continued to be encountered (3 basal cell carcinomas, 4 squamous cell carcinomas, and 10 AK), yet no new lesions developed subsequently (total follow-up period is not reported). The second report [9], probably more relevant to the present case, described a 50-year-old female with ET under HC for 26 years. After she had developed extensive AK fields resistant to multiple local treatment cycles for 6 years, she was switched to anagrelide in February 2017 with subsequent rapid improvement.

3. Discussion

Thus, including the present case, 3 patients have notable response of squamous dysplasia after switching of HC to anagrelide. In our case, the remission lasts already 20 months after drug switching (the longest follow-up period among reported patients). This sustainable effect indicates the existence of a protective action of anagrelide against the development of AK. The impressive clinical improvement of this patient contrasts the relative scarcity of reported cases with a similar outcome and raises the question of whether this was merely an isolated phenomenon or could represent a still underreported effect. To our opinion the latter explanation is probably more relevant for various reasons. Not all patients under HC will progress to the development of squamous dysplasia. The increase in the rates of nonmelanoma skin cancer development after significant cumulative HC doses is approximately 22% [5]. This points towards the existence of a susceptible subpopulation within HC treated patients that will develop overt "squamous dysplasia." As already mentioned, when these patients will require substitution of HC, the recommended 2nd-line medications are either IFN-α or busulfan, followed by anagrelide as a 3rd-line treatment option [2]. Both IFN-α and busulfan have distinct effects on skin cancers and skin carcinogenesis fields: IFN-α is employed as a treatment modality in selected cases of keratinocytic cancers [10], while busulfan increases the risk for the development of these neoplasms [6]. Thus, anagrelide will be used in a relative small proportion of patients with "squamous dysplasia" directly after HC to permit recording and attributing possible antineoplastic effects to this medication. It is worth noting that the only intricacy restricting exclusive attribution to anagrelide of the impressive AK clearance effect in our patient is that he received it together with acitretin for 3 months. A still unrecognized synergistic action of both substances against "squamous dysplasia" cannot be excluded, as well as the exact role of HC discontinuation in the regression of the induced AK fields. Retinoids do have a recognized action against carcinogenesis fields and are recommended, for example, in the treatment of multiple AK developing in transplanted patients under immunosuppression [11]. Yet, their prophylactic effect

stops after discontinuation. On the other hand, PDE3A, the target of anagrelide, is highly expressed in epithelial cancer cell lines, including lung, colon, and cervical cancer [12] and its targeted inhibition is evaluated for redirection of PDE3 inhibitors in anticancer treatment [13] as well as an intense search for new ones [14]. PDE3A is expressed ~ 40% more in sun-exposed (tibial) compared to sun-protected skin [14] underscoring the need to evaluate its expression in keratinocytic carcinomas, including AK. Likewise, in an experimental mouse model, cilostamide, a PDE3 inhibitor, increased apoptosis in UV damaged keratinocytes by 29%, while other PDE inhibitors (PDE2 inhibitors) demonstrated even more pronounced effects [15].

In conclusion, the rapid and sustained regression of HC induced AK fields draws attention to a possible role of the PDE 3 pathway, the major pharmacological target of anagrelide, as a promising intervention for keratinocytic cancers that warrants further investigation.

Conflicts of Interest

The authors declare that they have no conflicts of interest.

References

[1] C. Besses and A. Alvarez-Larrán, "How to Treat Essential Thrombocythemia and Polycythemia Vera," *Clinical Lymphoma, Myeloma & Leukemia*, vol. 16, pp. S114–S123, 2016.

[2] A. Tefferi, A. M. Vannucchi, and T. Barbui, "Essential thrombocythemia treatment algorithm 2018," *Blood Cancer Journal*, vol. 8, no. 1, 2018.

[3] B. Maurer-Schultze, M. Siebert, and I. D. Bassukas, "An in vivo study on the synchronizing effect of hydroxyurea," *Experimental Cell Research*, vol. 174, no. 1, pp. 230–243, 1988.

[4] O. H. Iversen, "Hydroxyurea enhances methylnitrosourea skin tumorigenesis when given shortly before, but not after, the carcinogen," *Carcinogenesis*, vol. 3, no. 8, pp. 891–894, 1982.

[5] C. Sanchez-Palacios and J. Guitart, "Hydroxyurea-associated squamous dysplasia.," *Journal of the American Academy of Dermatology*, vol. 51, no. 2, pp. 293–300, 2004.

[6] M. Gómez, V. Guillem, A. Pereira et al., "Risk factors for non-melanoma skin cancer in patients with essential thrombocythemia and polycythemia vera," *European Journal of Haematology*, vol. 96, no. 3, pp. 285–290, 2016.

[7] E. Antonioli, P. Guglielmelli, L. Pieri et al., "Hydroxyurea-related toxicity in 3,411 patients with Ph'-negative MPN," *American Journal of Hematology*, vol. 87, no. 5, pp. 552–554, 2012.

[8] P. J. M. Best and R. M. Petitt, "Multiple skin cancers associated with hydroxyurea therapy," *Mayo Clinic Proceedings*, vol. 73, no. 10, pp. 961–963, 1998.

[9] B. Bhoyrul, G. Brent, I. Abdul-Kadir, and J. Mikeljevic, "Multiple Treatment-Resistant Actinic Keratoses Secondary to Hydroxycarbamide," in *Skinmed*, vol. 15, pp. 489–494, 2017.

[10] A. Ismail and N. Yusuf, "Type i interferons: Key players in normal skin and select cutaneous malignancies," *Dermatology Research and Practice*, vol. 2014, Article ID 847545, 11 pages, 2014.

[11] B. S. Schreve, M. Anliker, A. W. Arnold et al., "Pre- and post-transplant management of solid organ transplant recipients:

Risk-adjusted follow-up," *Current Problems in Dermatology*, vol. 43, pp. 57–70, 2012.

[12] M. Nazir, W. Senkowski, F. Nyberg et al., "Targeting tumor cells based on Phosphodiesterase 3A expression," *Experimental Cell Research*, vol. 361, no. 2, pp. 308–315, 2017.

[13] D. H. Maurice, H. Ke, F. Ahmad, Y. Wang, J. Chung, and V. C. Manganiello, "Advances in targeting cyclic nucleotide phosphodiesterases," *Nature Reviews Drug Discovery*, vol. 13, no. 4, pp. 290–314, 2014.

[14] L. De Waal, T. A. Lewis, M. G. Rees et al., "Identification of cancer-cytotoxic modulators of PDE3A by predictive chemogenomics," *Nature Chemical Biology*, vol. 12, no. 2, pp. 102–108, 2016.

[15] J. J. Bernard, Y.-R. Lou, Q.-Y. Peng, T. Li, and Y.-P. Lu, "PDE2 is a novel target for attenuating tumor formation in a mouse model of UVB-induced skin carcinogenesis," *PLoS ONE*, vol. 9, no. 10, Article ID e109862, 2014.

35

Upfront Radiotherapy with Concurrent and Adjuvant Vismodegib is Effective and Well-Tolerated in a Patient with Advanced, Multifocal Basal Cell Carcinoma

Abigail I. Franco [ID],[1] **Gary Eastwick,**[2] **Ramsay Farah,**[2] **Marvin Heyboer** [ID],[2] **Mijung Lee** [ID],[2] **and Paul Aridgides** [ID][2]

[1]*St. Joseph's Hospital Health Center, 301 Prospect Avenue, Syracuse, NY 13203, USA*
[2]*Upstate University Hospital, 750 E. Adams Street, Syracuse, NY 13210, USA*

Correspondence should be addressed to Abigail I. Franco; abigail.francomd123@gmail.com

Academic Editor: Alireza Firooz

We present a case report of a male with multifocal and extensive basal cell carcinoma. Due to extremely large size and deep tumor infiltration, he was not a surgical candidate. Combined modality treatment of fractionated radiation with concurrent vismodegib was chosen. Concurrent treatment was previously reported in the *palliative* and *recurrent* setting. This is the first case of concurrent vismodegib and radiation therapy for *upfront definitive* management. The patient experienced complete response in all treated lesions.

1. Introduction

Basal cell carcinoma (BCC), the most common skin malignancy, has an estimated incidence of 226 cases per 100,0000 individuals yearly in the United States [1]. Surgical excision is extremely effective with <5% of patients developing local failure [2]. Radiation therapy (RT), while similarly curative for smaller tumors (95%), is more frequently used for larger tumors where size > 10 mm has been associated with lower efficacy (90%) [3]. As would be expected, even more advanced tumors are associated with higher rates of failure. In a retrospective review of 115 advanced BCCs treated with RT, where the median tumor size was 7 cm (range 3 to 32 cm), the 5-year cure rate dropped to 55% [4]. A recent consensus from a UK panel of experts has defined advanced BCC as being BCC stage II or above (as categorized by the American Joint Committee on Cancer as a tumor larger than 2 cm with no metastases), in which current treatment modalities may be contraindicated by clinical or patient-driven factors [4].

Vismodegib is a small molecule inhibitor of smoothened homologue (SMO) and has shown clinical efficacy in the treatment of locally advanced or metastatic BCC in patients who are not candidates for or have failed prior treatment with surgery and/or radiation [5]. In the Landmark phase II trial proving such efficacy, vismodegib led to treatment response in 43% of patients with locally advanced BCC, all of whom had previously failed RT [5]. Given the low cure rate using vismodegib alone following RT, and given the correlation of tumor size with local failure following primary radiotherapy alone [4, 6], we chose to administer vismodegib *concurrently* with electron beam radiation in the primary treatment of a patient with multiple extremely large BCC tumors of the torso. Previous reports have shown concurrent therapy to be effective in either the recurrent or metastatic setting [7, 8], but concurrent therapy has not been previously reported for upfront treatment until this case.

2. Case Presentation

2.1. Presentation. A male mason in his fifties presented with pain, shortness of breath, easy fatigability, generalized weakness, lightheadedness, and twenty-pound weight loss. He reported bleeding over several years from multiple skin lesions of the anterior (15 × 9 cm) and posterior (15 × 12.5 cm) right shoulder, right chest (6 × 7 cm), right neck (1 × 1 cm),

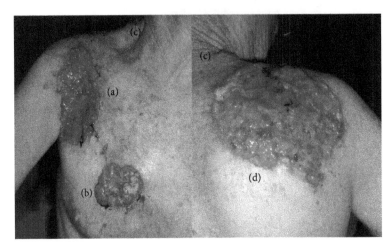

FIGURE 1: Large ulcerative lesions of the right thorax, with subcutaneous fat layer exposed, upon presentation: anterior upper ((a), size 15 × 9 cm), anterior lower ((b), 6 × 7 cm), and lower neck seen both in anterior and posterior views ((c), 1 × 1 cm) and the back ((d), 15 × 12.5 cm). One additional lesion in the left back (3.5 × 2 cm) is not shown. There is evidence of invasion to the underlying muscle (a, d) and pronounced nodularity (a, c, d).

and left back (3.5 × 2 cm) that correlated with significant occupational ultraviolet light exposure (see Figure 1). His hemoglobin on admission was 3.1 g/dL. The origin of the patient's severe anemia and associated constitutional symptoms was consistent with chronic bleeding from multifocal skin cancer. He was resuscitated with 7 units of packed red blood cells and metastatic work-up, consisting of computed tomography of the chest abdomen and pelvis, was negative. Pathologic biopsy of two lesions revealed ulcerated BCC, usual and infiltrating types. Surgical resection was not technically feasible due the extremely large skin surface area involved with deep muscle invasion. In multidisciplinary consultation with dermatology, radiation oncology, and medical oncology, concurrent radiation and vismodegib were recommended. The patient provided informed consent for the treatment modality as well as for being the subject for this case report.

2.2. Treatment. Radiotherapy was delivered using mixed six- and nine-mega-electron-volt (MeV) energy electrons to 66 Gray (Gy) in 2 Gy fractions (33 fractions) prescribed to the 90% isodose line to five separate lesions on the right and left back, right neck, and right anterior chest wall. Radiation was started urgently due to severe pain and bleeding. He was planned for upfront concurrent vismodegib (150 mg) which was initiated immediately following insurance approval, 3 weeks into his radiation treatment, on fraction 16 of 33. Following treatment, the patient reported nearly complete resolution of pain and bleeding, with significant regression of all treated lesions. One lesion, on the inferior right chest wall, had residual nodularity and was boosted to a total of 76 Gy with four additional 2.5 Gy fractions three weeks after finishing his initial radiation. During his course of radiation, the patient was treated with antibiotic therapy for secondary impetigo.

Vismodegib was continued adjuvantly for three months, until discontinuation due to development of grade 3 diarrhea.

His diarrhea was likely multifactorial since it resolved with discontinuation of vismodegib and successful treatment of *Clostridium difficile* colitis. Vismodegib was restarted after a 2-month break, initially on an every-other-day schedule for 1 month, and then increasing to once daily for 2 months, until GI upset recurred and the medication was discontinued.

By 6 months following radiation treatment, all lesions showed complete response with near-complete skin closure (Figure 2). The patient reported no residual pain but had moderate residual impairment in right shoulder abduction secondary to fibrosis of the skin/soft tissues and/or initial muscle involvement. Healing was achieved with the careful attention of a dedicated wound care service through the university hospital wound care center. The patient was followed for a period of 10 months. The largest ulcers on the right chest (a) and right upper back (d) were measured at 15 cm × 9 cm × 0.3 cm and 15 cm × 12.5 cm × 0.2 cm initially. They were treated with serial surgical debridement in the outpatient setting initially weekly and then biweekly. In addition, a moisture retentive dressing with antimicrobial/antifungal properties was applied every other day. Finally, a placenta derived tissue substitute application was used at 6 months. This resulted in objectively decreasing surface area to the point of complete healing. Following healing, the patient was to practice good skin care including application of moisturizing lotion twice daily.

3. Discussion

Radiation therapy (RT) is an extremely effective modality for BCC; however efficacy decreases with advanced lesions. Larger tumor size correlates with lower frequency of achieving complete remission (complete disappearance of the lesion upon first follow-up), showing only 70% complete remission for extensive BCCs [4]. Additionally, whereas typical BCC lesions treated with RT show a 5-year cure rate of 84–96%, this rate seems to decrease significantly with very large

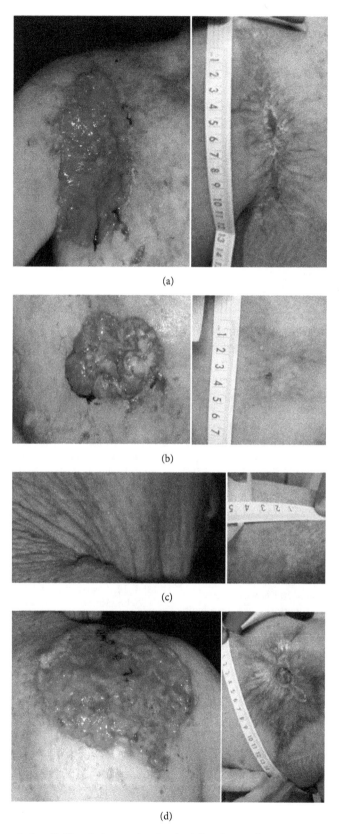

FIGURE 2: Lesions of the right thorax before (left) and six months after (right) radiation showing excellent response to radiation (66–76 Gy) with concurrent and adjuvant vismodegib: (anterior upper (a); anterior lower (b); lower neck (c); and back (d)). All lesions completely resolved with complete skin closure, including an additional left back lesion (not shown).

tumors to as low as 55%[4]. More aggressive types of BCC (including infiltrative BCC, as seen in our patient) are likely a contributing factor to the worse 5-year cure rates seen in advanced BCC [4].

Due to the aggressive nature of the BCC in our patient (size and histology) and the lower cure rates in such cases, we chose combined modality treatment using definitive radiotherapy with concurrent and adjuvant vismodegib. Vismodegib's efficacy following RT in locally advanced BCC is reported to be only 43% [5]. Our hope with this patient's treatment plan was that combining vismodegib and RT *concurrently* might prove more efficacious. We performed several PubMed searches to examine any evidence for concurrent vismodegib and RT and found one report (two patients) by Pollom et al. which showed efficacy for concurrent external beam radiation and vismodegib in the recurrent setting [7, 8]. Our case differs in its multifocal nature, higher burden of disease, and upfront (rather than recurrent) setting. To our knowledge, our case represents the first report of upfront definitive treatment for advanced BCC using concurrent RT and vismodegib. Even with the patient's extensive tumor volume, occupying an estimated 10–15% of the thorax skin surface area, complete remission and wound closure were achieved for all lesions.

Vismodegib is currently approved for patients with metastatic or locally advanced BCC who are not candidates for or who have had disease recurrence after surgery and/or radiation therapy [5]. Little is known about the interaction of radiation with vismodegib. Duration-limiting side effects have been well-documented with the use of vismodegib [5]. Combining treatment with radiation therapy may prove helpful since long-term treatment with vismodegib may not be realistic. This patient tolerated a total of six months of vismodegib with a two-month vismodegib-free vacation in the middle and using every-other-day dosing when restarting the treatment. The patient discontinued vismodegib twice due to GI upset. However, it is notable that the wounds showed significant improvement after vismodegib was restarted. The hedgehog pathway has been implicated in the wound healing process and it has previously been suggested that vismodegib may have potential to exacerbate radiation's side effect of slow wound healing [8, 9]. However this is contrary to our case, where the patient's extensive wounds healed entirely after combined vismodegib and radiation therapy. It is noted that this patient saw wound care first weekly and then twice monthly, which certainly contributed to his successful wound healing.

There is currently an open phase II trial investigating the safety and tolerability of combined vismodegib and radiotherapy in the setting of locally advanced head and neck basal cell carcinoma with neck nodal involvement. Our case report demonstrates the tolerability and efficacy of definitive doses of radiation to large areas of skin with concurrent vismodegib in treating multifocal large inoperable BCCs. It should be noted that the patient did not undergo rebiopsy or reimaging studies following his treatment; however, the patient was followed clinically until disappearance of all visible tumor and complete skin healing. This is our standard surveillance regimen for primary radiation, where we reserve biopsy for cases of incomplete response

Conflicts of Interest

The authors declare that there are no conflicts of interest regarding the publication of this article.

References

[1] G. Goldenberg, T. Karagiannis, J. B. Palmer et al., "Incidence and prevalence of basal cell carcinoma (BCC) and locally advanced BCC (LABCC) in a large commercially insured population in the United States: a retrospective cohort study," *Journal of the American Academy of Dermatology*, vol. 75, no. 5, pp. 957–966.e2, 2016.

[2] N. W. J. Smeets, G. A. M. Krekels, J. U. Ostertag et al., "Surgical excision vs Mohs' micrographic surgery for basal-cell carcinoma of the face: randomised controlled trial," *The Lancet*, vol. 364, no. 9447, pp. 1766–1772, 2004.

[3] M. K. Silverman, A. W. Kopf, C. M. Grin, R. S. Bart, and M. J. Levenstein, "Recurrence rates of treated basal cell carcinomas: part 1: overview," *The Journal of Dermatologic Surgery and Oncology*, vol. 17, no. 9, pp. 713–718, 1991.

[4] R. Piccinno, S. Benardon, F. M. Gaiani, M. Rozza, and M. Caccialanza, "Dermatologic radiotherapy in the treatment of extensive basal cell carcinomas: a retrospective study," *Journal of Dermatological Treatment*, vol. 28, no. 5, pp. 426–430, 2017.

[5] A. Sekulic, M. R. Migden, and A. E. Oro, "Efficacy and safety of vismodegib in advanced basal-cell carcinoma," *The New England Journal of Medicine*, vol. 366, no. 23, pp. 2171–2179, 2012.

[6] J. Locke, S. Karimpour, G. Young, M. A. Lockett, and C. A. Perez, "Radiotherapy for epithelial skin cancer," *International Journal of Radiation Oncology & Biology & Physics*, vol. 51, no. 3, pp. 748–755, 2001.

[7] E. L. Pollom, T. T. Bui, A. L. Chang, A. D. Colevas, and W. Y. Hara, "Concurrent vismodegib and radiotherapy for recurrent, advanced basal cell carcinoma," *JAMA Dermatology*, vol. 151, no. 9, pp. 998–1001, 2015.

[8] J. M. Strasswimmer, "Potential synergy of radiation therapy with vismodegib for basal cell carcinoma," *JAMA Dermatology*, vol. 151, no. 9, pp. 925-926, 2015.

[9] A. C. D. O. Gonzalez, Z. D. A. Andrade, T. F. Costa, and A. R. A. P. Medrado, "Wound healing—a literature review," *Anais Brasileiros de Dermatologia*, vol. 91, no. 5, pp. 614–620, 2016.

36

Drug Hypersensitivity due to Azathioprine with Elevated Procalcitonin

Tania Ahuja ⓘ,[1] Frank R. Chung,[2] and Tania Ruiz-Maya[3]

[1]New York University Langone Health, Department of Pharmacy, 550 First Avenue, New York, NY 10016, USA
[2]New York University School of Medicine, 550 First Avenue, New York, NY 10016, USA
[3]New York University Langone Health, Department of Medicine, 550 First Avenue, New York, NY 10016, USA

Correspondence should be addressed to Tania Ahuja; tania.ahuja@nyumc.org

Academic Editor: Alireza Firooz

We present a case of azathioprine hypersensitivity presenting as sepsis with elevated procalcitonin in a 68-year-old man with myasthenia gravis. The patient presented with fever, chills, nausea, vomiting, and headache. He developed numerous 1 cm erythematous papules over his upper torso. Infectious workup including bacteriological tests and microbial cultures was negative and a skin biopsy was performed which revealed suppurative folliculitis with eosinophils, consistent with drug hypersensitivity. Notably, acute phase reactants including C-reactive protein and procalcitonin were elevated upon presentation, likely secondary to drug hypersensitivity.

1. Background

Azathioprine is an immunosuppressant used in the treatment of various autoimmune conditions, including myasthenia gravis. Azathioprine immune hypersensitivity reaction is a rare adverse effect that has been reported in the literature relatively infrequently; however, the clinical presentation can often mimic sepsis [1, 2]. A review of case reports suggests that azathioprine-induced hypersensitivity reactions most commonly present with fever, chills, rigors, and/or gastrointestinal symptoms [1–7]. Clinicians should become familiar with the clinical presentation to recognize the symptoms and avoid early misdiagnosis.

2. Case Presentation

A 68-year-old man who was diagnosed with myasthenia gravis three months prior to admission presented with acute nonpruritic painless 1 cm erythematous papules over the upper torso, accompanied with subjective fevers, chills, nausea, vomiting, and frontal headache for 2 days. His past medical history was significant for heart failure with preserved ejection fraction of 65% and mechanical mitral valve replacement for which he was on warfarin. He was

started on prednisone 40 mg daily and pyridostigmine 120 mg four times daily, two and a half months prior to admission, and azathioprine 150 mg daily, 10 days prior to admission. Upon presentation, he was found to have a temperature of 102.7 degrees Fahrenheit, with a heart rate of 107 beats per minute, blood pressure of 159/87 mmHg, and oxygen saturation of 95% on room air.

A complete blood count with differential was remarkable for a white blood cell count of 15,000 cells/mm^3, with 89% neutrophils and venous lactate of 2.6 mmol/L. All other laboratory parameters including electrolytes, blood urea nitrogen, creatinine, blood glucose, and liver function tests were within normal limits. Given the fever, leukocytosis, and elevated lactate, the initial concern was for sepsis. Infectious workup included blood cultures, chest X-ray, urinalysis with urine culture, respiratory viral panel, Lyme titers, and procalcitonin. The chest X-ray showed a possible new left lower lobe basilar opacity, procalcitonin was 0.59 ng/mL, and the patient was started on antibiotics with ceftriaxone and azithromycin for suspected lower respiratory tract infection. Of note, his azathioprine was discontinued on presentation, due to concern for continued immunosuppression and possible infection. Two days after presentation, given the improvement in clinical symptoms the azathioprine 150 mg

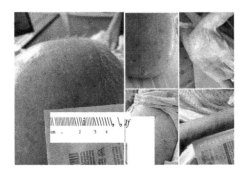

FIGURE 1: Clinical presentation: firm, indurated, erythematous papules, and nodules, with central pustules and vesicles on the head and scalp. Indurated papules on the palms of the hand. Erythematous pustules on the abdomen.

was reinitiated. Within a few hours, he became acutely ill, febrile to 103.7 degrees Fahrenheit and tachycardic to 115 beats per minute, with return of the initial presenting symptoms and new onset photophobia. Initially, there was concern for worsening sepsis; repeat procalcitonin was ordered along with C-reactive protein and erythrocyte sedimentation rate (ESR), with antimicrobial therapy broadened to vancomycin, piperacillin/tazobactam, and intravenous acyclovir. Notably, a diffuse 1 cm papulopustular rash erupted over the scalp, head, neck, thorax, abdomen, and upper and lower extremities including the palmar and dorsal aspects of the hand (Figure 1). As the cutaneous findings were nonspecific, the differential remained broad and infectious workup included bacterial, fungal, viral, or drug hypersensitivity. Drug hypersensitivity was suspected given the return of symptoms along with rash after rechallenge of azathioprine and the temporal response to the symptoms. The repeat procalcitonin was now elevated further to 5.36 ng/mL along with an elevated C-reactive protein of >270 mg/L and an ESR of 44 mm/hr.

The azathioprine was discontinued and the symptoms subsided with the pustules reduced in size and number. Biopsy of the pustule showed suppurative folliculitis, which is expected from a neutrophil driven process, consistent with azathioprine hypersensitivity (Figure 2). All pustule stains, bacterial, viral, including herpes zoster and varicella zoster, and periodic acid-Schiff-diastase (PAS-D) stains, were negative. Repeat liver function tests including AST/ALT remained within normal limits, and a complete blood count revealed a white blood cell count of 9,300 cells/mm^3 with 0% eosinophils. Antimicrobial therapy was deescalated. Over the next few days, the rash and symptoms resolved and the CRP decreased to 108 g/L. We utilized the Naranjo algorithm to estimate the probability of azathioprine causing hypersensitivity and found that our patient had a probable hypersensitivity reaction to azathioprine [8].

3. Discussion

Drug hypersensitivity syndrome (DHS) is often reported in patients treated with aromatic antiepileptic drugs and in rare cases with azathioprine [9]. The predominant cutaneous reaction reported in the literature is a neutrophilic dermatosis [9].

Other cutaneous effects may include an erythematous macular or maculopapular eruption and purpuric or petechial lesions [2, 7]. Azathioprine inhibits DNA and RNA synthesis and is used in a multitude of conditions from inflammatory bowel disease to autoimmune diseases such as connective tissue disease, rheumatoid arthritis, and myasthenia gravis amongst other things. It is a purine antagonist that is metabolized by thiopurine methyltransferase (TPMT) to the active compound, 6-mercaptopurine; however this metabolism seems to be unrelated to the incidence of hypersensitivity [10]. Furthermore, azathioprine has an inactive metabolite, methyl nitroimidazole, which may be responsible for the hypersensitivity reactions due to the generation of a hapten during metabolism [4, 9, 11, 12]. Although rare, there have been about 70 cases of azathioprine-induced hypersensitivity reported in the literature thus far, with concurrent corticosteroids at presentation being present in 39% of patients [9]. The onset of symptoms presented anywhere from 3-4 days of initiation of azathioprine, with 49% of patients exhibiting cutaneous findings suggesting a drug-induced acneiform and folliculitis eruption [9]. Although the systemic symptoms of azathioprine hypersensitivity include fever, chills, arthralgias, myalgias, leukocytosis, and cutaneous eruptions, other laboratory parameters may be unremarkable [1, 9]. Of note, the possibility of disseminated herpes or zoster should be considered in immunosuppressed patients hospitalized with acute folliculitis. It is critical to obtain a skin swab from the base of an intact unproofed pustule to submit for HSV and VZV PCR, as was done in our case, despite the pustular morphology. In addition, a bedside Tzanck smear is a rapid test and the dermatopathologist may find evidence of viral cytopathic changes. These findings were not found in our patient.

On initial presentation, azathioprine hypersensitivity may be confused with infection, as was the case in our patient. We observed an elevated procalcitonin in our patient, which has been identified as a biomarker to differentiate bacterial infections from viral infections and noninfectious inflammatory conditions [13]. For sepsis, procalcitonin, along with other diagnostic tools and physical examination, has been found to be more sensitive and more specific than other biomarkers, including CRP and lactate [13, 14]. Therefore, procalcitonin is often checked in patients that present with a sepsis like picture at our institution in the emergency room. However, elevations in acute phase reactants, such as procalcitonin, may lead to misdiagnosis and delay in management of drug related hypersensitivity reactions. In one retrospective review of drug reactions with eosinophilia and systemic symptoms, procalcitonin was found to be elevated to levels normally seen in bacterial infections or sepsis [15]. Similarly, we found that procalcitonin levels were elevated alongside other acute phase reactants, despite having a nonbacterial etiology and suspected drug hypersensitivity. This suggests that an elevated procalcitonin must be interpreted with caution in patients who may have proinflammatory etiologies beyond infections, such as hypersensitivity reactions, as this may result in anchoring and delay prompt diagnosis of the true etiology. While further studies are needed to determine the relationship between procalcitonin and drug hypersensitivity,

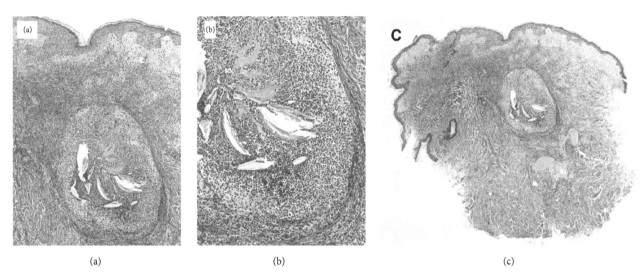

FIGURE 2: Histopathological features. (a) Lesion of acute ruptured suppurative folliculitis. Papillary dermal edema and neutrophilic dermal infiltration. (b) Dense netrophilic infiltrate in the follicle. (c) Lesion of acute suppurative folliculitis.

this report illustrates the need for clinical suspicion for a drug-induced hypersensitivity syndrome in patients started on azathioprine presenting with a sepsis like syndrome.

Other acute phase reactants that may be elevated with drug hypersensitivity include C-reactive protein and ESR, as was the case in our patient. Further, azathioprine hypersensitivity is often suspected upon resuming or rechallenge with azathioprine, where symptoms may recur within hours of the dose [16], consistent with our patient. Although he was not prescribed azathioprine on admission to the hospital, given the suspicion for sepsis, azathioprine was reinitiated in the hospital with return of symptoms. The timing of presentation with azathioprine hypersensitivity is critical to the diagnosis to distinguish from other idiosyncratic drug reactions such as DRESS (Drug Reaction with Eosinophilia and Systemic Symptom) [16]. Patients often present within 4 weeks of initiation of azathioprine and symptoms resolve within 7 days of drug cessation, with symptoms returning within hours of rechallenge [16], as was seen in our case. Given the severity of the reaction, patients that experience fever, hypotension, or a severe reaction should not be rechallenged [1, 16, 17].

In conclusion, we report a case of azathioprine hypersensitivity with cutaneous manifestations of neutrophilic dermatoses along with elevated serum CRP and procalcitonin. Early recognition of the signs and symptoms of azathioprine hypersensitivity may help clinicians in detecting and preventing further sequelae. Further analyses are required to determine the correlation of these acute phase reactants with the severity and outcome of hypersensitivity to medications.

Conflicts of Interest

All authors state that they have no conflicts of interest or financial disclosures.

Authors' Contributions

T. Ahuja, Frank R. Chung, and T. Ruiz-Maya were all clinical providers for the patient and major contributors in writing the manuscript. All authors read and approved the final manuscript.

References

[1] S. R. Knowles, A. K. Gupta, N. H. Shear, and D. Sauder, "Azathioprine hypersensitivity-like reactions - A case report and a review of the literature," *Clinical and Experimental Dermatology*, vol. 20, no. 4, pp. 353–356, 1995.

[2] M. E. C. Jeurissen, A. M. T. Boerbooms, L. B. A. Van De Putte, and M. W. M. Kruijsen, "Azathioprine induced fever, chills, rash, and hepatotoxicity in rheumatoid arthritis," *Annals of the Rheumatic Diseases*, vol. 49, no. 1, pp. 25–27, 1990.

[3] J. F. Assini, R. Hamilton, and J. M. Strosberg, "Adverse reactions to azathioprine mimicking gastroenteritis," *The Journal of Rheumatology*, vol. 13, no. 6, pp. 1117-1118, 1986.

[4] G. F. Watts and R. Corston, "Hypersensitivity to azathioprine in myasthenia gravis," *Postgraduate Medical Journal*, vol. 60, no. 703, pp. 362-363, 1984.

[5] B. E. Wilson and J. Parsonnet, "Azathioprine Hypersensitivity Mimicking Sepsis in a Patient with Crohn's Disease," *Clinical Infectious Diseases*, vol. 17, no. 5, pp. 940-941, 1993.

[6] P. Anthony Saway, L. W. Heck, J. R. Bonner, and J. K. Kirklin, "Azathioprine hypersensitivity. Case report and review of the literature," *American Journal of Medicine*, vol. 84, no. 5, pp. 960–964, 1988.

[7] S. M. Bergman, N. K. Krane, G. Leonard, M. C. Soto-Aguilar, and J. D. Wallin, "Azathioprine and Hypersensitivity Vasculitis," *Annals of Internal Medicine*, vol. 109, no. 1, pp. 83-84, 1988.

[8] C. A. Naranjo, U. Busto, and E. M. Sellers, "A method for estimating the probability of adverse drug reactions," *Clinical Pharmacology & Therapeutics*, vol. 30, no. 2, pp. 239–245, 1981.

[9] J. J. Bidinger, K. Sky, D. F. Battafarano, and J. S. Henning, "The cutaneous and systemic manifestations of azathioprine

hypersensitivity syndrome," *Journal of the American Academy of Dermatology*, vol. 65, no. 1, pp. 184–191, 2011.

[10] E. Yiasemides and G. Thom, "Azathioprine hypersensitivity presenting as a neutrophilic dermatosis in a man with ulcerative colitis," *Australasian Journal of Dermatology*, vol. 50, no. 1, pp. 48–51, 2009.

[11] M. Aleissa, P. Nicol, M. Godeau et al., "Azathioprine Hypersensitivity Syndrome: Two Cases of Febrile Neutrophilic Dermatosis Induced by Azathioprine," *Case Reports in Dermatology*, vol. 9, no. 1, pp. 6–11, 2017.

[12] M. Davis, A. L. Eddleston, and R. Williams, "Hypersensitivity and jaundice due to azathioprine.," *Postgraduate Medical Journal*, vol. 56, no. 654, pp. 274-275, 1980.

[13] C. Wacker, A. Prkno, F. M. Brunkhorst, and P. Schlattmann, "Procalcitonin as a diagnostic marker for sepsis: a systematic review and meta-analysis," *The Lancet Infectious Diseases*, vol. 13, no. 5, pp. 426–435, 2013.

[14] A. Kutz, B. Mueller, P. Schuetz et al., "Prognostic value of procalcitonin in respiratory tract infections across clinical settings," *Critical Care*, vol. 19, no. Suppl 1, p. P65, 2015.

[15] A. Taegtmeyer, A. Bravo, B. Zimmermanns, E. Liakoni, S. Kraehenbuehl, and M. Haschke, "C-reactive protein and procalcitonin in patients with DRESS syndrome," *Clinical and Translational Allergy*, vol. 4, no. Suppl 3, p. P12, 2014.

[16] A. James, J. Blagojevic, S. W. Benham, R. Cornall, and J. Frater, "Azathioprine hypersensitivity presenting as septic shock with encephalopathy," *BMJ Case Reports*, 2013.

[17] S. Knowles and N. H. Shear, "Azathioprine hypersensitivity reactions: Caution upon rechallenge," *Muscle & Nerve*, vol. 20, no. 11, pp. 1467-1468, 1997.

37

Skin Lesions Associated with Nutritional Management of Maple Syrup Urine Disease

Jaraspong Uaariyapanichkul,[1,2] Puthita Saengpanit,[2] Ponghatai Damrongphol,[3,4] Kanya Suphapeetiporn,[3,4] and Sirinuch Chomtho[1]

[1]Division of Nutrition, Department of Pediatrics, Faculty of Medicine, Chulalongkorn University, Bangkok 10330, Thailand
[2]Division of Nutrition, Department of Pediatrics, King Chulalongkorn Memorial Hospital, The Thai Red Cross Society, Bangkok 10330, Thailand
[3]Center of Excellence for Medical Genetics, Department of Pediatrics, Faculty of Medicine, Chulalongkorn University, Bangkok 10330, Thailand
[4]Excellence Center for Medical Genetics, King Chulalongkorn Memorial Hospital, The Thai Red Cross Society, Bangkok 10330, Thailand

Correspondence should be addressed to Sirinuch Chomtho; sirinuch.c@chula.ac.th

Academic Editor: Alireza Firooz

Introduction. Maple syrup urine disease (MSUD) is an inborn error of branched chain amino acids (BCAAs) metabolism. We report an infant with MSUD who developed 2 episodes of cutaneous lesions as a result of isoleucine deficiency and zinc deficiency, respectively. *Case Presentation.* A 12-day-old male infant was presented with poor milk intake and lethargy. The diagnosis of MSUD was made based on clinical and biochemical data. *Management and Outcome.* Specific dietary restriction of BCAAs was given. Subsequently, natural protein was stopped as the patient developed hospital-acquired infections which resulted in an elevation of BCAAs. Acrodermatitis dysmetabolica developed and was confirmed to be from isoleucine deficiency. At the age of 6 months, the patient developed severe lethargy and was on natural protein exclusion for an extended period. Despite enteral supplementation of zinc sulfate, cutaneous manifestations due to zinc deficiency occurred. *Discussion.* Skin lesions in MSUD patients could arise from multiple causes. Nutritional deficiency including isoleucine and zinc deficiencies can occur and could complicate the treatment course as a result of malabsorption, even while on enteral supplementation. Parenteral nutrition should be considered and initiated accordingly. Clinical status, as well as BCAA levels, should be closely monitored in MSUD patients.

1. Introduction

Maple syrup urine disease (MSUD; OMIM# 248600) is an autosomal recessive inborn error of metabolism, which can be managed by specific dietary modifications of branched chain amino acid intake. The incidence of MSUD is approximately 1 in 185,000 worldwide [1]. Although each disorder of inborn errors of metabolism is individually rare, their cumulative incidence is substantial (an incidence of 1 in 2,500–5,000 live births) and has been shown to be upwards of 1 in 800 [2].

We report an infant with MSUD who developed cutaneous lesions as a result of isoleucine deficiency while on dietary management. The skin lesions resolved after addition of isoleucine to the diet with normalization of isoleucine levels. We also report subsequent cutaneous lesions as a result of zinc deficiency during the following episode of treatment.

2. Case Report

A 12-day-old male Indian infant was referred to a tertiary care hospital due to poor milk intake and lethargy. The patient was a full-term neonate with an uncomplicated delivery, without any family history of metabolic disorder or consanguinity. The disease started 3 days earlier and the infant was previously admitted to a private hospital and received intravenous antibiotics for the treatment of presumed neonatal sepsis, but

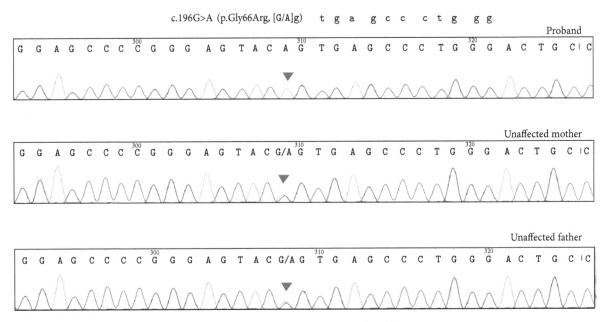

c.196G>A (p.Gly66Arg, [G/A]g)   t g a   g c c   c t g   g g

FIGURE 1: Electropherogram of the proband and his parents.

without any improvement. Initial biochemical investigations showed ketonuria, no metabolic acidosis, normoglycemia, and a mildly elevated level of ammonia (125 μmol/L). Microbiological examinations were all negative. Upon arrival, the patient had seizure and was intubated.

Further biochemical study with plasma amino acid analysis showed a leucine level of 4163.6 μmol/L (reference values: 42–133.1 μmol/L), isoleucine of 499.8 μmol/L (15.1–74.9 μmol/L), and valine of 784.3 μmol/L (73.6–273.1 μmol/L). Thus, the diagnosis of MSUD (maple syrup urine disease) was made based on clinical and biochemical data.

Whole exome sequencing revealed a novel homozygous missense variant c.196G>A (p.Gly66Arg) in the branched chain keto acid dehydrogenase E1 subunit beta *(BCKDHB)* gene. The variant was confirmed by PCR-Sanger sequencing to be homozygous in the patient and heterozygous in both parents (Figure 1).

Initial treatment included intravenous fluid and glucose with the aim to provide adequate energy to reduce catabolism and cessation of protein intake for 48–72 hours, administration of cofactors including thiamine, and adjunct treatment of neurological complications. Specific dietary restriction of branched chain amino acids (BCAAs) by using a branched chain-free amino acid supplement was given at the age of 17 days together with expressed breast milk as a source of natural protein via nasogastric tube.

On day 36, natural protein was stopped as the patient developed hospital-acquired pneumonia and diarrhea which resulted in an elevation of BCAAs. On day 45, multiple discrete erythematous macules and papules appeared on the skin of the forehead, hemorrhagic crusts at both upper and lower lips, as well as well-defined erythematous patches at both cheeks, flexor part of neck, forearms, upper anterior

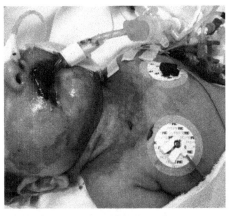

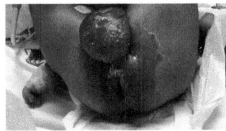

FIGURE 2: Skin lesions in the perioral, cheeks, neck, upper anterior chest wall, and perianal regions seen in an MSUD infant with isoleucine deficiency.

chest wall, and perianal regions which rapidly progressed (Figure 2).

The amino acid profile revealed an isoleucine level of 5.9 μmol/L, leucine of 1166 μmol/L, and valine of 159 μmol/L. The serum zinc level was normal (74 μg/dL). Mycological and microbiological examinations were performed and showed negative results. A final diagnosis of acrodermatitis dysmetabolica due to isoleucine deficiency was made based on the clinical findings and low isoleucine levels through this period. Expressed breast milk was added to the feeds with isoleucine supplementation of 100 mg/day. The patient had been on continuous venovenous hemofiltration for a 48-hour period to reduce elevated leucine levels. In addition, skin care with emollients was administered. The patient showed a rapid improvement in the skin lesions which started to recover within 2 days and healed in 10 days with no hyperpigmentation. Subsequent amino acid profile showed an increment of isoleucine to a normal level (45.97 μmol/L).

After hospital discharge, the feeding regimens were continued with branched chain-free amino acid supplement and expressed breast milk with supplementation of isoleucine 100 mg/day and valine 50 mg/day to prevent the deficiency, which yielded total energy of 130 kcal/kg/day, total protein of 3 g/kg/day, leucine, isoleucine, and valine of 50 mg/kg/day each.

A subsequent episode of cutaneous manifestations occurred at the age of 6 months. The patient developed severe lethargy. Leucine encephalopathy was initially suspected and dietary management with cessation of natural protein intake was started as a part of the MSUD emergency protocol. Despite receiving seemingly adequate energy (110 kcal/kg/day) and protein intake from branched chain-free amino acid supplement (3 g/kg/day), the patient's level of consciousness was slow to improve and he was on natural protein exclusion for an extended period despite continuing isoleucine and valine supplementation. A complication of parainfluenza infection and a significant period of diarrhea soon followed and he had been on enteral supplementation of zinc sulfate 2 mg/kg/day together with other micronutrients supplementation. Ten days after admission, disseminated brown maculopapular exanthem appeared on the skin of the extremities, as well as well-defined erythematous patches on the perianal region (Figure 3).

Isoleucine deficiency was initially suspected; however, the amino acid profile later still showed elevated levels of branched chain amino acids with leucine of 533.25 μmol/L (41.63–189.6 μmol/L), isoleucine of 490.53 μmol/L (18.37–72.26 μmol/L), and valine of 400.05 μmol/L (78.57–263.66 μmol/L). Hence, in this subsequent episode of cutaneous manifestation, zinc deficiency causing acrodermatitis enteropathica was confirmed as the serum zinc level was low (56.9 μg/dL) despite continued supplementation.

Skin lesions showed no significant improvement after an increased dosage of enteral chelated zinc to 4 mg/kg/day. Parenteral nutrition with added zinc was then given intravenously due to suspected malabsorption. However, the skin lesions continued to worsen with desquamation in the following week. The patient became edematous, also suspected to be from protein deficiency as a result of malabsorption during the course of treatment (Figure 4). Albumin transfusion, parenteral nutrition containing limited amount of amino acids (based on leucine intake), and extra zinc were given along with branched chain-free amino acid supplement and led to his recovery.

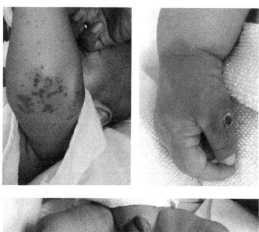

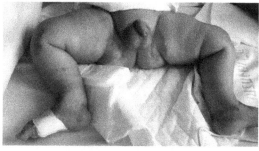

FIGURE 3: Skin lesions on the extremities and perianal region seen in an MSUD patient with zinc deficiency.

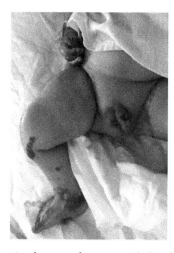

FIGURE 4: The patient became edematous with skin desquamation in the extremities and perianal region during the course of treatment.

3. Discussion

Dietary restriction of BCAAs (leucine, valine, and isoleucine) while avoiding their deficiency, maintaining growth and nutritional status, and avoiding catabolism is the mainstay of nutritional therapy in MSUD [3]. The aim is to maintain plasma BCAA concentrations within a target treatment range that is not associated with neurotoxicity [3].

The patient developed isoleucine deficiency and presented with skin lesions of acrodermatitis dysmetabolica. These cutaneous lesions have been described during treatment of aminoacidopathies (MSUD) [4, 5] and organic acidemias (methylmalonic acidemia, glutaric aciduria, and propionic acidemia) [6, 7] due to deficiency of isoleucine. It has been called acrodermatitis acidemica [6–10] or acrodermatitis dysmetabolica [10, 11]. Other nutritional causes have also been described such as biotin and free fatty acid deficiency [12]. Moreover, inadequate intake of BCAAs can also induce exfoliative erythroderma in MSUD infants [13].

In Thailand, MSUD patients have been diagnosed; however, there is no report in details regarding the complication of skin manifestations. Our patient had the clinical profile and responded to treatment similar to the cases with isoleucine deficiency described previously. Treatment options to prevent deficiency of branched chain amino acids include supplementation with specific amino acid powder, supplementation of expressed breast milk, or infant formula with known amino acid concentration as sources of natural protein. It is also necessary to frequently monitor the patients to optimize their growth and dietary intake and ensure normal levels of branched chain amino acids.

During the treatment course, skin lesions can develop. It is essential to be aware of their causes such as zinc deficiency and specific amino acid deficiency despite enteral supplementation. Malabsorption can occur, especially during and after an episode of diarrhea or infection. For this patient, parenteral nutrition is delayed during the turnaround time for laboratory reports of plasma amino acids and zinc which were not readily available in Thailand. We believe that this scenario is still pertinent with other developing countries as well. Nevertheless, we do hope that, by learning from this case, caregivers will become more aware of these complications and may lead to better care for patients with inborn errors of metabolism, especially regarding earlier initiation of parenteral nutrition.

4. Learning Points

(i) Skin lesions in MSUD patients could arise from multiple causes.

(ii) Nutritional deficiency including isoleucine, zinc, and protein deficiency can occur and could complicate the treatment course, even while on enteral supplementation as a result of malabsorption. Parenteral nutrition should be considered and initiated accordingly.

(iii) Clinical status, as well as BCAA levels, should be closely monitored in MSUD patients.

Conflicts of Interest

The authors declare that there are no conflicts of interest regarding the publication of this paper.

References

[1] L. J. Elsas and P. B. Acosta, "Inherited metabolic disease: Amino acids, Organic acids, and Galactose," in *Modern Nutrition in Health and Disease*, A. C. Ross, B. Caballo, R. J. Cousins, K. L. Tucker, and T. R. Ziegler, Eds., pp. 906–969, Lippincott Williams & Wilkin, Philadelphia, Pa, USA, 11th edition, 2014.

[2] C. M. Mak, H.-C. H. Lee, A. Y.-W. Chan, and C.-W. Lam, "Inborn errors of metabolism and expanded newborn screening: Review and update," *Critical Reviews in Clinical Laboratory Sciences*, vol. 50, no. 6, pp. 142–162, 2013.

[3] F. White, "Disorders of amino acid metabolism, organic acidaemias and urea cycle defects; Maple syrup urine disease," in *Clinical Paediatric Dietetics*, V. Shaw and M. Lawson, Eds., pp. 399–403, Blackwell Publishing, Oxford, UK, 4th edition, 2015.

[4] B. Ross, M. Kumar, H. Srinivasan, and A. V. Ekbote, "Isoleucine deficiency in a neonate treated for maple syrup urine disease masquerading as acrodermatitis enteropathica," *Indian Pediatrics*, vol. 53, no. 8, pp. 738–740, 2016.

[5] I. Templier, J.-L. Reymond, M.-A. Nguyen et al., "Acrodermatitis enteropathica-like syndrome secondary to branched-chain amino acid deficiency during treatment of maple syrup urine disease," *Annales de Dermatologie et de Venereologie*, vol. 133, no. 4, pp. 375–379, 2006.

[6] S. Niiyama, S. Koelker, I. Degen, G. F. Hoffmann, R. Happle, and R. Hoffman, "Acrodermatitis acidemica secondary to malnutrition in glutaric aciduria type I," *European Journal of Dermatology*, vol. 11, no. 3, pp. 244–246, 2001.

[7] L. De Raeve, L. De Meirleir, J. Ramet, Y. Vandenplas, and E. Gerlo, "Acrodermatitis enteropathica-like cutaneous lesions in organic aciduria," *Journal of Pediatrics*, vol. 124, no. 3, pp. 416–420, 1994.

[8] A. M. Bosch, J. H. Sillevis Smitt, A. H. Van Gennip et al., "Iatrogenic isolated isoleucine deficiency as the cause of an acrodermatitis enteropathica-like syndrome," *British Journal of Dermatology*, vol. 139, no. 3, pp. 488–491, 1998.

[9] J. J. Domínguez-Cruz, M. Bueno-Delgado, J. Pereyra, J. Bernabeu-Wittel, and J. Conejo-Mir, "Acrodermatitis enerophatica-like skin lesions secondary to isoleucine deficiency," *European Journal of Dermatology*, vol. 21, no. 1, pp. 115-116, 2011.

[10] D. Tabanlioğlu, S. Ersoy-Evans, and A. Karaduman, "Acrodermatitis enteropathica-like eruption in metabolic disorders: Acrodermatitis dysmetabolica is proposed as a better term," *Pediatric Dermatology*, vol. 26, no. 2, pp. 150–154, 2009.

[11] K. Flores, R. Chikowski, and D. S. Morrell, "Acrodermatitis dysmetabolica in an infant with maple syrup urine disease," *Clinical and Experimental Dermatology*, vol. 41, no. 6, pp. 651–654, 2016.

[12] K. A. Gehrig and J. G. H. Dinulos, "Acrodermatitis due to nutritional deficiency," *Current Opinion in Pediatrics*, vol. 22, no. 1, pp. 107–112, 2010.

[13] H. Northrup, E. S. Sigman, and A. A. Hebert, "Exfoliative Erythroderma Resulting From Inadequate Intake of Branched-Chain Amino Acids in Infants With Maple Syrup Urine Disease," *JAMA Dermatology*, vol. 129, no. 3, pp. 384-385, 1993.

38

Different Clinical Features of Acral Abortive Hemangiomas

N. Vega Mata,[1] **J. C. López Gutiérrez,**[2] **B. Vivanco Allende,**[3] **and M. S. Fernández García**[1,3]

[1]*Department of Pediatric Surgery, Hospital Universitario Central de Asturias, Oviedo, Spain*
[2]*Department of Pediatric Surgery, Hospital La Paz, Madrid, Spain*
[3]*Department of Pathology, Hospital Universitario Central de Asturias, Oviedo, Spain*

Correspondence should be addressed to N. Vega Mata; natalizvm@gmail.com

Academic Editor: Masatoshi Jinnin

Some infantile hemangiomas called in literature "minimal or arrested growth hemangiomas" or "abortive hemangiomas" are present at birth and have a proliferative component equaling less than 25% of its total surface area. Often, they are mistaken for vascular malformation. We present five patients (three girls and two boys) with abortive hemangiomas diagnosed between January 2010 and December 2015 localized in acral part of the extremities. They were congenital lesions resembling precursor of hemangiomas but did not show proliferation phase. Immunohistochemical Glut-1 was performed in all of them as a way to confirm the abortive hemangioma diagnosis. The most common appearance was a reticulated erythematous patch with multiple fine telangiectasias on the surface. We remark that one of them presented a segmental patch with two different morphologies and evolutions. The proximal part showed pebbled patches of bright-red hemangioma and presented proliferation and the distal part with a reticulated network-like telangiectasia morphology remained unchanged. We detected lower half of the body preference and dorsal region involvement preference without ventral involvement. The ulceration occurred in three patients with two different degrees of severity.

1. Introduction

Infantile hemangiomas (IH) are the most common tumour of infancy and childhood, usually absent at birth or present as a premonitory mark (e.g., pink macule, telangiectatic patches, or bruise-like area). The hallmarks of IH are their 3 clearly defined stages: they appear in the first weeks of life and undergo a rapid growth phase, followed by a period of slow involution with possible residual lesions [1, 2]. This typical evolution makes them easy to diagnose clinically in most cases. In addition, IH express an erythrocyte-type glucose transport protein (GLUT-1) in their endothelial cells, which is a highly specific marker of IH [1, 3].

Some IH have a proliferative component equaling less than 25% of its total surface area. They resemble premonitory marks and they have been called in medical literature "minimal or arrested growth hemangioma"(IH-MAG) or "abortive hemangiomas." Diagnosis of IH-MAGs can be difficult because they can present as a macular infantile hemangioma with a network-like and blotchy appearance and they are often mistaken for vascular malformation [4]. We describe the clinical, histological, and evolution data of five patients IH-MAGs involving the lower extremities showing atypical and characteristic clinical course. The immunohistochemical Glut-1 confirmed the IH diagnosis. Clinical features, complications, and evolution are analyzed.

2. Methods

We report five patients seen between January 2010 and December 2015 with IH that did not show postnatal proliferation. All patients did not have family history of similar lesions and the rest of their physical examination was normal. We performed a punch biopsy and immunohistochemistry in all cases. GLUT-1 positive immunostaining was seen and it confirmed that it was IH-MAG.

3. Case 1

An 11-month-old Caucasian boy presented at birth an erythematous patch with a network-like and blotchy appearance in the dorsal surface of his right foot that extended onto the

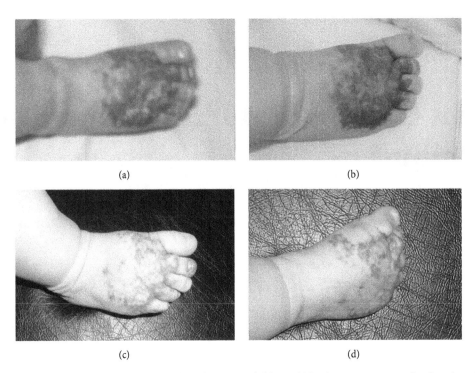

(a)

(b)

(c)

(d)

Figure 1: Case 1. (a) Ulceration on an erythematous patch with a network-like and blotchy appearance in the dorsal surface of the foot of a boy of 3 months. (b) Resolution of the ulceration after 1 month with propranolol treatment. Progressive regression of the lesion at 9 months (c) and 11 months (d).

digits but not to the distal tip (Figure 1). He was born full-term weighing 3240 g, the result of the mother's second pregnancy and an eutocic delivery. The lesion did not proliferate but he was referred to our centre at 3 months of life for a deep ulceration within the erythematous patch. The ulceration did not respond to topical and systemic antibiotic and it produced an important pain. So, a skin biopsy of 5 mm was carried out and the histopathology revealed ectatic vessels in the dermis without lobular pattern. Endothelial cells of these vessels were positive for anti-Glut-1 immunostaining compatible as abortive hemangioma. We initiated treatment with propranolol (3 mg/Kg/day) and the patient presented a good response. The ulcerative lesion healed and the erythematous patch started an involutive evolution without complication.

4. Case 2

A 4-month-old Caucasian baby girl presented at birth an erythematous scaly plaque with geometric border covering all lateral aspect of her right ankle as a sock-like distribution was seen. She was born full-term weighing 3.270 g, the result of the mother's first pregnancy and an eutocic delivery, with no personal or family history of interest. This plaque had bright-red papules, telangiectatic in appearance with a surrounding area darker in colour (Figure 2). The rest of the physical examination was normal. The lesions remained stable and there was no sign of proliferation but over the first week of life the lesion presented numerous superficial ulcerations, resulting in severe pain. A skin biopsy of 5 mm was carried out and the histopathology revealed a hyperkeratosis

epidermis and ectatic vessels in the papillary and reticular dermis without lobular pattern. In the reticular dermis, there were plump endothelial cells and ectatic thin-walled vascular spaces. Endothelial cells were positive for anti-GLUT-1 immunostaining. Due to ulceration, we initiated treatment with propranolol (3 mg/Kg/day) and the patient presented a quick involution of hemangioma for four months. After, she had to discontinue the treatment because of an episode of bronchiolitis and the hemangioma continued with a slowly spontaneous involution. In this moment, she is one and a half years old and she still has residual lesions composed of a reticulated patch with a network-like telangiectasia, a darker periphery with anemic areas, and spontaneous involution is present.

5. Case 3

A 2-month-old Caucasian girl presented at birth an erythematous scaly patch in the dorsal and lateral surface of the left foot extending onto the digits (Figure 3). She was born full-term weighing 3460 g. The plaque did not present proliferation but, as case 2, over the first week of life it presented numerous superficial ulcerations, resulting in severe pain. A skin biopsy of 5 mm was carried out and the histopathology revealed ectatic vessels in the papillary and superficial reticular dermis without a lobular pattern and the anti-GLUT-1 antibody was positive. We initiated treatment with propranolol (3 mg/Kg/day) for 6 months and the patient presented a good response. The ulcerative lesion scared and it started an involutive evolution. In this moment, she presents

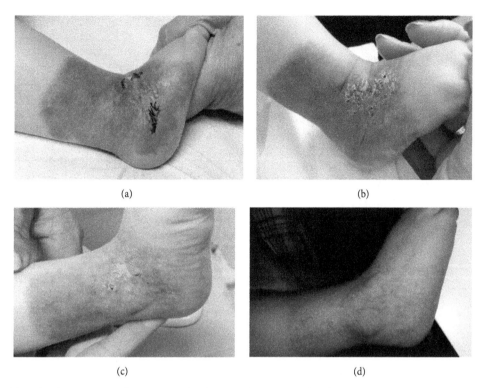

(a)

(b)

(c)

(d)

FIGURE 2: Case 2. (a) A skin biopsy on erythematous scaly plaque with geometric border covering all lateral aspect of her right ankle as a sock-like distribution. (b) Numerous superficial ulcerations of this erythematous scaly plaque. (c) Progressive regression of the lesion and the ulceration with propranolol treatment. (d) Spontaneous involution of the lesion.

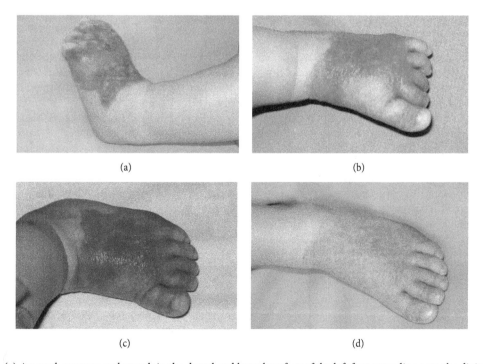

(a)

(b)

(c)

(d)

FIGURE 3: Case 3. (a) An erythematous scaly patch in the dorsal and lateral surface of the left foot extending onto the digits which presented multiple and superficial ulcerations. (b) Response to propranolol after the first month of treatment. (c) Response to propranolol at sixth months of treatment. (d) Spontaneous involution.

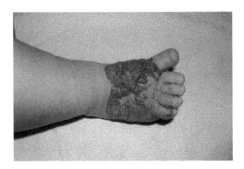

FIGURE 4: Case 4. Pebbled patches of bright-red hemangioma and the distal part extending onto the digits presenting reticulated network-like telangiectasia morphology.

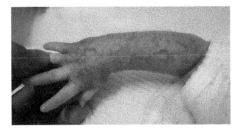

FIGURE 5: Case 5. An erythematous patch with prominent surface telangiectases on the dorsal arm of a 3-month girl.

a residual lesion composed of a reticulated patch with a network-like telangiectasia and spontaneous involution is present.

6. Case 4

An 8-month-old Caucasian boy was referred to our centre for a segmental patch with two different morphologies. The proximal part presented pebbled patches of bright-red hemangioma and the distal part extending onto the digits presented a reticulated network-like telangiectasia morphology (Figure 4). He was born in the 40th week of an uncomplicated pregnancy. The lesion had been present from birth, the proximal part presented proliferation, but the distal part remained unchanged. A proximal and a distal 4 mm punch biopsy were performed and both revealed ectatic vessels in the papillary and superficial reticular dermis with lobular pattern. The endothelial cells of both superficial and deep vessels were positive for anti-GLUT-1 immunostaining. The lesion did not present ulceration. We initiated treatment with propranolol (3 mg/Kg/day) and the hemangioma started a progressive involution but we did not have pictures to show the involution of the lesion because the patient missed the follow-up.

7. Case 5

A 3-month-old Caucasian girl presented at birth an erythematous patch with prominent surface telangiectases on her dorsal arm (Figure 5). She was born at 39 weeks of gestation after an uncomplicated pregnancy. The telangiectatic macule

had remained unchanged but due to family anxiety a biopsy was performed. Histology showed ectatic vessels in the papillary dermis without a lobular pattern and GLUT-1-positive vessels were seen. Then, a reticular abortive hemangioma was diagnosed. The patient was asymptomatic so we decided to maintain an expectant management and wait for a slowly spontaneous involution.

8. Discussion

The characteristic clinical features at birth of IH and of congenital haemangioma are well established. HI are usually absent at birth or present in one-third as a premonitory mark in the form of telangiectatic papules, pale pinkish maculae, or mottled vascular stain. Its hallmark is its rapid postnatal growth beginning 2 weeks after birth and followed by slow involution [2]. However, congenital hemangiomas, both major subtypes RICH and NICH, are fully grown at birth. The regression in RICH usually starts a few days to a few weeks after birth, and complete resolution usually occurs by 14 months. The NICH do not resolve spontaneously and the tumour grows proportionately with the child [5].

In our five cases, the lesions were present at birth and showed neither the typical morphology present in a RICH nor NICH. Then as the clinical presentation was not typical for either a congenital haemangioma or an IH, vascular malformation was considered in the differential diagnosis. A biopsy for histology study and Glut-1 antibody staining was performed in all cases. Glut-1-positive immunostaining was seen, confirming that it was true IH and not congenital hemangioma (RICH or NICH) or vascular malformation [5]. In particular, those lesions present at birth that do not exhibit a postnatal growth were IH-MAG a subtype of IH. GLUT-1 is an established specific marker for IH and is useful in terms of distinguishing it from other paediatric vascular tumours or vascular malformations. It would have been very difficult to differentiate them from vascular malformation without the aid of GLUT-1 staining [3, 4, 6].

We present these five cases of IH-MAGs with three different morphologies localized on acral part of the extremities. The most common appearance was as reticulated erythematous patches with multiple fine telangiectasias on the surface as in cases 2, 3, and 5. The first patient had an erythematous patch with a network-like and blotchy appearance in the dorsal surface of his right foot that extended onto the digits. The fourth case presented a segmental patch with two different morphologies. The proximal part exhibiting pebbled patches of bright-red hemangioma and the distal part extending onto the digits had a reticulated network-like telangiectasia morphology. This last morphology had not been described before and in our experience we have not seen the other two morphologies described in IH-MAGs: grouped telangiectasias overlying normal-appearing skin or bluish plaques with normal or a pale peripheral halo [1].

We reviewed the literature and we detected that IH-MAG frequently involved the lower half of the body (57% [1], 100% [5], 41% [7], 64% [8], and 68% [9]), and a high percentage of them affected acral part. In addition, these acral IH were more likely to have a predominantly reticular morphology.

Suh and Frieden have reported that IH-MAGs were 26 times more likely than IH to appear on the lower half of the body compared with the upper half of the body [10]. Our experience supports this hypothesis as 4 of our 5 cases were located on the foot. We emphasize that all our patients had the dorsal region involved. If we review the literature we realize that hemangiomas in the ventral part of acral extremities present neither arrested growth nor ulceration. Perhaps, the different characteristics of the skin in the dorsal or ventral surface of acral extremities change the evolution of these lesions. Another important characteristic of this subtype of IH was its predominance in girls and Caucasian race. We also support this predilection for the female sex and Caucasian race because three of our patients were females and all of them were Caucasians [10].

The higher incidence of hemangiomas in Caucasian population, females, and premature infants could be related to higher level of renin found in these groups of populations [6]. In fact, some authors have demonstrated the involvement of the renin-angiotensin system (RAS) in the biology of IH. This is based on the expression of angiotensin-converting enzyme and angiotensin II receptor 2 on the endothelium of proliferating IH-derived blast cell proliferation [7]. Certainly, RAS play an important role in the biology of IH and potentially to IH-MAG but more research is still needed in order to elucidate the exact role of RAD in IH-MAG.

A subtype of IM-MAG with a predominantly reticular pattern was described by Mulliken as reticular hemangioma (RIH-MAG). It is characterized by severe complications including intractable ulceration, tissue, and bone destruction. Additionally it can be associated with structural anomalies [8, 11]. Ulceration was a common finding in our group. It occurred in two patients with reticular morphology and in one patient without this reticular pattern [9, 12]. We detected two different degrees of involvement: ulcerations in two patients (cases 2 and 3) were numerous and superficial but in another patient (case 1) the ulceration was focal, deep, and difficult to heal.

The presence of ulceration in an IH-MAG suggests that proliferation alone may not be the sole reason and that other mechanisms such as hypoxia or local environment may have a role.

The natural history of IH-MAG is regression as other forms of infantile hemangioma. We detected that the involution phase is slower than usual and begins by about 1 year of age. Some of them do not require any treatment other than observation. The need for treatment in acral IH-MAG comes from ulceration showing a good response to propranolol as normal IH. They can leave residual lesions composed of a slightly puffy skin and telangiectasias.

9. Conclusion

We present a subtype of infantile haemangioma with similar clinical course: present at birth, located on the dorsum of feet, and showing minimal and arrested growth and developing characteristic ulceration. We highlight the importance of performing immunohistochemical Glut-1 examination in order to confirm diagnosis when clinical features are atypical.

IH-MAGs were more likely than IH to appear in girls, on the lower half of the body and on dorsal surface. Acral abortive hemangiomas were more likely to have a predominantly reticular morphology. Ulceration is a frequent complication of acral abortive hemangiomas.

Conflicts of Interest

The authors declare that there are no conflicts of interest regarding the publication of this paper.

References

[1] F. Corella, X. Garcia-Navarro, A. Ribe, A. Alomar, and E. Baselga, "Abortive or minimal-growth hemangiomas: Immunohistochemical evidence that they represent true infantile hemangiomas," *Journal of the American Academy of Dermatology*, vol. 58, no. 4, pp. 685–690, 2008.

[2] F. Toledo-Alberola, I. Betlloch-Mas, L. Cuesta-Montero et al., "Abortive hemangiomas. Description of clinical and pathological findings with special emphasis on dermoscopy," *European Journal of Dermatology*, vol. 20, no. 4, pp. 497–500, 2010.

[3] P. E. North, M. Waner, A. Mizeracki, and M. C. Mihm Jr., "GLUT1: A newly discovered immunohistochemical marker for juvenile hemangiomas," *Human Pathology*, vol. 31, no. 1, pp. 11–22, 2000.

[4] A. Martín-Santiago, A. Bauzá, L. del Pozo, and P. Carrillo, "Abortive or Minimal-Growth Hemangiomas. A Review of 14 Cases," *Actas Dermosifiliogr*, vol. 103, no. 3, pp. 246–250, 2012.

[5] M. G. Liang and I. J. Frieden, "Infantile and congenital hemangiomas," *Seminars in Pediatric Surgery*, vol. 23, no. 4, pp. 162–167, 2014.

[6] T. Itinteang, A. H. Withers, P. F. Davis, and S. T. Tan, "Biology of Infantile Hemangioma," *Frontiers in Surgery*, vol. 1, no. 38, 2014.

[7] T. Itinteang, R. Marsh, P. F. Davis, and S. T. Tan, "Angiotensin II causes cellular proliferation in infantile haemangioma via angiotensin II receptor," *Journal of Clinical Pathology*, vol. 68, no. 5, pp. 346–350, 2015.

[8] J. B. Mulliken, J. J. Marler, P. E. Burrows, and H. P. W. Kozakewich, "Reticular infantile hemangioma of the limb can be associated with ventral-caudal anomalies, refractory ulceration, and cardiac overload," *Pediatric Dermatology*, vol. 24, no. 4, pp. 356–362, 2007.

[9] D. Bessis, M. Bigorre, and C. Labrèze, "Reticular infantile hemangiomas with minimal or arrested growth associated with lipoatrophy," *Journal of the American Academy of Dermatology*, vol. 72, no. 5, Article ID 10002, pp. 828–833, 2015.

[10] K.-Y. Suh and I. J. Frieden, "Infantile hemangiomas with minimal or arrested growth: A retrospective case series," *Archives of Dermatology*, vol. 146, no. 9, pp. 971–976, 2010.

[11] N. A. Weitz, M. L. Bayer, E. Baselga et al., "The biker-glove pattern of segmental infantile hemangiomas on the hands and feet," *Journal of the American Academy of Dermatology*, vol. 71, no. 3, pp. 542–547, 2014.

[12] C. Koh, E. Sugo, and O. Wargon, "Unusual presentation of GLUT-1 positive infantile haemangioma," *Australasian Journal of Dermatology*, vol. 50, no. 2, pp. 136–140, 2009.

39

A Tale of Two Cysts: Steatocystoma Multiplex and Eruptive Vellus Hair Cysts

Rachel J. Waldemer-Streyer and Ellen Jacobsen

College of Medicine, University of Illinois-Chicago, Urbana Campus, 506 South Mathews Ave., 190 Medical Sciences Building, MC-714, Urbana, IL 61801, USA

Correspondence should be addressed to Ellen Jacobsen; ellenj@volo.net

Academic Editor: Alireza Firooz

Background. Steatocystoma multiplex (SM) and eruptive vellus hair cysts (EVHC) are uncommon benign tumors of the pilosebaceous unit. Both SM and EVHC are characterized by smooth, asymptomatic papules or nodules, most commonly presenting on the chest, limbs, and abdomen. Most cases of SM and EVHC are sporadic, although less common autosomal dominant inherited forms have been reported. *Main Observation.* In this report we present two cases of cutaneous cysts exhibiting characteristics of either SM or EVHC. Both patients presented with numerous 1-2 mm asymptomatic papules and responded well to surgical expression by incision and drainage (I&D). *Conclusion.* SM and EVHC are similar in clinical presentation and management. Previously reported "hybrid-type" tumors present strong evidence for a relationship between the two lesions pathologically. Due to potential similarity of EVHC and SM cyst contents, I&D and subsequent microscopic examination cannot definitely differentiate between EVHC, SM, and hybrid cysts.

1. Introduction

Steatocystoma multiplex (SM) and eruptive vellus hair cysts (EVHC) are uncommon benign tumors of the pilosebaceous unit. SM is characterized by multiple smooth asymptomatic papules or nodules, usually presenting on the chest, limbs and axillae, back, or abdomen. Facial involvement is less frequently noted but has been reported [1, 2]. Eruptive vellus hair cysts (EVHC) are a related cutaneous tumor and feature a similar clinical presentation with regard to appearance and spatial distribution, although facial EVHCs are a noted variant [3]. Both SM and EVHC are most likely to emerge during adolescence or early adulthood [1, 3]. Clinical diagnosis of these disorders can be a challenge due to their relative rarity of occurrence. Here we describe two patients with cutaneous cysts exhibiting the features of either SM or EVHC.

2. Case Reports

2.1. Case Report #1. A 15-year-old Caucasian male presented with a six-year history of multiple noninflamed, nonumbilicated papules on his anterior chest and abdomen. The initial eruption in 2009 of white and pink perifollicular 1-2 mm papules was especially numerous (>25) over the sternum, where they developed in a diamond-shaped pattern. No family history of similar dermatological disorders was noted. This eruption was clinically diagnosed as steatocystoma multiplex and showed significant improvement after five years of treatment with a topical 10% glycolic acid lotion. I&D expression of the few remaining lesions resulted in oily, curd-like material containing multiple vellus hairs (Figure 1). While this patient's lesions were not biopsied, a representative photomicrograph of a steatocystoma is shown in Figure 2. Interestingly, the lesions were preceded by a severe case of molluscum contagiosum that spanned the patient's chest, abdomen, back, and buttocks and was treated with 5% imiquimod cream. In addition to molluscum contagiosum, the patient's history was positive for atopic eczema and pityriasis alba on other areas of his body. Concomitant dermatological disorders included acne in the form of open and closed comedones on his face, neck, and chest. The SM lesions were distinct from the

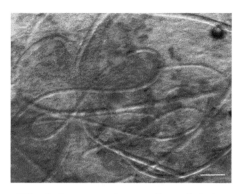

FIGURE 1: Vellus hairs present in cysts from clinical presentation case #1, a 15-year-old male patient. Cyst contents were expressed via incision and drainage and mounted with a coverslip without KOH. Scale bar = 100 microns.

acne lesions, the latter of which were erythematous and inflamed.

2.2. Case Report #2. A 67-year-old Caucasian female presented with numerous 1-2 mm white and yellow papules in a bilateral periorbital distribution (Figure 3(a)), which had emerged over the course of 15 years. Favre-Racouchot syndrome was initially suspected due to her age, cyst location, and concomitant solar elastosis. However, the papules that present with Favre-Racouchot syndrome are often yellow or brown in appearance and accompanied by open comedones, in contrast to our patient. Thus, several of these papules were removed and evaluated pathologically, revealing a mixture of milia and small cysts consistent with the diagnosis of eruptive vellus hair cysts; these contained multiple small lumenal degenerating hair shafts. A representative photomicrograph of an EVHC lesion is shown in Figure 4. Several of this patient's cysts were removed surgically for cosmetic reasons. One year after surgery, no recurrence of the expressed cysts was noted (Figure 3(b)). The patient's history was significant for milia, actinic keratoses, and discoid lupus erythematosus lesions on the scalp.

3. Discussion

Many similarities exist between SM and EVHC in terms of clinical presentation. Both SM and EVHC are most likely to emerge during adolescence or early adulthood [1, 3]. However, in their review of EVHC cases, Torchia et al. noted the presence of an interesting subgroup of patients that developed EVHC after age 35. Many of the individuals in this subgroup were women who presented with facial cysts rather than more common sites on the trunk and limbs [3], similar to our second patient. Our female patient also exhibited numerous milia, benign keratinous cysts that commonly present periorbitally. However, current literature does not seem to suggest a general correlation between milia and EVHC formation [3].

Most cases of SM and EVHC are sporadic, although familial cases of each have been reported and are transmitted in an autosomal dominant fashion [1–6]. It is notable that, in our first patient, SM developed shortly after a severe case of molluscum contagiosum and a general history of atopy. As the causes of nonhereditary SM are unknown, it is tempting to speculate that the imiquimod treatment and subsequent robust immune response may have played a role in the development of his cysts.

The true differentiation between SM and EVHC occurs at the histological level. Histological examination of a biopsied SM cyst will reveal thin walls of stratified squamous epithelium without a granular layer, typically with abundant sebaceous input (Figure 2). The cyst is frequently connected to the epidermis by a tissue cord originating from the infundibulum of the pilosebaceous unit [1]. Each steatocystoma is associated with a hair follicle, which can result in retention of trapped vellus hairs in the cystic lumen, as seen in our first patient [1, 2, 7]. Notably, the lesions seen in SM are bona fide tumors, rather than retention cysts caused by blockage of a sebaceous gland [1, 7]. The lining of the cystic cavity typically retains the undulated eosinophilic structure characteristic of the sebaceous duct, from which these hamartomas originate [2].

EVHCs originate from the isthmus or infundibulum of the pilosebaceous unit and thus are often lined by squamous epithelium containing a granular layer, in contrast to SM. These cysts also typically contain laminated keratin and multiple vellus hairs (Figure 4). Due to their different origins in the pilosebaceous unit, SM and EVHC cysts also differ in the classes of keratin found in their walls; while both cysts express keratin 17, only steatocystomas demonstrate expression of keratin 10 [8]. Interestingly, I&D and subsequent microscopic examination of cyst contents have been suggested as a less-invasive alternative to punch biopsy to diagnose EVHC, based on the presence of vellus hairs [9–11]. We disagree with this assertion, as SM lesions can also exhibit vellus hair inclusion, as shown in Figure 1 and reported in other sources [1, 2, 7]. Thus, histologic examination of the biopsied cyst wall and contents remains the gold standard to definitively differentiate between SM and EVHC. However, given the relative ease of examining cyst contents after I&D and the general rule that EVHC lesions are likely to contain a higher number of vellus hairs than those of SM, this procedure may still be useful in a clinical setting.

Intriguingly, there have been various reports of patients presenting with both SM and EVHC concurrently, or with hybrid cysts that exhibit features of both disorders [2, 6, 12–15]. Such reports have prompted speculation that SM and EVHC may be related and on the continuum of one unified disease process [2, 6, 14]. Ohtake et al. were the first to suggest that these hybrid-type tumors may be the result of cystic changes near the junction of the pilosebaceous duct, rather than discrete zones of the hair follicle [15]. Further investigations into the biological mechanisms regulating pilosebaceous tumor development may prove rewarding for our scientific understanding of the relationship between SM and EVHC.

Ultimately, the distinction between SM and EVHC may be primarily an academic one. Both lesions respond to similar treatment modalities and the problems they present are predominantly cosmetic, as they are rarely correlated to any serious genetic syndromes. Noted interventions with a

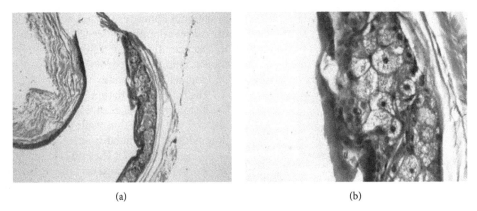

(a)   (b)

FIGURE 2: Representative photomicrograph of a steatocystoma stained with hematoxylin and eosin (H&E) at 100x (a) and 400x (b) magnification. Abundant sebaceous input is clearly visible in the cyst wall.

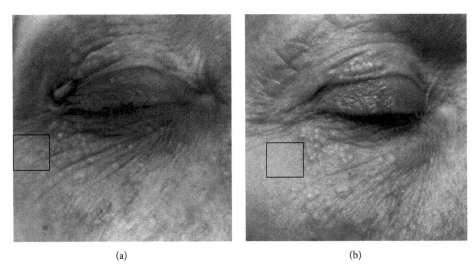

(a)   (b)

FIGURE 3: (a) Clinical presentation case #2, a 67-year-old female patient, presurgery. Numerous periorbital 1-2 mm white and yellow papules are shown. Papules inside the highlighted region (black box) were removed surgically. (b) Clinical presentation case #2, one year after surgery. No recurrence of removed papules was observed (boxed region).

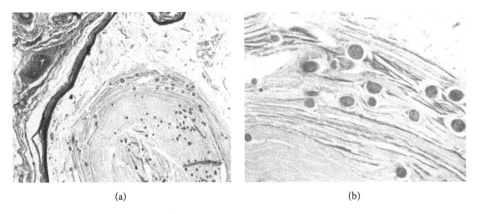

(a)   (b)

FIGURE 4: Representative photomicrograph of EVHC stained with H&E at 100x (a) and 400x (b) magnification. Keratin and numerous vellus hair shafts are visible in the cyst lumen.

history of efficacy include expression via surgical incision, excision, or needle aspiration; retinoic acid; and Erbium:YAG or CO_2 lasers [3, 12, 16]. While there have been some reports of spontaneous resolution of EVHC [3], this appears to be a minority of cases.

4. Conclusion

Our report details two cases of uncommon pilosebaceous tumors, steatocystoma multiplex, and eruptive vellus hair cysts. Despite clear histological differences between these lesions, SM and EVHC are similar in clinical presentation and management. "Hybrid-type" tumors present strong evidence for a relationship between the SM and EVHC pathologically. Due to their relative rarity of occurrence, familiarity with cyst presentation in these lesions will prove useful for accurate clinical diagnosis.

Conflicts of Interest

The authors declare no conflicts of interest regarding the publication of this paper.

Acknowledgments

The authors would like to thank Michael Rabkin, M.D., Ph.D., and Milena Kozovska, M.D., Ph.D. (both of the Rabkin Dermatopathology Laboratory in Tarentum, PA) for the photomicrograph images of representative SM and EVHC histology. The authors also gratefully acknowledge the University of Illinois-Chicago Research Open Access Article Publishing (ROAAP) Fund for financial support in publishing this case report.

References

[1] G. Plewig, H. H. Wolff, and O. Braun-Falco, "Steatocystoma multiplex: anatomic reevaluation, electron microscopy, and autoradiography," *Archives of Dermatological Research*, vol. 272, no. 3-4, pp. 363–380, 1982.

[2] S. Cho, S.-E. Chang, J.-H. Choi, K.-J. Sung, K.-C. Moon, and J.-K. Koh, "Clinical and histologic features of 64 cases of steatocystoma multiplex," *Journal of Dermatology*, vol. 29, no. 3, pp. 152–156, 2002.

[3] D. Torchia, J. Vega, and L. A. Schachner, "Eruptive vellus hair cysts: a systematic review," *American Journal of Clinical Dermatology*, vol. 13, no. 1, pp. 19–28, 2012.

[4] H. T. Kamra, P. A. Gadgil, A. G. Ovhal, and R. R. Narkhede, "Steatocystoma multiplex-a rare genetic disorder: a case report and review of the literature," *Journal of Clinical and Diagnostic Research*, vol. 7, no. 1, pp. 166–168, 2013.

[5] A. S. Antal, D. Kulichova, S. Redler, R. C. Betz, and T. Ruzicka, "Steatocystoma multiplex: keratin 17—the key player?" *British Journal of Dermatology*, vol. 167, no. 6, pp. 1395–1397, 2012.

[6] E. Sánchez-Yus, A. Aguilar-Martínez, M. C. Cristóbal-Gil, F. Urbina-González, and P. Guerra-Rodríguez, "Eruptive vellus hair cyst and steatocystoma multiplex: two related conditions?" *Journal of Cutaneous Pathology*, vol. 15, no. 1, pp. 40–42, 1988.

[7] A. M. Kligman and J. D. Kirschbaum, "Steatocystoma multiplex: a dermoid tumor," *The Journal of Investigative Dermatology*, vol. 42, pp. 383–387, 1964.

[8] H. Tomková, W. Fujimoto, and J. Arata, "Expression of keratins (K10 and K17) in steatocystoma multiplex, eruptive vellus hair cysts, and epidermoid and trichilemmal cysts," *The American Journal of Dermatopathology*, vol. 19, no. 3, pp. 250–253, 1997.

[9] S. D. Hong and I. J. Frieden, "Diagnosing eruptive vellus hair cysts," *Pediatric Dermatology*, vol. 18, no. 3, pp. 258–259, 2001.

[10] T. I. Kaya, C. Tataroglu, U. Tursen, and G. Ikizoglu, "Eruptive vellus hair cysts: an effective extraction technique for treatment and diagnosis," *Journal of the European Academy of Dermatology and Venereology*, vol. 20, no. 3, pp. 264–268, 2006.

[11] A. Karadag, E. Cakir, and A. Pelitli, "Eruptive vellus hair cysts: an alternative diagnosing method," *Indian Journal of Dermatology, Venereology and Leprology*, vol. 75, no. 5, pp. 537–538, 2009.

[12] E. Papakonstantinou, I. Franke, and H. Gollnick, "Facial steatocystoma multiplex combined with eruptive vellus hair cysts: a hybrid?" *Journal of the European Academy of Dermatology and Venereology*, vol. 29, no. 10, pp. 2051–2053, 2015.

[13] A. Yamada, K. Saga, and K. Jimbow, "Acquired multiple pilosebaceous cysts on the face having the histopathological features of steatocystoma multiplex and eruptive vellus hair cysts," *International Journal of Dermatology*, vol. 44, no. 10, pp. 861–863, 2005.

[14] P. Kiene, A. Hauschild, and E. Christophers, "Eruptive vellus hair cysts and steatocystoma multiplex. Variants of one entity?" *British Journal of Dermatology*, vol. 134, no. 2, pp. 365–367, 1996.

[15] N. Ohtake, Y. Kubota, O. Takayama, S. Shimada, and K. Tamaki, "Relationship between steatocystoma multiplex and eruptive vellus hair cysts," *Journal of the American Academy of Dermatology*, vol. 26, no. 5, pp. 876–878, 1992.

[16] W. Bakkour and V. Madan, "Carbon dioxide laser perforation and extirpation of steatocystoma multiplex," *Dermatologic Surgery*, vol. 40, no. 6, pp. 658–662, 2014.

40

Repigmentation of Tenacious Vitiligo on Apremilast

Sara B. Huff[1] and Lorie D. Gottwald[2]

[1]University of Toledo College of Medicine and Life Sciences, 3000 Arlington Avenue, Toledo, OH 43614, USA
[2]Department of Dermatology, University of Toledo Medical Center, 3000 Arlington Avenue, Toledo, OH 43614, USA

Correspondence should be addressed to Sara B. Huff; sara.monroe@utoledo.edu

Academic Editor: Kowichi Jimbow

Vitiligo is a common pigment disorder characterized by acquired loss of function or absence of melanocytes, leading to distinct areas of depigmentation. Physical exam reveals sharply demarcated, depigmented macules or patches on otherwise normal skin. Vitiligo can present at any age, in any skin color. There is no specific serologic marker for diagnosis, but patients often have other autoimmune problems. Treatment options are limited and are difficult given the fact that the pathogenesis of the disease is not well elucidated. We present the case of a 52-year-old woman with vitiligo for over 2 decades. The patient's medical history reveals a lack of response to many different approaches. This case highlights the ability of apremilast, an FDA-approved drug for the treatment of psoriasis and psoriatic arthritis, to achieve repigmentation in a case a vitiligo that has been extremely recalcitrant.

1. Introduction

Vitiligo is a common pigment disorder characterized by acquired development of white macules on the skin due to the loss of functioning melanocytes in the skin, the hair, or both [1]. Although the pathogenesis is not known, it is thought to be a cumulative effect of different mechanisms, including autoimmune, neurohormonal, genetic, oxidative stress, and cytotoxic [1–3]. The areas of depigmentation are usually symmetrical, sharply demarcated, and enlarged over time. Vitiligo affects all ages, races, and ethnic groups [2]. Considering the distinct contrast in white patches with the normal skin, vitiligo is more prominent in darker skinned persons. Vitiligo can greatly impact the quality of life for anyone afflicted, no matter what age. Patients report feeling stigmatized, being isolated, and having low self-esteem [1, 4].

Although topical and systemic glucocorticoids, topical calcineurin inhibitors, and narrowband ultraviolet B phototherapy are used to promote repigmentation, they all have varying degrees of success [2, 5, 6]. The response to treatments is lengthy and may be highly different among patients and even inconsistent in different body areas in the same patient. Vitiligo is a chronic disease with a highly unpredictable progression. Studies regarding these treatment options are generally poor or uncontrolled, resulting in the inability to amalgamate conclusions because of the considerable heterogeneity in study design and outcome measure. Hence, alternative and more efficacious therapies are needed for the study and treatment of vitiligo.

2. Case Report

A 52-year-old woman presented for a follow-up of chronic vitiligo. No other concomitant autoimmune diseases are known in this patient. She developed vitiligo in 1995 and has been seen in this clinic since 1998. She used topical tacrolimus, pimecrolimus, mometasone furoate cream, clobetasol propionate cream, topical psoralen combined with photochemotherapy with UVA, intramuscular triamcinolone acetonide, intramuscular alefacept, subcutaneous etanercept, oral cyclosporine, oral dapsone, and oral prednisone in the past. The patient stopped the use of medications for 5 years prior to re-presenting due to lack of success with repigmentation with the previously listed medications. Her attempt at multiple non-FDA-approved medications illustrates her frustration. At the first visit, the diagnosis of chronic vitiligo was readdressed. The recent data suggesting that apremilast may have a broad effect on inflammation was reviewed and

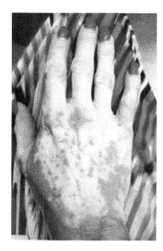

FIGURE 1: Clinical appearance of the right dorsal hand 5 and a half months after beginning apremilast.

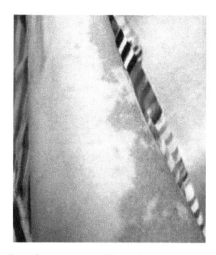

FIGURE 2: Clinical appearance of the right anterior forearm 5 and a half months after beginning apremilast.

the patient was willing to try apremilast in a non-FDA-approved fashion [7]. After six weeks of apremilast treatment, she reported she believed she was starting to repigment. She continued treatment with apremilast at 30 mg twice daily. Three months after initiating treatment, the patient presented for a follow-up with mild improvement. The patient was bolstered at this time with 60 mg intramuscular triamcinolone acetonide and apremilast 30 mg twice daily was maintained. Note that many years of attempts at steroids as a solo therapy had yielded no improvement. Six weeks following this visit she started to note repigmentation of hands, but felt that normal skin was darkening as well, secondary to ambient sunlight, and she had a bit more pronounced hypopigmentation of perioral area. She received a repeat 60 mg intramuscular triamcinolone acetonide injection and maintained apremilast 30 mg twice daily. Five and a half months after beginning the apremilast treatment, she continued to have areas of improvement, but with a few new areas of hypopigmentation on her feet. The patient felt that repigmentation of hands and forearms was progressing slowly as seen in Figures 1 and 2. At follow-up, 6 and a half months after beginning apremilast treatment, the patient reports repigmentation in bilateral arms, legs, hands, feet, chest, and face. The areas appear red before repigmenting. She had no sun exposure in the interim. At her next follow-up, 8 months after beginning apremilast treatment, the patient experienced fairly significant repigmentation. It was important to continue following the patient without steroids to monitor her progress. At her last visit, 5 months without triamcinolone acetonide supplementation and 11 months after beginning apremilast 30 mg twice daily treatment, the patient was doing extremely well. She is tolerating the apremilast and is repigmenting on her chest and arms 60–70% and now also on her face. The patient provided images of 7 months without triamcinolone acetonide and 13 months after beginning apremilast 30 mg twice daily as shown in Figures 3 and 4. Side effects and rationale regarding apremilast treatment were reviewed at each visit. The patient reported no side effects throughout.

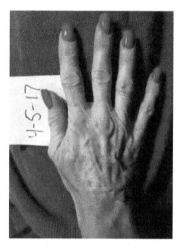

FIGURE 3: Clinical appearance of the right dorsal hand 13 months after using apremilast 30 mg twice daily.

3. Discussion

The treatment of vitiligo is challenging given the lack of well controlled studies and inability to pool results based on considerable heterogeneity in study design and outcome measure. Apremilast has been shown to help in autoimmunity from alopecia areata [7]. Our case shows a patient who was treated with apremilast 30 mg twice daily and achieved significant repigmentation in the presence of initial steroid bolstering and continued repigmentation without steroids.

Apremilast is a phosphodiesterase-4 enzyme (PDE-4) inhibitor. Apremilast is FDA-approved for the treatment of patients with moderate to severe plaque psoriasis who are candidates for phototherapy or systemic therapy, as well as for use in psoriatic arthritis. PDE-4 normally degrades cyclic adenosine monophosphate (cAMP) into $5'$-adenosine monophosphate. By inhibiting the PDE-4 enzyme specific for cAMP degradation, this results in increased intracellular cAMP levels and thereby regulation of numerous inflammatory mediators through the cAMP second messenger effect

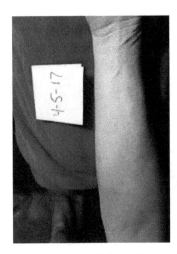

FIGURE 4: Clinical appearance of the right anterior forearm 13 months after using apremilast 30 mg twice daily.

(e.g., decreased expression of TNF-α, and interleukin- (IL-) 17, IL-23, and interferon gamma, as well as increased IL-10) [8]. When intracellular cAMP is elevated, inflammatory signaling and cytokines are suppressed and anti-inflammatory modulators, such as IL-10, are increased. Vitiligo, like psoriasis, is linked to a dysregulated immune system governed by a proinflammatory cytokine network, involving local and systemic chronic inflammatory processes [8–10]. Melanocytes cultured from vitiligo patient skin samples have been shown to express high levels of cytokines including IL-6 and IL-17 [9]. Positive correlations between levels of IL-17 and disease extent and activity have been found [9]. IL-6 and IL-8 can attract immune components to the skin and may be the link between the triggering event and the initiation of the autoimmune response that results in vitiligo progression [9]. Recent observations have indicated the critical role of altered cellular immunity, autoimmunity, and cytokines in the etiopathogenesis of vitiligo [11]. The use of apremilast, an oral PDE-4 inhibitor for chronic inflammatory diseases, which does not target any single mediator, but rather has a broad range of effects, has been shown to be helpful in the treatment of vitiligo in our patient [8]. There are possible risks to every intervention for vitiligo. Common side effects of apremilast are diarrhea, headache, nausea, vomiting, weight loss, and depression; these adverse events typically present early and are self-limiting. The advantages of using apremilast include ease of oral administration, minimal drug interaction potential, and safety adverse event profile. It should be noted that vitiligo can spontaneously be repigmented. Spontaneous repigmentation would be unlikely in this case, given the chronicity of disease. A PubMed search of articles indexed for MEDLINE using the terms *vitiligo, apremilast,* and *repigmentation* revealed that there currently are no known cases of repigmentation in patients with vitiligo on apremilast that have been reported. Our patient presented with chronic vitiligo that was extremely recalcitrant to many different classes of drugs and modalities of delivery.

4. Conclusion

Psoriasis, alopecia areata, and vitiligo share a common pathway of autoimmunity, inflammatory signals, and cytokines present, although their pathogenesis is not completely understood. Apremilast is FDA-approved for psoriasis and psoriatic arthritis. Apremilast has also been shown to inhibit the development of alopecia areata [7]. We present this case to demonstrate the ability of apremilast to allow for repigmentation in a patient with chronic recalcitrant vitiligo in conjunction with initial systemic glucocorticoids. More clinical studies, ideally a randomized placebo-controlled trial, would be needed to prove that apremilast leads to repigmentation in vitiligo.

Conflicts of Interest

The authors declare that there are no conflicts of interest regarding the publication of this paper.

References

[1] G. F. Mohammed, A. H. Gomaa, and M. S. Al-Dhubaibi, "Highlights in pathogenesis of vitiligo," *World Journal of Clinical Cases*, vol. 3, no. 3, pp. 221–230, 2015.

[2] C. K. Sharma, M. Sharma, B. Aggarwal, and V. Sharma, "Different advanced therapeutic approaches to treat vitiligo," *Journal of Environmental Pathology, Toxicology and Oncology*, vol. 34, no. 4, pp. 321–334, 2015.

[3] J. F. Rork, M. Rashighi, and J. E. Harris, "Understanding autoimmunity of vitiligo and alopecia areata," *Current Opinion in Pediatrics*, vol. 28, no. 4, pp. 463–469, 2016.

[4] C. M. Nguyen, K. Beroukhim, M. J. Danesh, A. Babikian, J. Koo, and A. Leon, "The psychosocial impact of acne, vitiligo, and psoriasis: A review," *Clinical, Cosmetic and Investigational Dermatology*, vol. 9, pp. 383–392, 2016.

[5] B. S. Daniel and R. Wittal, "Vitiligo treatment update," *Australasian Journal of Dermatology*, vol. 56, no. 2, pp. 85–92, 2015.

[6] K. Ezzedine, V. Eleftheriadou, M. Whitton, and N. van Geel, "Vitiligo," *The Lancet*, vol. 386, no. 9988, pp. 74–84, 2015.

[7] A. Gilhar, A. G. Schrum, A. Etzioni, H. Waldmann, and R. Paus, "Alopecia areata: Animal models illuminate autoimmune pathogenesis and novel immunotherapeutic strategies," *Autoimmunity Reviews*, vol. 15, no. 7, pp. 726–735, 2016.

[8] P. Schafer, "Apremilast mechanism of action and application to psoriasis and psoriatic arthritis," *Biochemical Pharmacology*, vol. 83, no. 12, pp. 1583–1590, 2012.

[9] P. Manga, N. Elbuluk, and S. J. Orlow, "Recent advances in understanding vitiligo," *F1000Research*, vol. 5, 2016.

[10] P. H. Schafer, A. Parton, L. Capone et al., "Apremilast is a selective PDE4 inhibitor with regulatory effects on innate immunity," *Cellular Signalling*, vol. 26, no. 9, pp. 2016–2029, 2014.

[11] M. Kidir, A. A. Karabulut, M. E. Ercin, and P. Atasoy, "Regulatory T-cell cytokines in patients with nonsegmental vitiligo," *International Journal of Dermatology*, vol. 56, no. 5, pp. 581–588, 2017.

41

Granulosis Rubra Nasi Response to Topical Tacrolimus

Farhana Tahseen Taj,[1] **Divya Vupperla,**[2] **and Prarthana B. Desai**[1]

[1]Department of Dermatology, Venereology & Leprosy, Jawaharlal Nehru Medical College and KLE's Dr. Prabhakar Kore Hospital and Medical Research Centre, Belgaum, Karnataka 590 010, India
[2]Department of Dermatology, Venereology & Leprosy, Government District Headquarters Hospital, Khammam, Andhra Pradesh 507 002, India

Correspondence should be addressed to Farhana Tahseen Taj; farhanahaveri@gmail.com

Academic Editor: Jacek Cezary Szepietowski

Granulosis Rubra Nasi (GRN) is a rare disorder of the eccrine glands. It is clinically characterized by hyperhidrosis of the central part of the face, most commonly on the tip of the nose, followed by appearance of diffuse erythema over the nose, cheeks, chin, and upper lip. It is commonly seen in childhood but it can present in adults. Here we report a case of GRN in an adult patient with very unusual histopathological presentation.

1. Introduction

Granulosis Rubra Nasi (GRN) is also known as "Acne papulo-rosacea of the nose.". In 1901, a German dermatologist, Jadassohn, had described the first case of GRN as "Nasi hyperhidrotic Erythematosa micropapules Dermatosis Infantum" [1]. It is an inflammatory dermatosis involving eccrine sweat glands of central face and clinically presents with hyperhidrosis, erythema, papules, pustules, and vesicles. Rarely small comedo like lesions may be present [2].

It is usually limited to the front and sides of the nose. It may also affect the eyebrow, upper lip, and cheek. Presentation is common in childhood with a peak age of presentation at 7–12 years, but adolescent and adult onset is also possible. It has a chronic course and resolves at puberty without any sequelae. It is described as a focal form of hyperhidrosis which differs from the other forms, as it does not depend on the hypothalamic or emotional stimuli [3].

2. Case Report

A 33-year-old male patient presented with asymptomatic lesion over nose since 2 years to the outpatient department of dermatology and leprosy. The patient gave no history of any treatment taken before. There was no history of any fluid or cheesy material coming out of the lesions and no history of itching or burning (Figure 1). Clinically, we made a diagnosis of Granulosis Rubra Nasi, Lymphangioma Circumscriptum, Nevus Comedonicus, and sebaceous gland hyperplasia.

A biopsy of the skin lesion was done. The histopathology report showed epidermal hyperplasia with spongiosis. Dermis shows dilated eccrine sweat glands. The infundibular and sebaceous ducts are plugged with stratum corneum and villous hair follicles. There is moderately peri-infundibular infiltrate of lymphocytes and plasma cells. Papillary dermis shows dilated capillaries with extravasation of hemosiderin (Figure 2).

The patient has been treated with topical tacrolimus 0.03% and systemic corticosteroids. After 15 days of follow-up, the patient has shown good response (Figure 3).

3. Discussion

This is a chronic, benign condition of unknown etiology [2, 4]. It is rare with autosomal dominant or autosomal recessive pattern of inheritance. The gene locus remains unidentified [5]. Persistent localized hyperhidrosis of central face is the main cause for this condition [6]. GRN usually starts in early childhood and resolves spontaneously at puberty, but rarely it may persist [7] Males are most commonly affected. 6 out of 7 patients described by Jadassohn were boys [1]. This condition is usually asymptomatic except for mild pruritus.

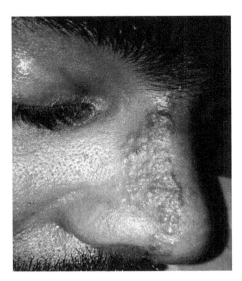

FIGURE 1: Multiple hyperpigmented papules and some vesicles present over the right side of the nose.

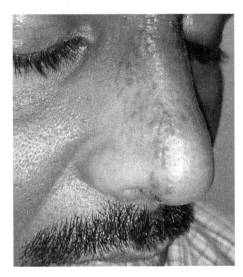

FIGURE 3: Three weeks after treatment with topical tacrolimus.

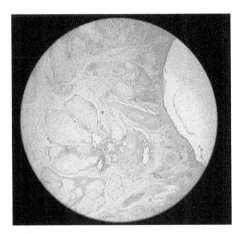

FIGURE 2: Histopathology: epidermal hyperplasia with spongiosis. Dermis shows villous hair follicle with sebaceous gland hyperplasia with peri-infundibular infiltrate of lymphocytes and plasma cells with dilated capillaries and extravasation of hemosiderin.

Hyperhidrosis is the initial conspicuous feature of GRN which tends to worsen in summer. Excessive sweating may precede other changes by several years. Small beads of sweat can be seen at the tip of the nose. As a result of persistent hyperhidrosis, diffuse erythema develops over the tip of the nose. Erythema may gradually extend to involve upper lip, cheeks, and chin with sweat droplets studded over, giving glistening appearance. Small erythematous macules, papules, vesicles, or pustules lesions can also be seen [2, 8]. These lesions disappear on diascopy and reappear on relieving pressure [2].

The pathogenesis is unknown. It is an inflammatory dermatosis involving eccrine sweat glands of central face involving nose, cheeks, or chin, representing a unique sweat retention form [2]. Some authors have suggested a defect in vasomotor and secretory functions of the nose. Presence of significant increase in sweating on the nose and central

face appears to be responsible for the secondary changes like erythema and erythematous papules [9].

The differential diagnosis like rosacea or perioral dermatitis can be considered. But, in rosacea, there is erythema over nose and cheeks along with telangiectasias but there is no hyperhidrosis of the central part of the face. Perioral dermatitis can present with erythema, small monomorphic papules, and pustules with or without scaling involving the perioral area without hyperhidrosis. Other differential diagnoses include acne vulgaris, lupus pernio, lupus erythematosus, lupus vulgaris, leishmaniasis, actinic keratosis or skin cancer, miliaria crystallina, and hidrocystoma [2, 4, 10]. Acne vulgaris presents with comedones, papules, and pustules without hyperhidrosis and telangiectasia. Lupus pernio or chilblain lupus presents with dusky papules and plaques on the nose, toes, and fingers. Lupus erythematosus has history of photosensitivity. In acute lupus erythematosus, there is a malar rash with mouth ulcers but there is no hyperhidrosis. Miliaria crystallina presents with vesicles mainly over the areas occluded by clothes.

Association with primary palmoplantar hyperhidrosis, acrocyanosis, and poor peripheral circulation was observed. Kumar et al. had reported an association with another eccrine gland disorder, hidrocystoma [8]. Heid et al. had reported an association with rhinorrhea [11]. Heid et al. reported pheochromocytoma with GRN in a 19-year-old woman who showed regression of hyperhidrosis and the nasal dermatosis after surgical removal of the tumor [11]. Barber had suggested involvement of adenoids, which can provide a source of irritation at the tip of the nose [12]. Topical indomethacin, drying lotions like calamine, tetracycline, cryotherapy, and X-rays (temporary benefit) have been described in the treatment of GRN [13]. Recently, use of botulinum toxin A that induced long-term remission in a patient with GRN was described by Grazziotin et al. [14]; botulinum toxin A improves GRN by decreasing hyperhidrosis.

Granulosis Rubra Nasi presents with three stages: initial hyperhidrosis followed by erythema and papular lesions and late vesicular stage. Our patient presented with late vesicular stage, so topical tacrolimus 0.03% was advised with good clinical response. There are no complications associated with the condition and the disease has excellent prognosis with self-resolution. Systemic corticosteroids help by reducing the inflammatory infiltrate around sweat glands. Topical tacrolimus has been used in low dose, 0.03%, with excellent response [8].

The diagnosis is usually clinical. Histology shows dilation of dermal blood vessels and lymphatics with perivascular lymphocytic infiltration and dilation of sweat ducts. Eccrine hidrocystoma also shows dilatation of sweat glands with solitary or multiple cysts lined by a double layer of cuboidal cells on histology, but dilatation of dermal vessels and perivascular mononuclear infiltrate is not seen [4, 10].

4. Conclusion

GRN is a rare disorder. One should remember that it could be a complication of hyperhidrosis. Treatment is symptomatic and cosmetic. Counseling the patients about the self-limiting nature of the condition is of paramount importance. To the best of our knowledge, there are not any case reports showing GRN with sebaceous gland hyperplasia.

Conflicts of Interest

The authors declare that they have no conflicts of interest.

References

[1] J. Jadassohn, "Ueber eine eigenartige Erkrankung der Nasen- haut bei Kindern ("Granulosis rubra nasi")," *Archiv für Derma- tologie und Syphilis*, vol. 58, no. 1-2, pp. 145–158, 1901.

[2] P. J. Mendoza, L. S. Saldana, and A. R. Patricia, "Nasi rubra granulosis," *Dermatol Peru*, vol. 13, pp. 125–127, 2003.

[3] C. Sargunam, J. Thomas, and N. Ahmed, "Granulosis rubra nasi," *Indian Dermatology Online Journal (IDOJ)*, vol. 4, no. 3, p. 208, 2013.

[4] B. M. Hantash and R. M. Rashid, *Granulosis rubra nasi*, http://emedicine.medscape.com/article/1072459-overview.

[5] F. Grinoni, "Contributo clinico allo studio dell'etiopatogenesi della Granulosis Rubra Nasi," *G Dermatol Sif*, vol. 96, p. 227, 1955.

[6] O. P. Kreiden, R. Boni, and G. Burg, "Hyperhidrosis and botulinum toxic in dermatology," *Curr Probi Dermato*, vol. 30, pp. 178–187, 2002.

[7] G. Zuccati, C. Filippeschi, A. Mastrolorenzo, A. L. Rapaccini, L. Tiradritti, and C. Staderini, "Granulosis Rubra Nasi," *Giornale Italiano di Dermatologia e Venereologia*, vol. 125, no. 6, pp. 275- 276, 1990.

[8] P. Kumar, A. Gosai, A. K. Mondal, N. R. Lal, and R. C. Gharami, "Granulosis rubra nasi: A rare condition treated successfully with topical tacrolimus," *Dermatology Reports*, vol. 4, no. 1, article no. e5, 2012.

[9] B. Piotr and P. Katarzyna, "Granulosis rubra nasi -a case report, a literature review," *Dermatol Online*, vol. 2, no. 3, pp. 144–146, 2011.

[10] J. L. Miller and H. J. Hurley, "Diseases of the eccrine and apocrine sweat glands," in *Dermatology*, J. L. Bolognia, J. L. Jorizzo Joseph, and R. P. Rapini, Eds., pp. 531–548, Mosby: Elsevier, 2nd edition, 2008.

[11] E. Heid, F. Samain, G. Jelen, and S. Boivin, "Granulosis rubra nasi and pheochromocytoma," *Annales de Dermatologie et de Venereologie*, vol. 123, no. 2, pp. 106–108, 1996.

[12] H. W. Barber, "Two cases of granulosis rubra nasi in boys," *Proceedings of the Royal Society of Medicine*, vol. 12, no. 40, 1919.

[13] F. F. Hellier, "Granulosis rubra nasi in a mother and daughter," *British Medical Journal*, vol. 2, no. 1068, 1937.

[14] T. C. Grazziotin, R. B. Buffon, A. P. D. Da Silva Manzoni, A. S. Libis, and M. B. Weber, "Treatment of granulosis rubra nasi with botulinum toxin type a," *Dermatologic Surgery*, vol. 35, no. 8, pp. 1298-1299, 2009.

42

Concurrent Diagnoses of Cutaneous Sarcoidosis and Recurrent Metastatic Breast Cancer: More than a Coincidental Occurrence?

Jacqueline Deen [D],[1] Nick Mellick,[2] and Laura Wheller[3]

[1]Department of Dermatology, Sunshine Coast University Hospital, 6 Doherty Street, Birtinya, Queensland 4575, Australia
[2]Department of Pathology, Medlab Pathology, 280 Newmarket Road, Wilston, Queenslan 4051, Australia
[3]Department of Dermatology, Mater Misercordiae Hospital, Raymond Terrace, South Brisbane, Queensland 4101, Australia

Correspondence should be addressed to Jacqueline Deen; jacqui.deen@gmail.com

Academic Editor: Jaime A. Tschen

Sarcoidosis is a rare, chronic, multisystem disease of unknown aetiology, characterised by non-caseating epithelioid cell granulomas. Its association with internal malignancy, in particular haematological cancers has been strongly documented in the literature, while its link with solid organ malignancies is less extensively reported. We present an atypical case of cutaneous sarcoidosis occurring in association with breast cancer recurrence in a 49-year-old female. Physician recognition of this link between sarcoidosis and internal malignancy is vital because many cases of sarcoidosis in association with neoplasia present initially, or even exclusively, with cutaneous sarcoidal lesions that may precede the development of cancer by several years, or as in our case, present as a cutaneous marker of concomitant underlying malignancy. Our case highlights the importance of age-appropriate cancer screening in additional to a routine work-up for systemic sarcoidosis in a patient with cutaneous sarcoidosis.

1. Introduction

Sarcoidosis is a chronic, idiopathic, multisystem disease, characterised by non-caseating epithelioid cell granulomas. The lungs are involved in more than 90% of cases, but the lymphatic system, eyes, and skin may also be affected. Less common but usually more severe forms can involve the liver, spleen, central nervous system, heart, upper respiratory tract, and bones. Its pathogenesis appears to correspond to an aberrant immune response in a susceptible host. Sarcoidosis typically affects young adults, with a slight female general predominance [1, 2].

Various diseases have been associated with sarcoidosis, including autoimmune disorders such as rheumatoid arthritis, psoriasis, vasculitis, thyroid disease, systemic sclerosis, and Sjogren syndrome. Haematological malignancies, in particular lymphoproliferative disorders such as Hodgkin lymphoma, are most strongly associated with sarcoidosis compared to solid organ malignancies [2, 3]. We present a rare case of cutaneous sarcoidosis occurring in association with breast carcinoma.

2. Case Report

A 49-year-old female presented with a 2-month history of asymptomatic lesions on the left knee found incidentally on routine full skin examination. The patient was otherwise well, with no pulmonary or systemic symptoms.

She had a past history of breast cancer diagnosed 4 years ago, managed by lumpectomy and adjuvant chemoradiotherapy achieving remission. The patient had regular cancer surveillance and was currently on adjuvant tamoxifen, with a planned duration of 10 years. Her other notable medical history included lifelong asthma, gastrooesophageal reflux disease, depression, subacute thyroiditis and previous shoulder, and knee arthroscopies. Her regular medications included tamoxifen, pantoprazole, venlafaxine, budesonide/formoterol, and terbutaline. She was a lifetime non-smoker and rarely consumed alcohol. The patient had no family history of autoimmune conditions.

Examination revealed numerous erythematous-to-brown, non-tender papules occurring on the anterior left knee (Figure 1). On the right foot, at the site of a scar

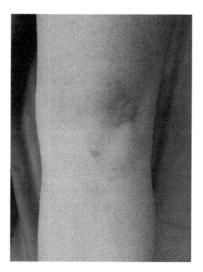

FIGURE 1: Clinical photograph showing numerous erythematous-to-brown papules on the anterior left knee.

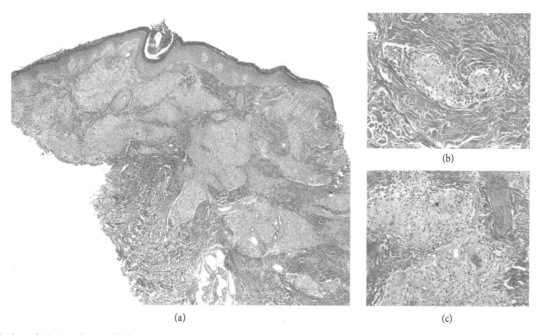

(a)　　　　　　　　　　　　　　　　　(b)

(c)

FIGURE 2: (a, b and c) Histology of left knee lesion showing a sarcoidal-type granulomatous reaction. (a) Much of the reticular dermis is occupied by a granulomatous infiltrate (hematoxylin and eosin staining, original magnification x40). (b and c) Individual granulomas are sarcoidal in type, i.e., non-necrotising with a minimal associated lymphocytic infiltrate (so-called "naked" granulomas) (hematoxylin and eosin staining, original magnification x200).

from prior cryotherapy for plantar warts, the patient had a similar area of firm indurated erythematous-to-brown change. Dermoscopy of both sites showed orange and yellow translucent globules ("apple-jelly" sign). There were no skin lesions detected on full skin examination suspicious for malignancy. There was no lymphadenopathy and systemic examination was otherwise unremarkable.

Skin biopsy showed multiple, variably sized naked sarcoidosis type granulomas scattered throughout the dermis (Figure 2). Chest radiograph showed bilateral hilar lymphadenopathy and serum angiotensin-converting enzyme was elevated at 107 U/L. Other laboratory tests were within normal limits (full blood count, liver and renal function tests, and calcium and inflammatory markers). Further investigations excluded systemic sarcoidosis (cardiac MRI and CT-PET scan). The CT PET ordered during systemic work-up, however, showed a solitary lesion in the T10 vertebra and subsequent biopsy proved recurrent metastatic breast cancer.

The patient's management was then deferred to a medical oncologist for ongoing care of her metastatic breast cancer. She received stereotactic radiation to her spinal lesion and was commenced on a special access program with ribociclib. Following breast cancer treatment, cutaneous sarcoidal lesions completely resolved.

TABLE 1: Previous literature cases of breast cancer and sarcoidosis.

Reference	Sex	Patient age (years)	Interval b/t diseases (years)	Sarcoidosis onset*	Tumour type
Prior et al. (1952) [6]	F	59	5	P	Breast adenocarcinoma
Brincker et al. (1974) [5]	F	NS	NS	P	NS
	F			P	
	F			P	
	M			P	
Suen JS et al (1990) [7]	F	50	0.7	A	Breast cancer (stage II)
Shah AK et al (1990) [8]	F	36	3	P	Invasive ductal carcinoma
Von Knorring et al. (1976) [9]	F	74	5	P	Non-metastasizing breast carcinoma
Whittington R et al. (1986) [10]	F	52	0.6	A	Infiltrating ductal carcinoma
	F	42	5	P	Metastatic breast cancer
Reich J et al. (1995) [11]	F	47	10	A	Intraductal breast carcinoma
	F	55	9	P	Infiltrating ductal breast carcinoma
Brechtek B et al. (1996) [4]	F	58	1	P	NS
Seersholm N et al. (1997) [12]	NS	NS	NS	P	NS
Romer FK et al. (1998) [13]	F	Between 19-78 years	NS	P	NS
	F			P	
	F			P	
	F			P	
	F			P	
	F			P	
Askling J et al. (1999) [14]	NS	NS	NS	P	NS
	NS			P	NS
Lower EE et al. (2001) [15]	F	25	5	P	Invasive ductal carcinoma
	F	57	5	P	Infiltrating ductal carcinoma
	F	58	8	P	Invasive ductal carcinoma
	F	40	2	A	Invasive ductal carcinoma
	F	49	1	A	Invasive ductal carcinoma
	F	38	2	A	Invasive ductal carcinoma
	F	36	1	A	Invasive ductal carcinoma
	F	57	8	A	Invasive ductal carcinoma
	F	55	0	C	Invasive ductal carcinoma
	F	43	0	C	Intraductal carcinoma
Garcia et al. (2003) [16]	F	44	3	P	Invasive lobular breast carcinoma with ductal and mucinous features
Chen W et al. (2004) [17]	F	NS	NS	P	NS
	F	NS	0	C	NS
Van der Hoeven JJ et al. (2004) [18]	F	NS	0	C	Ductal carcinoma of breast
Gusakova I et al. (2007) [19]	F	69	6	A	Infiltrating ductal carcinoma of breast
	F	60	4	A	Infiltrating ductal carcinoma of breast

Concurrent Diagnoses of Cutaneous Sarcoidosis and Recurrent Metastatic Breast Cancer: More than...

161

TABLE 1: Continued.

Reference	Sex	Patient age (years)	Interval b/t diseases (years)	Sarcoidosis onset*	Tumour type
Tolaney SM et al. (2007) [20]	F	47	0	C	Invasive lobular carcinoma of breast
	F	51	2	A	Invasive ductal carcinoma
	F	31	0	C	Invasive ductal carcinoma
Ataergin S et al. (2009) [21]	F	75	12	A	Breast cancer (T3N1M0)
Viswanath L et al. (2009) [22]	F	50	2	A	Infiltrating ductal carcinoma breast
Ito T et al. (2010) [23]	F	90	6	A	Metastatic breast cancer
	F	52	4	A	Invasive ductal carcinoma breast
Alexandrescu DT et al. (2011) [1]	F	72	8	P	NS
	F	46	4	P	NS
	F	46	5	P	Infiltrating ductal carcinoma of breast
Bush E et al. (2011) [24]	F	42	0	C	Infiltrating ductal carcinoma of breast
Nishioka M et al (2012) [25]	F	79	0	C	Recurrent breast cancer (local)
DeFilippis EM et al (2013) [26]	F	63	0	C	Stage 1 breast cancer
Akhtari et al. (2014) [27]	F	47	0	C	Ductal invasive carcinoma
Kim et al. (2014) [28]	F	44	2	A	Ductal invasive carcinoma
Zivin et al. (2014) [29]	F	32	0	C	Ductal invasive carcinoma
Altinkaya et al. (2015) [30]	F	70	0	C	Ductal invasive carcinoma
Conte et al. (2015) [31]	F	50	0	C	Ductal invasive carcinoma
El Hammoumi (2015) [32]	F	51	3	A	Lobular carcinoma breast
Chen J et al. (2015) [33]	F	62	7	A	Infiltrating ductal carcinoma
	F	54	0	C	Infiltrating ductal carcinoma
	F	50	24	P	Infiltrating ductal carcinoma
	F	63	34	P	Infiltrating ductal carcinoma
	F	77	9	P	Infiltrating ductal carcinoma
Present case	F	49	0	C	Recurrent metastatic breast cancer

F: female, patient age: age at concurrent disease diagnosis, interval b/t diseases: interval between both diseases (sarcoidosis and breast cancer).
*P: **preceded** breast cancer diagnosis; C: occurred **concomitantly** with breast cancer diagnosis; A: occurred **after** breast cancer diagnosis.

3. Discussion

Cutaneous involvement presents in 25% of patients with systemic sarcoidosis and may be the only manifestation [4]. Dermatologists are frequently the first clinicians to identify sarcoidosis as specific skin lesions are often the presenting sign and skin biopsy enables early diagnosis. Skin lesions are extremely variable and may be specific or nonspecific. Specific lesions are those that histologically display noncaseating granulomas, which manifest clinically as maculopapules, plaques, lupus pernio, scar-sarcoidosis, and subcutaneous sarcoidosis. Nonspecific lesions lack histological evidence of sarcoid granulomas and the most significant lesions are erythema nodosum. In isolated cutaneous disease, further evaluation is essential as transformation into systemic sarcoidosis occurs in approximately one-third of patients within three years [1, 2].

Various diseases have been associated with sarcoidosis. Previously, an association between sarcoidosis and malignancy has been described, although no clear relationship has been identified. In most cases, sarcoidosis was diagnosed before the detection of an associated neoplasm. Haematological malignancies remain most strongly associated compared to solid tumours [1–3]. Brincker and Wilbek in 1974 were first to describe this association, reporting that, in patients with sarcoidosis, lymphoma occurred 11 times more frequently and lung cancer occurred three times more frequently compared with the general population [5].

Previous literature cases of sarcoidosis occurring with breast cancer are summarised in Table 1. The average patient age was 53 years, with 98.3% being female. In 30 (48.4%) patients the identification of sarcoidosis preceded the diagnosis of breast cancer; in 18 (29.0%) patients breast cancer diagnosis preceded sarcoidosis; and in 14 (22.6%) patients both diseases occurred concomitantly. The average time interval between the diagnosis of sarcoidosis and breast cancer was 8.3 years (range 1-34 years). When breast cancer predated sarcoidosis, the average interval was 4.1 years (range 0.6-12 years). In our case, the patient age at diagnosis was 49 years, which is similar to what was described in the literature.

Our case is unique in that the cutaneous sarcoidosis most likely occurred around the same time the patient's breast cancer recurrence was diagnosed and investigation for systemic sarcoidosis revealed her metastatic disease. This may be an incidental finding or indicate that dysregulation of the immune system mediated by either the breast cancer or sarcoidosis lead to the granulomatous inflammation of sarcoidosis or neoplasm, respectively [3, 4, 34]. In addition, there was complete resolution of the cutaneous sarcoidal lesions following treatment of the patient's metastatic breast cancer, strengthening the correlation between both entities.

Recognition by physicians of this link between sarcoidosis and internal malignancy is vital because many cases of sarcoidosis in association with neoplasia present initially, or even exclusively, with cutaneous sarcoidal lesions that may precede the development of cancer by several years or as in our case, present as a cutaneous marker of concomitant underlying malignancy. Thus, in addition to routine screening for systemic sarcoidosis, patients diagnosed with cutaneous sarcoidosis should be closely followed up, particularly including age-appropriate cancer screening to exclude the development of associated malignancy [1].

Conflicts of Interest

The authors declare that there are no conflicts of interest.

References

[1] D. T. Alexandrescu, C. Lisa Kauffman, T. E. Ichim, N. H. Riordan, F. Kabigting, and C. A. Dasanu, "Cutaneous sarcoidosis and malignancy: An association between sarcoidosis with skin manifestations and systemic neoplasia," *Dermatology Online Journal*, vol. 17, no. 1, 2011.

[2] A. Grados, M. Ebbo, E. Bernit et al., "Sarcoidosis occurring after solid cancer: a nonfortuitous association: report of 12 cases and review of the literature," *Medicine (United States)*, vol. 94, no. 28, article no. e928, 2015.

[3] M. D. Schweitzer, O. Salamo, G. Holt, E. Donna, and M. Mirsaeidi, "Sarcoidosis onset after breast cancer; a potential association," *European Journal of Internal Medicine*, vol. 44, pp. e11–e12, 2017.

[4] B. Brechtel, N. Haas, B. M. Henz, and G. Kolde, "Allopurinol: A therapeutic alternative for disseminated cutaneous sarcoidosis," *British Journal of Dermatology*, vol. 135, no. 2, pp. 307–309, 1996.

[5] H. Brincker and E. Wilbek, "The incidence of malignant tumours in patients with respiratory sarcoidosis," *British Journal of Cancer*, vol. 29, no. 3, pp. 247–251, 1974.

[6] J. T. Prior, "Boeck's sarcoid with coexisting carcinoma," *The American Journal of Surgery*, vol. 83, no. 2, pp. 201–204, 1952.

[7] J. S. Suen, M. S. Forse, R. H. Hyland, and C. K. Chan, "The malignancy-sarcoidosis syndrome," *CHEST*, vol. 98, no. 5, pp. 1300–1302, 1990.

[8] A. K. Shah, L. Solomon, and M. A. Gumbs, "Sarcoidosis of the breast coexisting with mammary carcinoma," *New York State journal of medicine*, vol. 90, no. 6, pp. 331–333, 1990.

[9] J. von Knorring and O. Selroos, "Sarcoidosis with thyroid involvement, polymyalgia rheumatica and breast carcinoma: A case report," *Scandinavian Journal of Rheumatology*, vol. 5, no. 2, pp. 77–80, 1976.

[10] R. Whittington, A. Lazarus, S. Nerenstone, and A. Martin, "Sarcoidosis developing during therapy for breast cancer," *CHEST*, vol. 89, no. 5, pp. 762-763, 1986.

[11] J. M. Reich, J. P. Mullooly, and R. E. Johnson, "Linkage analysis of malignancy-associated sarcoidosis," *CHEST*, vol. 107, no. 3, pp. 605–613, 1995.

[12] N. Seersholm, J. Vestbo, and K. Viskum, "Risk of malignant neoplasms in patients with pulmonary sarcoidosis," *Thorax*, vol. 52, no. 10, pp. 892–894, 1997.

[13] F. K. Rømer, P. Hommelgaard, and G. Schou, "Sarcoidosis and cancer revisited: a long-term follow-up study of 555 Danish sarcoidosis patients," *European Respiratory Journal*, vol. 12, no. 4, pp. 906–912, 1998.

[14] J. Askling, J. Grunewald, A. Eklund, G. Hillerdal, and A. Ekbom, "Increased risk for cancer following sarcoidosis," *American Journal of Respiratory and Critical Care Medicine*, vol. 160, no. 5, part 1, pp. 1668–1672, 1999.

[15] E. E. Lower, H. H. Hawkins, and R. P. Baughman, "Breast disease in sarcoidosis," *Sarcoidosis Vasculitis and Diffuse Lung Diseses*, vol. 18, no. 3, pp. 301–306, 2001.

[16] C. A. Garcia, R. J. Rosenberg, and R. P. Spencer, "FDG-Positron Emission Tomographic Imaging in Carcinoma of the Breast: Interference by Massive Sarcoidosis," *Clinical Nuclear Medicine*, vol. 28, no. 3, pp. 218-219, 2003.

[17] W. Chen, R. A. Miller, and K. A. Hebbe, "Sarcoidosis and breast carcinoma: three case reports and review," *Journal of Clinical Oncology*, pp. 22–867, 2004.

[18] J. J. M. Van Der Hoeven, N. C. Krak, O. S. Hoekstra et al., "18F-2-fluoro-2-deoxy-D-glucose positron emission tomography in staging of locally advanced breast cancer," *Journal of Clinical Oncology*, vol. 22, no. 7, pp. 1253–1259, 2004.

[19] I. Gusakova, K. Lavrenkov, S. Ariad, and W. Mermershtain, "Pulmonary sarcoidosis mimicking metastases in breast cancer patients," *Onkologie*, vol. 30, no. 6, pp. 327-328, 2007.

[20] S. M. Tolaney, Y. L. Colson, R. R. Gill et al., "Sarcoidosis mimicking metastatic breast cancer," *Clinical Breast Cancer*, vol. 7, no. 10, pp. 804–810, 2007.

[21] S. Ataergin, N. Arslan, A. Ozet, and M. A. Ozguven, "Abnormal 18F-FDG Uptake Detected with Positron Emission Tomography in a Patient with Breast Cancer: A Case of Sarcoidosis and Review of the Literature," *Case Reports in Medicine*, vol. 2009, Article ID 785047, 4 pages, 2009.

[22] L. Viswanath, S. Pallade, B. Krishnamurthy et al., "Darier-Roussy Sarcoidosis Mimicking Metastatic Breast Cancer," *Case Reports in Oncology*, vol. 2, no. 3, pp. 251–254, 2009.

[23] T. Ito, T. Okada, K. Murayama et al., "Two cases of sarcoidosis discovered accidentally by positron emission tomography in patients with breast cancer," *The Breast Journal*, vol. 16, no. 5, pp. 561–563, 2010.

[24] E. Bush, D. Lamonica, and T. O'Connor, "Sarcoidosis mimicking metastatic breast cancer," *The Breast Journal*, vol. 17, no. 5, pp. 533–535, 2011.

[25] M. Nishioka, K. Igawa, Y. Yahata, M. Tani, and I. Katayama, "Simultaneous occurrence of dermatomyositis and systemic

sarcoidosis with recurrent breast cancer," *The Journal of Dermatology*, vol. 39, no. 5, pp. 485-486, 2012.

[26] E. M. DeFilippis and E. K. Arleo, "New diagnosis of sarcoidosis during treatment for breast cancer, with radiologic-pathologic correlation," *Clinical Imaging*, vol. 37, no. 4, pp. 762–766, 2013.

[27] M. Akhtari, J. R. Quesada, M. R. Schwartz, S. B. Chiang, and B. S. Teh, "Sarcoidosis presenting as metastatic lymphadenopathy in breast cancer," *Clinical Breast Cancer*, vol. 14, no. 5, pp. e107–e110, 2014.

[28] H. S. Kim, S.-Y. Lee, S. C. Oh, C. W. Choi, J. S. Kim, and J. H. Seo, "Case report of pulmonary sarcoidosis suspected to be pulmonary metastasis in a patient with breast cancer," *Cancer Research and Treatment*, vol. 46, no. 3, pp. 317–321, 2014.

[29] S. Zivin, O. David, and Y. Lu, "Sarcoidosis mimicking metastatic breast cancer on FDG PET/CT," *Internal Medicine*, vol. 53, no. 21, pp. 2555-2556, 2014.

[30] M. Altinkaya, N. Altinkaya, and B. Hazar, "Sarcoidosis mimicking metastatic breast cancer in a patient with early-stage breast cancer," *Turkish Journal of Surgery*, vol. 32, no. 1, pp. 71–74, 2016.

[31] G. Conte, F. Zugni, M. Colleoni, G. Renne, M. Bellomi, and G. Petralia, "Sarcoidosis with bone involvement mimicking metastatic disease at ^{18}F-FDG PET/CT: Problem solving by diffusion whole-body MRI," *ecancermedicalscience*, vol. 9, 2015.

[32] M. El Hammoumi, M. El Marjany, D. Moussaoui, A. Doudouh, H. Mansouri, and E. H. Kabiri, "Mediastinal sarcoidosis mimicking lymph malignancy recurrence after anti-neoplastic therapy," *Archivos de Bronconeumología*, vol. 51, no. 7, pp. e33–e35, 2015.

[33] J. Chen, R. Carter III, D. Maoz, A. Tobar, E. Sharon, and F. Greif, "Breast cancer and sarcoidosis: Case series and review of the literature," *Breast Care*, vol. 10, no. 2, pp. 137–140, 2015.

[34] P. R. Cohen and R. Kurzrock, "Sarcoidosis and malignancy," *Clinics in Dermatology*, vol. 25, no. 3, pp. 326–333, 2007.

43

Squamous Cell Carcinoma Arising within Verruca Vulgaris on the Nipple

Araya Zaesim [ID],[1] Amanda C. Jackson [ID],[1] Sang Wook Lee [ID],[1] and Shaun A. Price[1,2]

[1]Mercer University School of Medicine, Columbus, GA, USA
[2]Department of General Surgery, St. Francis Center for Surgical Care, Columbus, GA, USA

Correspondence should be addressed to Araya Zaesim; zaesim.araya@gmail.com

Academic Editor: Jacek Cezary Szepietowski

Cutaneous squamous cell carcinoma (SCC) is a common form of skin cancer and often appears as a hard, scaly lump that occasionally ulcerates. It is usually associated with cumulative exposure to ultraviolet light, although prior scarring, chronic wounds, exposure to radiation, HPV infection, and immunosuppression are also associated risk factors. Primary SCC of the nipple is very rare and only a few cases have been reported. We present a case of a 49-year-old female with concerns of a right nipple lesion with erythema and pain. She was initially evaluated for Paget's disease with an underlying malignancy and cellulitis, but, after biopsy and investigation, she was found to have a well-differentiated SCC arising from a verruca vulgaris. Current literature does not provide distinct guidelines on management of SCC or its variants on the nipple, and the case was managed based off of SCC at other cutaneous sites as well as other cases of SCC on the nipple.

1. Introduction

Squamous cell carcinoma (SCC) of the skin and basal cell carcinoma of the skin are the most common cancers diagnosed annually in the United States [1]. Exact numbers are unknown as these common nonmelanoma skin cancers are not required to be reported to cancer registries. SCC arises from malignant transformation of epidermal keratinocytes. Examination of a suspected lesion typically reveals a hard and scaly plaque or nodule that occasionally ulcerates [2]. The most common reported risk factor for SCC is cumulative exposure to ultraviolet light [3]. Other risk factors include scarring, chronic wounds, ionizing radiation, HPV infection, and immunosuppression. Cutaneous SCC is usually not fatal, but it is associated with invasion causing local disfigurement and occasionally distant metastases. Primary SCC of the nipple is extremely rare and is noted in English literature only ten times [4–13]. Management of SCC of the nipple is derived from the understanding of cutaneous SCC in more common areas, although a wide variety of treatment modalities has been reported.

2. Case Report

A 49-year-old Caucasian woman was referred to a general surgeon by her primary care physician for a right nipple lesion. She reports no past medical history, and social history is notable for tobacco use. The patient stated that she first noticed a small, yellow, and fleshy bump on her right nipple approximately two years prior. She became concerned due to its rapid growth in the last year. Four months prior, she visited her primary care provider who performed a shave biopsy of the lesion. Initial pathology results suggested squamous cell carcinoma, but this was thought to be discordant with the clinical picture. At consultation, she reported that her right breast had also started feeling hot and tender for two weeks duration. On examination, her right breast was erythematous and rigid with a 2.2 cm lesion consuming the right nipple. Her nipple also drained yellow pus. The patient was placed on a course of antibiotics due to concerns for an abscess.

An MRI was ordered to investigate possible underlying breast malignancy. Results of the MRI showed no solid mass underlying the nipple. A wedge biopsy of the nipple was

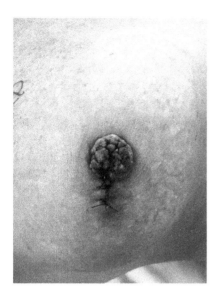

FIGURE 1: A wedge biopsy was taken from the nipple which appeared to have a 2.2 cm lesion.

performed to confirm the initial shave biopsy pathology (Figure 1). Pathology showed verrucous histologic features with chronic inflammation and underlying abscess with concerns for a possible cutaneous malignancy. Specifically, there was marked papillomatosis with hypergranulomatosis between the papillae as well as a lack of granules at the papillary surfaces. Immunohistochemical testing was also positive for HPV L1 capsid protein. Because the initial shave biopsy showed SCC with positive margins, this clinical picture suggested that an inadequate sample was taken during the wedge biopsy. After consultation of literature, excision with wide margins was determined to be appropriate for removal of the lesion.

The patient underwent a wide excision of the right nipple-areola complex for removal of the growth. A 6.2 cm x 3.2 cm skin ellipse was excised encompassing the 2.2 cm nipple lesion. On final histologic examination, the lesion was found to be a large tumor with verrucous features, hyperkeratosis, dyskeratosis, and nests of keratin pearl formation (Figure 2). Two areas showed microinvasion of the dermis with loss of the basal lamina. There were also significant acute and chronic inflammatory responses in the deep dermis representing an underlying abscess. These findings are congruent with the diagnosis of a well-differentiated squamous cell carcinoma with arising within verruca vulgaris. All margins were found to be clear of tumor cells. The post-op course was uneventful. She continues to follow up to monitor potential recurrence of the growth.

3. Discussion

Although cutaneous SCC is a very common diagnosis, to have it occur on the nipple is unlikely. This is primarily due to risk factors associated with the disease. They are usually associated with cumulative exposure to ultraviolet light although prior scarring, chronic wounds, exposure to

radiation, HPV infection, smoking, and immunosuppression are also associated risk factors. Ultraviolet light exposure is by far the most important risk factor [3]. Thus, in a location such as the nipple which does not see as much cumulative lifetime ultraviolet exposure as other skin locations, it is no wonder that the occurrence of SCC there is rare.

In the case of the presented patient, minor sun damage to the upper chest was noted. The patient also reported infrequent use of tanning beds, which could have induced pathology in the presenting location. However, she has never had any previous history of skin pathology to date. It would be expected that this patient presenting with a nonmelanoma skin cancer would have had pathology in areas with more cumulative ultraviolet exposure such as the face, hands, arms, and upper chest. Of previously reported cases of cutaneous SCC of the nipple, most patients had previous history of multiple nonmelanoma skin cancers in other locations. It is strange that this patient's presentation of her first diagnosed nonmelanoma skin cancer was on the nipple-areola complex. Patients with their first nonmelanoma skin cancer have a 3-year mean cumulative risk of 47% for development of another nonmelanoma skin cancer highlighting the need for adequate follow-up and monitoring [14].

The patient presented represents a unique instance of SCC of the nipple. No previous literature accounts for SCC of the nipple arising within a biopsy proven verruca vulgaris. Verruca vulgaris, or more commonly warts, is primarily caused by viruses within the family of human papilloma viruses (HPV). HPV is a group of approximately 100 strains of viruses that can cause disordered epithelial growth. This often results in the growth of warts on the hands, plantar surface of the feet, or anogenital region [15]. HPV strains are well-recognized contributors to SCC arising in anogenital, penile, cervical, and oropharyngeal areas of the body. The mutagenic properties of HPV are due to encoded viral oncoproteins that inhibit host tumor suppressor genes [16]. Immunosuppressive disorders, sun exposure, and tobacco use increase risk of HPV-related SCC. The presented patient is immunocompetent and has no prior history of HPV-related pathologies (i.e., abnormal pap smear, anogenital warts, etc.). However, chronic tobacco use combined with HPV exposure could have increased her risk of developing SCC. Literature searches reveal that while HPV may increase risk of SCC, it is still quite rare to have a verruca vulgaris arise from the nipple let alone transform into cutaneous SCC.

Although SCC can arise de novo and contain verrucoid features, confidence regarding the diagnosis of verruca vulgaris is gained from the initial biopsy at the lesion edge which strongly appeared as a verruca vulgaris and stained positively for an HPV capsid protein. Also, the patient's history of an initial, fleshy lesion on the nipple must be taken into account as a verruca vulgaris is often diagnosed by patient history.

One major differential diagnosis physicians must consider when a patient presents with a lesion of the nipple is Paget's disease of the breast (PDB). PDB is an uncommon diagnosis, but it is the most common lesion of the nipple [17]. It is crucial that this diagnosis be ruled out as PDB is often associated with an underlying breast cancer [18, 19]. Described as being a thickened, crusted lesion with irregular

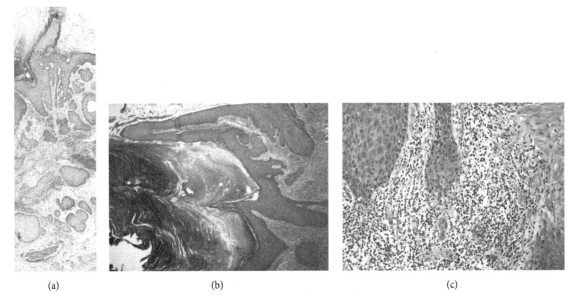

<table>
</table>

(a) (b) (c)

FIGURE 2: Histologic examination of a large section of tissue at 10x magnification (a) demonstrates the verrucoid top of the lesion and the invasive deep edge. Wide nests of tumor cells can be seen invading as well as a desmoplastic reaction to the nests and the lymphoplasmacytic host response. A low power image of the verrucous surface at 4x magnification (b) shows the verrucous surface with peaking hyperkeratosis and subtle koilocytotic changes. A high power image at 20x (c) shows dissolution of the basal lamina and invasion of the dermis. There is invasion by a small cluster of keratinocytes with the expected lymphoplasmacytic host response and desmoplastic host response (samples stained with hematoxylin and eosin).

borders usually limited to the nipple-areola complex, it can be hard to visually distinguish from a possible SCC. Suggested management of PDB includes an initial biopsy which can confirm the lesion or lead to an alternative diagnosis such as SCC. Guidelines also suggest further investigation using a mammogram or MRI to rule out any underlying breast malignancy. Such a distinction is important as it can guide differing management techniques.

As SCC of the nipple has a very low incidence, no standard management guidelines have been established. Many of the current examples in literature suggest wide local excision as the primary mode of treatment, but some patients have been offered mastectomy and radiation [4–13]. Two of the cases reported local recurrence, of which one had local resection with unclear margins. The other case was treated with novel photodynamic therapy with cryotherapy. With surgical resection, as with resection of cutaneous carcinomas on other areas of the skin, clear margins provide the best prognosis. One case which was treated with mastectomy was last reported as having no recurrence at the five-year point [7]. More data is still needed to determine the best mode of treatment.

Conflicts of Interest

The authors declare that there are no conflicts of interest regarding the publication of this paper.

Acknowledgments

The authors would like to thank Dr. Frank Willett for

providing insight about the pathology for the tissue samples shown.

References

[1] American Cancer Society, *Cancer Facts & Figs*, American Cancer Society, Atlanta, Ga, USA, 2018.

[2] A. Reszko, S. Z. Aasi, L. D. Wilson et al., "Cancer of the skin," in *Cancer: Principles and Practice of Oncology*, V. T. DeVita Jr., T. S. Lawrence, and S. A. Rosenberg, Eds., pp. 1610–1633, Lippincott Williams & Wilkins, Philadelphia, Pa, USA, 9th edition, 2011.

[3] S. A. Gandhi and J. Kampp, "Skin Cancer Epidemiology, Detection, and Management," *Medical Clinics of North America*, vol. 99, no. 6, pp. 1323–1335, 2015.

[4] K. Dye, M. Saucedo, D. Raju, and N. Aydin, "A common cancer in an uncommon location: A case report of squamous cell carcinoma of the nipple," *International Journal of Surgery Case Reports*, vol. 36, pp. 94–97, 2017.

[5] A. A. Pendse and S. M. O'Connor, "Primary invasive squamous cell carcinoma of the nipple," *Case Reports in Pathology*, vol. 2015, 5 pages, 2015.

[6] P. T. Brookes, S. Jhawar, C. P. Hinton, S. Murdoch, and T. Usman, "Bowen's disease of the nipple—a new method of treatment," *The Breast*, vol. 14, no. 1, pp. 65–67, 2005.

[7] N. Hosaka, K. Uesaka, T. Takaki, Y. Zhang, K. Takasu, and S. Ikehara, "Poorly differentiated squamous cell carcinoma of the nipple: a unique case for marked exophytic growth, but little invasion with neuroendocrine differentiation," *Medical Molecular Morphology*, vol. 44, no. 3, pp. 174–178, 2011.

[8] C. E. Loveland-Jones, F. Wang, R. R. Bankhead, Y. Huang, and K. J. Reilly, "Squamous cell carcinoma of the nipple following radiation therapy for ductal carcinoma in situ: a case report," *Journal of Medical Case Reports*, vol. 4, no. 186, 2010.

[9] J. King and H. Kremer, "Squamous cell carcinoma of the nipple: an unusual location in a male patient," *The American Surgeon*, vol. 78, no. 2, pp. E101–E102, 2012.

[10] S. S. Sofos, H. Tehrani, N. Lymperopoulos, J. Constantinides, and M. I. James, "Primary squamous cell carcinoma of the nipple: a diagnosis of suspicion," *Journal of Plastic, Reconstructive & Aesthetic Surgery*, vol. 66, no. 11, pp. 315–317, 2013.

[11] V. S. Venkataseshan, D. C. Budd, D. U. Kim, and R. V. P. Hutter, "Intraepidermal squamous carcinoma (Bowen's disease) of the nipple," *Human Pathology*, vol. 25, no. 12, pp. 1371–1374, 1994.

[12] S. P. Upasham, M. Vinodkiri, and S. Sudhamani, "One more common tumor in an uncommon location: squamous cell carcinoma on nipple areola complex," *Indian Journal of Cancer*, vol. 51, no. 3, pp. 376-377, 2014.

[13] R. Sharma and M. Iyer, "Bowen's disease of the nipple in a young man with AIDS: a case report," *Clinical Breast Cancer*, vol. 9, no. 1, pp. 53–55, 2009.

[14] I. Marcil and R. S. Stern, "Risk of developing a subsequent nonmelanoma skin cancer in patients with a history of non-melanoma skin cancer: a critical review of the literature and meta-analysis," *JAMA Dermatology*, vol. 136, no. 12, pp. 1524–1530, 2000.

[15] Y. Kurisu, M. Tsuji, E. Yasuda, M. Fujiwara, and S. Moriwaki, "Immunohistochemical findings and differential diagnosis of papillary-type cutaneous verrucous carcinoma of the neck: A case report," *Oncology Letters*, vol. 10, no. 6, pp. 3823–3825, 2015.

[16] B. Aldabagh, J. G. Angeles, A. R. Cardones, and S. T. Arron, "Cutaneous Squamous Cell Carcinoma and Human Papillomavirus: Is There an Association?" *Dermatologic Surgery*, vol. 39, no. 1, pp. 1–23, 2013.

[17] H. S. Lim, S. J. Jeong, J. S. Lee et al., "Paget disease of the breast: mammographic, US, and MR imaging findings with pathologic correlation," *RadioGraphics*, vol. 31, no. 7, pp. 1973–1987, 2011.

[18] C. Karakas, "Paget's disease of the breast," *Journal of Carcinogenesis*, vol. 10, no. 1, p. 31, 2011.

[19] G. H. Sakorafas, K. Blanchard, M. G. Sarr, and D. R. Farley, "Paget's disease of the breast," *Cancer Treatment Reviews*, vol. 27, no. 1, pp. 9–18, 2001.

44

Erythema Dyschromicum Perstans in an 8-Year-Old Indian Child

Alexander K. C. Leung (iD)[1,2] **and Joseph M. Lam**[3,4]

[1]*Clinical Professor of Pediatrics at The University of Calgary, Canada*
[2]*Pediatric Consultant at The Alberta Children's Hospital, Calgary, Alberta, Canada T2M 0H5*
[3]*Clinical Associate Professor of Pediatrics at the University of British Columbia, Canada*
[4]*Associate Member at the Department of Dermatology and Skin Sciences at the University of British Columbia, Vancouver, British Columbia, Canada*

Correspondence should be addressed to Alexander K. C. Leung; aleung@ucalgary.ca

Academic Editor: Jaime A. Tschen

We report an 8-year-old East Indian boy with erythema dyschromicum perstans. The condition has very rarely been reported in prepubertal Indian children. A perusal of the literature revealed but two cases, to which we add another one. Recognition of erythema dyschromicum perstans in prepubertal Indian children is important for proper diagnosis and to prevent unnecessary investigations.

1. Introduction

Erythema dyschromicum perstans, also known as ashy dermatosis or dermatosis cenicienta, is an acquired, chronic pigmentary disorder characterized by slowly progressive, ashy gray-colored macules/patches distributed symmetrically on the trunk and proximal extremities [1]. The condition was first described in 1957 by Oswaldo Ramirez in Salvadorans [2]. Ramirez called patients with this condition *los cenicienta* which in Spanish means the ash-colored ones because of the characteristic ashy color of the lesions [2]. The term "erythema dyschromicum perstans" was coined by Convit et al. in 1961 when they reported five patients with numerous macules of grayish color with slightly raised, firm erythematous border [3]. The disorder has very rarely been reported in prepubertal Indian children. A perusal of the literature revealed but two cases, to which we add another.

2. Case Report

An 8-year-old East Indian boy with Fitzpatrick skin type IV phototype complexion presented with numerous blue-gray macules and patches over the back, anterior trunk, arms, and legs of 8 months' duration. The lesions first appeared on the back and then spread to the anterior trunk, arms, and legs. Some of the lesions were mildly pruritic and some with preceding erythematous borders. The lesions were progressive and increased in size and number with time. There were no identifiable triggers. His past medical history was significant for Berry syndrome (a complex aortopulmonary malformation). The aortopulmonary malformation was repaired surgically at 10 days of life. The surgical repair was successful and the postoperative course was uneventful. Otherwise, his health was unremarkable and he was not on any medications. There was no history of previous skin eruption. He had no known family history of autoimmune disorder or similar skin disease.

On physical examination, there were numerous well-demarcated, oval, ash-brown macules and patches symmetrically distributed over the back, anterior trunk, arms, and legs (Figures 1–3). The lesions measured 0.5 to 6 cm and some lesions were confluent. There were no erythematous borders and no desquamation. Darier's sign was negative. The mucous membranes, face, scalp, palms, soles, and nails were spared. A well-healed scar from previous sternotomy was noted on the chest. The rest of the physical examination was unremarkable.

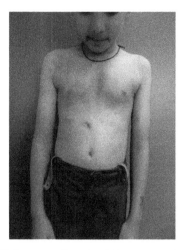

FIGURE 1: Well-demarcated oval ash-brown macules and patches symmetrically distributed over the anterior chest and abdomen.

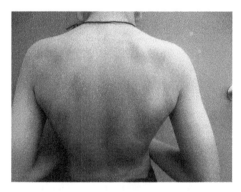

FIGURE 2: Well-demarcated oval ash-brown macules and patches symmetrically distributed over the upper back.

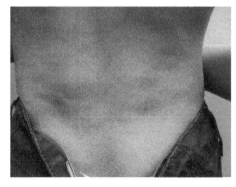

FIGURE 3: Well-demarcated oval blue-gray macules and patches symmetrically distributed over the lower back.

Dermoscopy of a lesion showed faint gray-blue to bluish small dots over a bluish background, corresponding to melanin-laden melanophages in deeper dermis (Tyndall effect) (Figure 4). The patient was diagnosed to have erythema dyschromicum perstans based on the clinical and dermoscopic findings.

Parents were reassured of the benign nature of the disorder and that the lesions would resolve with time. A skin biopsy was declined by the parents.

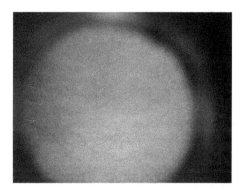

FIGURE 4: Dermoscopy of a lesion showed gray-blue to bluish small dots over a bluish background, corresponding to melanin-laden melanophages in deeper dermis (Tyndall effect).

3. Discussion

Typically, erythema dyschromicum perstans presents as ashy gray to grayish brown oval macules/patches symmetrically distributed over the body [4–7]. Sites of predilection include the trunk, followed by the proximal extremities, neck, and face [8]. The mucosal surfaces, genitals, scalp, palms, soles, and nails are generally spared [9]. The size of the lesions ranges from a few millimeters to several centimeters in diameter [9]. A slightly raised, erythematous border may be present in the early stage which, when present, is characteristic [10, 11]. The erythematous border tends to resolve with time [6]. In one study, an erythematous border is found only in 17.6% of cases [9]. The condition is typically asymptomatic, but mild pruritus may occur [5, 7, 9]. Dermoscopy of the lesion typically shows gray-blue to bluish small dots over a bluish background, corresponding to melanin-laden melanophages in deeper dermis (Tyndall effect), as is illustrated in the present case [12].

Our patient had typical clinical and dermoscopic features of erythema dyschromicum perstans. A skin biopsy was declined by the parents given the benign nature of the disorder and that the lesions tend to resolve with time.

Erythema dyschromicum perstans occurs most commonly in individuals under 30 years of age with a peak in the second decade of life [7, 9]. The disorder is rare in prepubertal children, especially in the Asian population [13]. In adults, the disorder is more prevalent in the Latin American and Asian population [1, 7, 9]. Dark-skinned individuals (Fitzpatrick types IV and V) are most commonly affected [1, 8, 9]. In contrast to the adult population, children with this disorder are usually Caucasians [6, 13, 14]. Erythema dyschromicum perstans has very rarely been reported in prepubertal Indian children. A perusal of the literature revealed but two cases. In 1996, Umap reported the first case of erythema dyschromicum perstans in a 10-year-old Indian child with multiple lesions of erythema dyschromicum perstans over the face and upper limbs of 10 months' duration [15]. In 2013, Keisham et al. reported another case of erythema dyschromicum perstans in an 8-year-old Indian child who presented with asymptomatic, gradually progressive ashy gray-colored, confluent, symmetrical macules over the entire trunk, proximal limbs, posterior neck, forehead, and left upper eyelid [13]. Herein, we report an 8-year-old East Indian boy with erythema dyschromicum perstans.

The exact etiology of erythema dyschromicum perstans is not known. Most cases are idiopathic [7]. Erythema dyschromicum perstans has been reported in association with exposure to drugs (penicillin, benzodiazepines, ethambutol, fluoxetine, and omeprazole), radiographic contrast media (barium sulfate), parasitic infestations (whipworm), fungicide (chlorothalonil), chemicals (ammonium nitrate), herbal consumption (Tokishakuyakusa), endocrinopathies (hypothyroidism, diabetes mellitus), dyslipidemia, infections (human immunodeficiency virus, hepatitis C, and enterovirus), and cobalt allergy [16–20]. Our patient did not have any identifiable triggers. Appropriate laboratory investigations should be performed if an underlying cause is suspected.

Erythema dyschromicum perstans should be differentiated from idiopathic eruptive macular pigmentation and lichen planus pigmentosus. In idiopathic eruptive macular pigmentation, lesions are ashy brown, nonconfluent, and smaller in size and tend to regress with time. In lichen planus pigmentosus, lesions are brown to gray-brown macules/patches, pruritic, and without an active erythematous border. The lesions often occur in sun-exposed and intertriginous areas and may involve mucous membranes. Other differential diagnoses include maculopapular mastocytosis, postinflammatory hyperpigmentation, morphea, pityriasis rosea, Addison disease, hemochromatosis, arsenism, contact dermatitis, multiple fixed drug eruption, confluent and reticulated papillomatosis of Gougerot and Carteaud, tuberculoid leprosy, and pinta.

Erythema dyschromicum perstans can be cosmetically distressing and socially embarrassing, especially if the lesion occurs in a visible area such as the face [1, 21]. The cutaneous eruption tends to resolve in 2 to 3 years in prepubertal children but tends to persist in adults [4, 6]. Our patient and family were reassured of the benign nature of the condition and that the lesions would resolve with time.

4. Conclusion

In adults, erythema dyschromicum perstans is more prevalent in the Latin American and Asian population. Dark-skinned individuals are most commonly affected. In contrast to the adult population, children with this disorder are usually Caucasians. Erythema dyschromicum perstans has very rarely been reported in prepubertal Indian children. A perusal of the literature revealed but two cases, to which we are going to add another one. Erythema dyschromicum perstans should be included in the differential diagnosis of pigmentary disorders in prepubertal Indian children. Recognition of erythema dyschromicum perstans in prepubertal Indian children is important so that a proper diagnosis can be made.

Conflicts of Interest

Professor Leung and Dr. Lam have disclosed no relevant financial relationship. They have received no external funding for the preparation of this manuscript.

References

[1] J. A. Wolfshohl, E. R. C. Geddes, A. B. Stout, and P. M. Friedman, "Improvement of erythema dyschromicum perstans using a combination of the 1,550-nm erbium-doped fractionated laser and topical tacrolimus ointment," *Lasers in Surgery and Medicine*, vol. 49, no. 1, pp. 60–62, 2017.

[2] C. O. Ramirez, "Los cenicientos: problema clinica," in *Proceedings of the First Central American Congress of Dermatology*, pp. 122–130, 1957.

[3] J. Convit, F. Kerdel-Vegas, and G. Rodríguez, "Erythema Dyschromicum Perstans," *Journal of Investigative Dermatology*, vol. 36, no. 6, pp. 457–462, 1961.

[4] N. K. Antonov, I. Braverman, A. Subtil, and C. L. Halasz, "Erythema dyschromicum perstans showing resolution in an adult," *JAAD Case Reports*, vol. 1, no. 4, pp. 185–187, 2015.

[5] C. Raquel Ferrão de Melo, S. Carvalho, and M. C. de Sá, "Erythema dyschromicum perstans in a child following an enteroviral meningitis," *Anais Brasileiros de Dermatologia*, vol. 92, no. 1, pp. 137-138, 2017.

[6] N. B. Silverberg, J. Herz, A. Wagner, and A. S. Paller, "Erythema Dyschromicum Perstans in Prepubertal Children," *Pediatric Dermatology*, vol. 20, no. 5, pp. 398–403, 2003.

[7] F. Wang, Y.-K. Zhao, Z. Wang, J.-H. Liu, and D.-Q. Luo, "Erythema dyschromicum perstans response to isotretinoin," *JAMA Dermatology*, vol. 152, no. 7, pp. 841-842, 2016.

[8] M. Pinheiro Gaio Seabra Rato, A. F. Monteiro, J. Aranha, and E. Tavares, "Ashy dermatosis with involvement of mucous membranes," *Anais Brasileiros de Dermatologia*, vol. 92, no. 5, pp. 17–20, 2017.

[9] S. E. Chang, H. W. Kim, J. M. Shin et al., "Clinical and histological aspect of erythema dyschromicum perstans in Korea: A review of 68 cases," *The Journal of Dermatology*, vol. 42, no. 11, pp. 1053–1057, 2015.

[10] S. Bahadir, Ü. Çobanoglu, G. Çimsit, S. Yayli, and K. Alpay, "Erythema dyschromicum perstans: Response to dapsone therapy," *International Journal of Dermatology*, vol. 43, no. 3, pp. 220–222, 2004.

[11] T. Numata, K. Harada, R. Tsuboi, and Y. Mitsuhashi, "Erythema dyschromicum perstans: Identical to ashy dermatosis or not," *Case Reports in Dermatology*, vol. 7, pp. 146–150, 2015.

[12] E. Errichetti, V. Angione, and G. Stinco, "Dermoscopy in assisting the recognition of ashy dermatosis," *JAAD Case Reports*, vol. 3, no. 6, pp. 482–484, 2017.

[13] R. Sarkar, S. Chugh, V. Garg, and C. Keisham, "Ashy dermatosis in an 8-year-old Indian child," *Indian Dermatology Online Journal (IDOJ)*, vol. 4, no. 1, p. 30, 2013.

[14] A. M. Tisack, R. H. Huggins, and H. W. Lim, "Erythema dyschromicum perstans in a Caucasian pediatric patient," *Journal of Drugs in Dermatology (JDD)*, vol. 12, no. 7, pp. 819-820, 2013.

[15] P. S. Umap, "Erythema dyschromicum perstans," *Indian Journal of Dermatology*, vol. 41, no. 2, pp. 68-69, 1996.

[16] S. Chua, M. M. F. Chan, and H. Y. Lee, "Ashy dermatosis (erythema dyschromicum perstans) induced by omeprazole: A report of three cases," *International Journal of Dermatology*, vol. 54, no. 10, pp. e435–e436, 2015.

[17] S. Jablonska, "Ingestion of ammonium nitrate as a possible cause of erythema dyschromicum perstans (ashy dermatosis)," *Dermatologica Sinica*, vol. 150, no. 5, pp. 287–291, 1975.

[18] G. J. Kontochristopoulos, K. Aroni, G. Anagnostopoulos, L. Nakopoulou, and N. C. Tassopoulos, "Erythema dyschromicum perstans and hepatitis C virus infection," *International Journal of Dermatology*, vol. 40, no. 5, pp. 346–348, 2001.

[19] J. Molinero, J. J. Vilata, E. Nagore, L. Obón, C. Grau, and A. Aliaga, "Ashy dermatosis in an HIV antibody-positive patient," *Acta Dermato-Venereologica*, vol. 80, no. 1, pp. 78-79, 2000.

[20] P. Zenorola, M. Bisceglia, and M. Lomuto, "Ashy dermatosis associated with cobalt allergy," *Contact Dermatitis*, vol. 31, no. 1, pp. 53-54, 1994.

[21] V. Mahajan, P. Chauhan, K. Mehta, and A. Sharma, "Erythema dyschromicum perstans: Response to topical tacrolimus," *Indian Journal of Dermatology*, vol. 60, no. 5, p. 525, 2015.

45

Clinical Manifestation, Dermoscopy, and Scanning Electron Microscopy in Two Cases of Contagious Ecthyma (Orf Nodule)

Ana Laura Rosifini Alves Rezende,[1] **Fred Bernardes Filho ⓘ,**[1] **Natália Aparecida de Paula,**[1] **Loan Towersey,**[2] **Roderick Hay,**[3] **and Marco Andrey Cipriani Frade ⓘ**[1]

[1]*Dermatology Division, Department of Internal Medicine, Ribeirão Preto Medical School, University of São Paulo, Ribeirão Preto, São Paulo, Brazil*
[2]*AIDS Division, Carlos Tortelly Municipal Hospital, Ministry of Health, Niterói, Rio de Janeiro, Brazil*
[3]*International Foundation for Dermatology, London, UK*

Correspondence should be addressed to Marco Andrey Cipriani Frade; mandrey@fmrp.usp.br

Academic Editor: Alireza Firooz

Orf is a highly contagious skin disease commonly seen in goats and sheep that can be transmitted to people who have direct contact with infected animals. Here, we report the clinical manifestation, dermoscopy, and scanning electron microscopy in two women who developed skin lesions on their hands after handling goats with wounds in the udders. Human orf is usually self-limiting and no specific treatment is needed.

1. Introduction

Contagious ecthyma also called contagious pustular dermatitis or scabby mouth is a zoonotic disease, called orf in humans, which is caused by a double-stranded DNA virus, ORFV, and usually affects sheep and goats [1, 2]. Human infection occurs through inoculation of broken or abraded skin from infected animals or contaminated fomites [1, 3].

The clinical manifestation, dermoscopy, and scanning electron microscopy in two women, who developed skin lesions on their hands after handling goats with wounds on the udders, are presented herein.

2. Case Report

A 63-year-old female came for consultation presenting with an erythematous violaceous plaque on the right index finger that had started 7 days previously. On examination a central necrotic area (Figure 1(a)) was observed. Fracture and acute vascular occlusion were excluded. Laboratory tests were unremarkable. A consultation with the dermatology department was then requested.

The patient raised goats on her farm. The animals had some udder lesions, so she needed to daily bottle-feed milk to the kids. She did not wear gloves while performing this task. During the evaluation of the patient, it was observed that the patient's daughter presented with a similar skin lesion on the left thumb, and she reported that she also helped to feed the little goats. Dermatology exam showed an indurated nodule with central umbilication covered by crust and surrounded by a reddish halo (Figure 1(b)). Dermoscopy of the finger nodule showed an erythematous area, central ulceration, yellow crust, brown dots, a white structureless area partially surrounding the lesion, and dotted vessels (Figure 2). The diagnosis of orf was suspected.

Upon domiciliary visit to the patient's farm, goats with udder lesions (Figure 3(a)) were found. The electron microscope has been used for the diagnosis of orf. In this case, it showed ovoid particles with a crisscross appearance due to viral particles (Figure 4); polymerase chain reaction was positive for the specific virus (ORFV) (Figure 4). The patient was advised to feed the kids using gloves (Figure 5) and to commence local wound care for the lesions, because the disease was showing spontaneous regression.

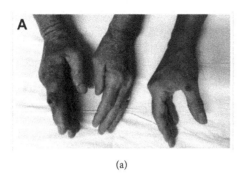
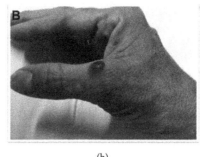

(a)   (b)

FIGURE 1: (a) Erythematous-violaceous papules and an ulcerated violaceous nodule on the patient's (left) and her daughter's (right) fingers; (b) a violaceous erythematous lesion with red outer ring, and erythematous border on the right thumb of patient's daughter.

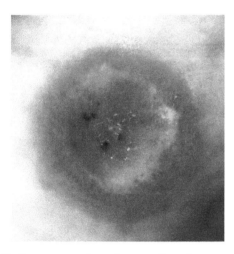

FIGURE 2: Dermoscopy showed an erythematous area, central ulceration, yellow crust, brown dots, a white structureless zone partially surrounding it, and dotted vessels; original magnification x10 (DermLite II Pro 3Gen, San Juan Capistrano, CA, USA).

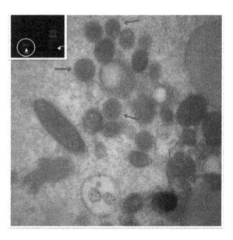

FIGURE 4: Electron microscopy showing numerous viral particles (DNA core surrounded by double layered capsid) (red arrow). Insert: polymerase chain reaction (PCR) orf virus result. 2% agarose gel, with PCR product with ORF1/ORF2 primers, specific for orf virus; 140pb positive fragment (white circle); DNA ladder (100pb).

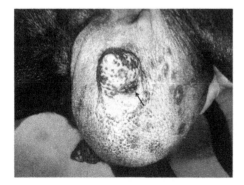

FIGURE 3: (a) Udder lesions (arrow) on the patient's goat.

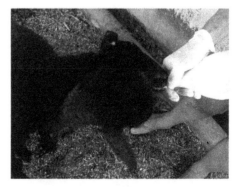

FIGURE 5: Patient feeding the kids using gloves.

3. Discussion

Orf is characterized by one or multiple nodules on the hands and fingers, but also on the feet, legs, neck, and face [1–3]. The disease passes through different phases. The first phase occurs after a brief incubation period of 3 to 5 days and presents with a small papule. Then, the lesions enlarge and progress to nodules that ulcerate and form crusts. The disease usually does not require specific treatment, because the lesions show spontaneous regression within 4–8 weeks [1–3]. Besides dermatologic features, the patient may experience some systemic symptoms and signs, such as fever and, less commonly, lymphangitis, lymphadenitis, and ocular damage [2, 3]. Orf may also trigger erythema multiforme [4].

The diagnosis is based on the history, physical examination, and some complementary investigations, such as dermoscopy, histopathology, PCR detection, and electron microscopy [1, 5–7].

Occupational skin diseases are particularly important in dermatology, because they can lead to high morbidity in workers and can also reduce their productivity. Moreover, they also represent a public health risk.

The case of orf nodules in relatives shows the importance of disseminating knowledge about this skin disease, because the patient was sent to the emergency room due to suspected necrosis of the finger, but actually she had a benign and self-resolving disease.

Although no person-to-person spread occurs, people in the same environment may be contaminated by the same source (infected animal). Differential diagnoses include, depending on the phase of the disease, anthrax, atypical mycobacteriosis, cowpox, pseudocowpox (Milker's nodule), pyoderma, herpetic whitlow, tularemia, keratoacanthoma, fish-tank granuloma, and sporotrichosis [1, 2, 8]. Dermoscopy is a very helpful tool to diagnose orf and Milker's nodule, but it cannot differentiate between them, so further diagnostic tools are required. We used both electron microscopy and PCR detection to confirm the orf virus diagnosis.

We emphasize the importance of using more specific techniques to confirm the diagnosis, especially when dealing with an occupational skin disease which has repercussions on public system.

Disclosure

All authors meet the criteria for authorship, including acceptance of responsibility for its scientific content. All authors have contributed to prepare and they approved the final manuscript.

Conflicts of Interest

The authors declare no conflicts of interest regarding this manuscript or the work described herein.

Acknowledgments

The authors thank Electron Microscopy Multiuser Laboratory, Department of Cell and Molecular Biology and Pathogenic Bioagents, Ribeirão Preto Medical School, University of São Paulo, Brazil.

References

[1] J. V. Caravaglio and A. Khachemoune, "Orf virus infection in humans: A review with a focus on advances in diagnosis and treatment," *Journal of Drugs in Dermatology (JDD)*, vol. 16, no. 7, pp. 684–689, 2017.

[2] J. A. Bala, K. N. Balakrishnan, A. A. Abdullah et al., "The re-emerging of orf virus infection: a call for surveillance, vaccination and effective control measures," *Microbial Pathogenesis*, vol. 120, pp. 55–63, 2018.

[3] C. Bergqvist, M. Kurban, and O. Abbas, "Orf virus infection," *Reviews in Medical Virology*, vol. 27, no. 4, Article ID e1932, 2017.

[4] R. H. Joseph, F. A. Haddad, A. L. Matthews, A. Maroufi, B. Monroe, and M. Reynolds, "Erythema multiforme after orf virus infection: A report of two cases and literature review," *Epidemiology and Infection*, vol. 143, no. 2, pp. 385–390, 2015.

[5] E. Ayhan and H. Aktaş, "Dermoscopic features and types of orf and milker's nodule," *Postepy Dermatologii i Alergologii*, vol. 34, no. 4, pp. 357–362, 2017.

[6] S. Chavez-Alvarez, L. Barbosa-Moreno, A. Villarreal-Martinez, O. T. Vazquez-Martinez, and J. Ocampo-Candiani, "Dermoscopy of contagious ecthyma (orf nodule)," *Journal of the American Academy of Dermatology*, vol. 74, no. 5, pp. e95–e96, 2016.

[7] F. Peng, Z. Chen, S.-Y. Zheng, H.-M. Li, J. Du, and J.-Z. Zhang, "A case of orf identified by transmission electron microscopy," *Chinese Medical Journal*, vol. 129, no. 1, pp. 108-109, 2016.

[8] A. López-Cedeño, G. Cañedo, N. Knöpfel, I. Colmenero, E. Pérez-Pastrana, and A. Torrelo, "Erythema multiforme after orf virus infection," *Pediatric Dermatology*, vol. 35, no. 4, pp. e237–e238, 2018.

Permissions

All chapters in this book were first published in CRDM, by Hindawi Publishing Corporation; hereby published with permission under the Creative Commons Attribution License or equivalent. Every chapter published in this book has been scrutinized by our experts. Their significance has been extensively debated. The topics covered herein carry significant findings which will fuel the growth of the discipline. They may even be implemented as practical applications or may be referred to as a beginning point for another development.

The contributors of this book come from diverse backgrounds, making this book a truly international effort. This book will bring forth new frontiers with its revolutionizing research information and detailed analysis of the nascent developments around the world.

We would like to thank all the contributing authors for lending their expertise to make the book truly unique. They have played a crucial role in the development of this book. Without their invaluable contributions this book wouldn't have been possible. They have made vital efforts to compile up to date information on the varied aspects of this subject to make this book a valuable addition to the collection of many professionals and students.

This book was conceptualized with the vision of imparting up-to-date information and advanced data in this field. To ensure the same, a matchless editorial board was set up. Every individual on the board went through rigorous rounds of assessment to prove their worth. After which they invested a large part of their time researching and compiling the most relevant data for our readers.

The editorial board has been involved in producing this book since its inception. They have spent rigorous hours researching and exploring the diverse topics which have resulted in the successful publishing of this book. They have passed on their knowledge of decades through this book. To expedite this challenging task, the publisher supported the team at every step. A small team of assistant editors was also appointed to further simplify the editing procedure and attain best results for the readers.

Apart from the editorial board, the designing team has also invested a significant amount of their time in understanding the subject and creating the most relevant covers. They scrutinized every image to scout for the most suitable representation of the subject and create an appropriate cover for the book.

The publishing team has been an ardent support to the editorial, designing and production team. Their endless efforts to recruit the best for this project, has resulted in the accomplishment of this book. They are a veteran in the field of academics and their pool of knowledge is as vast as their experience in printing. Their expertise and guidance has proved useful at every step. Their uncompromising quality standards have made this book an exceptional effort. Their encouragement from time to time has been an inspiration for everyone.

The publisher and the editorial board hope that this book will prove to be a valuable piece of knowledge for researchers, students, practitioners and scholars across the globe.

List of Contributors

Georgios Gaitanis, Theodora Tsironi and Ioannis D Bassukas
Department of Skin and Venereal Diseases, Faculty of Medicine, School of Health Sciences, University of Ioannina, Ioannina, Greece

Panagiota Spyridonos
Laboratory of Medical Physics, Faculty of Medicine, School of Health Sciences, University of Ioannina, Ioannina, Greece

Araya Zaesim, Amanda C. Jackson and Sang Wook Lee
Mercer University School of Medicine, Columbus, GA, USA

Grigorios Theodosiou
Specialist in Dermatology-Venereology, Department of Dermatology, Sk ane University Hospital, Jan Waldenstroms gata 16, 20502, Malmo, Sweden

Marina Papageorgiou and Ioanna Mandekou-Lefaki
Specialist in Dermatology-Venereology, State Clinic of Dermatology, Hospital for Skin and Venereal Diseases, Delfon 124, 54643, Thessaloniki, Greece

Shaun A. Price
Mercer University School of Medicine, Columbus, GA, USA Department of General Surgery, St. Francis Center for Surgical Care, Columbus, GA, USA

Alexander K. C. Leung
Clinical Professor of Pediatrics at the University of Calgary, Canada
Pediatric Consultant at The Alberta Children's Hospital, Calgary, Alberta, Canada T2M 0H5

Joseph M. Lam
Clinical Associate Professor of Pediatrics at the University of British Columbia, Canada
Associate Member at the Department of Dermatology and Skin Sciences at the University of British Columbia, Vancouver, British Columbia, Canada

Abigail I. Franco
St. Joseph's Hospital Health Center, 301 Prospect Avenue, Syracuse, NY 13203, USA

Gary Eastwick, Ramsay Farah, Marvin Heyboer, Mijung Lee and Paul Aridgides
Upstate University Hospital, 750 E. Adams Street, Syracuse, NY 13210, USA

Sara B. Huff
University of Toledo College of Medicine and Life Sciences, 3000 Arlington Avenue, Toledo, OH 43614, USA

Lorie D. Gottwald
Department of Dermatology, University of Toledo Medical Center, 3000 Arlington Avenue, Toledo, OH 43614, USA

Farhana Tahseen Taj and Prarthana B. Desai
Department of Dermatology, Venereology & Leprosy, Jawaharlal Nehru Medical College and KLE's Dr. Prabhakar Kore Hospital and Medical Research Centre, Belgaum, Karnataka 590 010, India

Divya Vupperla
Department of Dermatology, Venereology & Leprosy, Government District Headquarters Hospital, Khammam, Andhra Pradesh 507 002, India

Tania Ahuja
New York University Langone Health, Department of Pharmacy, 550 First Avenue, New York, NY 10016, USA

Frank R. Chung
New York University School of Medicine, 550 First Avenue, New York, NY 10016, USA

Tania Ruiz-Maya
New York University Langone Health, Department of Medicine, 550 First Avenue, New York, NY 10016, USA

Jacqueline Deen
Department of Dermatology, Sunshine Coast University Hospital, 6 Doherty Street, Birtinya, Queensland 4575, Australia
Department of Pathology, Medlab Pathology, 280 Newmarket Road, Wilston, Queenslan 4051, Australia

Farahnaz Bidari-Zerehpoosh, Shahram Sabeti, Farid Arman and Hania Shakeri
Shahid Beheshti University of Medical Sciences, Tehran, Iran

Roxana Mititelu
Department of Dermatology, McGill University Health Centre, Montreal, QC, Canada

Nick Mellick
Department of Pathology, Medlab Pathology, 280 Newmarket Road, Wilston, Queenslan 4051, Australia

Laura Wheller
Department of Dermatology, Mater Misercordiae Hospital, Raymond Terrace, South Brisbane, Queensland 4101, Australia

Georgios Gaitanis and Ioannis D. Bassukas
Department of Skin and Venereal Diseases, Faculty of Medicine, School of Health Sciences, University of Ioannina, Ioannina, Greece

Dora Gougopoulou and Eleni Kapsali
Hematology Clinic, Department of Internal Medicine, Faculty of Medicine, School of Health Sciences, University of Ioannina, Ioannina, Greece

N. Vega Mata
Department of Pediatric Surgery, Hospital Universitario Central de Asturias, Oviedo, Spain

M. S. Fernández García
Department of Pediatric Surgery, Hospital Universitario Central de Asturias, Oviedo, Spain
Department of Pathology, Hospital Universitario Central de Asturias, Oviedo, Spain

J. C. López Gutiérrez
Department of Pediatric Surgery, Hospital La Paz, Madrid, Spain

B. Vivanco Allende
Department of Pathology, Hospital Universitario Central de Asturias, Oviedo, Spain

Dharshini Sathishkumar, Dincy Peter, Susanne Pulimood and Meera Thomas
Department of Dermatology Venereology and Leprosy, Christian Medical College, Vellore, India

Henning Wiegmann, Frederic Valentin and Vinzenz Oji
Auckland University of Technology, Auckland 1142, New Zealand

Hans Christian Hennies
Center for Dermatogenetics, Division of Human Genetics, Medical University of Innsbruck, Innsbruck, Austria
Cologne Center for Genomics, Division of Dermatogenetics, University of Cologne, Germany
Cologne Excellence Cluster on Cellular Stress Responses in Aging-Associated Diseases (CECAD), University of Cologne, Cologne, Germany

Department of Biological and Geographical Sciences, University of Huddersfield, Huddersfield, UK

Aslı Bilgiç Temel and Şoner Uzun
Dermatology and Venereology Department, Akdeniz University Faculty of Medicine, Antalya, Turkey

Betül Unal
Pathology Department, Akdeniz University Faculty of Medicine, Antalya, Turkey

Hatice Erdi Şanlı
Dermatology and Venereology Department, Ankara University Faculty of Medicine, Ankara, Turkey

Şeniz Duygulu
Dermatology and Venereology Department, Pamukkale University Faculty of Medicine, Denizli, Turkey

Sezin Fıcıcıoğlu
Department of Dermatology, Trakya University Faculty of Medicine, Balkan Yerleskesi, Edirne, Turkey

Selma Korkmaz
Department of Dermatology, Suleyman Demirel University Faculty of Medicine, Isparta, Turkey

Ranran Zhang and William Nicholas Rose
Department of Pathology and Laboratory Medicine, University of Wisconsin, Madison, WI, USA

Sara Ghoneim
Saba University School of Medicine, the Bottom, Netherlands

Alvaro J. Ramos-Rodriguez and Fernando Vazquez de Lara
Icahn School of Medicine at Mount Sinai West, New York, NY, USA

Lauren Bonomo
Icahn School of Medicine at Mount Sinai, New York, NY, USA

Michael P. Salna
Department of Cardiothoracic Surgery, Stanford University School of Medicine, Stanford, CA, USA

Hannah M. Singer
Columbia University College of Physicians and Surgeons, New York City, NY, USA

Ali N. Dana
Dermatology Service, James J. Peters VA Medical Center, Bronx, NY, USA
Department of Dermatology, Columbia University College of Physicians and Surgeons, New York City, NY, USA

Ugur Uslu, Franz Heppt and Michael Erdmann
Department of Dermatology, Friedrich-Alexander-University Erlangen Nurnberg (FAU), Universit at sklinikum Erlangen, Erlangen, Germany

Elena Vargas-Laguna, Adrián Imbernón-Moya and Antonio Aguilar-Martínez
Department of Dermatology, Hospital Universitario Severo Ochoa, Avenida de Orellana, Leganes, 28911, Madrid, Spain

Fernando Burgos
Department of Pathology, Hospital Universitario Severo Ochoa, Avenida de Orellana, Leganes, 28911, Madrid, Spain

Amal A. Kokandi
Department of Dermatology, Faculty of Medicine, King Abdulaziz University, Jeddah, Saudi Arabia

Sakunee Niranvichaiya and Daranporn Triwongwaranat
Department of Dermatology, Faculty of Medicine Siriraj Hospital, Mahidol University, Bangkok, Thailand

R. M. Ngwanya, B. Kakande and N. P. Khumalo
Groote Schuur Hospital and the University of Cape Town, Cape Town, South Africa

Rachel J. Waldemer-Streyer and Ellen Jacobsen
College of Medicine, University of Illinois-Chicago, Urbana Campus, 506 South Mathews Ave, 190 Medical Sciences Building, MC-714, Urbana, IL 61801, USA

Sirinuch Chomtho
Division of Nutrition, Department of Pediatrics, Faculty of Medicine, Chulalongkorn University, Bangkok 10330, Thailand

Jaraspong Uaariyapanichkul
Division of Nutrition, Department of Pediatrics, Faculty of Medicine, Chulalongkorn University, Bangkok 10330, Thailand
Division of Nutrition, Department of Pediatrics, King Chulalongkorn Memorial Hospital, The Thai Red Cross Society, Bangkok 10330, Thailand

Puthita Saengpanit
Division of Nutrition, Department of Pediatrics, King Chulalongkorn Memorial Hospital, the Thai Red Cross Society, Bangkok 10330, Thailand

Ponghatai Damrongphol and Kanya Suphapeetiporn
Center of Excellence for Medical Genetics, Department of Pediatrics, Faculty of Medicine, Chulalongkorn University, Bangkok 10330, Thailand

Excellence Center for Medical Genetics, King Chulalongkorn Memorial Hospital, the Thai RedCross Society, Bangkok 10330, Thailand

Bader Alharbi, Samer Alamri and Ahmed Mahdi
King Abdullah International Medical Research Center, King Saud bin Abdulaziz University for Health Sciences, Jeddah 21423, Saudi Arabia

Siham Marghalani
King Abdullah International Medical Research Center, King Saud bin Abdulaziz University for Health Sciences, Jeddah 21423, Saudi Arabia
Department of Dermatology, King Khaled National Guard Hospital, National Guard Health Affairs, Jeddah 21423, Saudi Arabia

Gerhard Eichhoff
Wellington Regional Hospital, Wellington 6242, New Zealand

Noriko Soffi Harun
Department of Rheumatology, Hutt Hospital, Lower Hutt, New Zealand

Vanessa Di Palma and Jeffrey C. Dawes
Department of Obstetrics and Gynecology, University of Calgary, Calgary, AB, Canada

Jill P. Stone
Division of Plastic Surgery, Department of Surgery, University of Calgary, Calgary, AB, Canada

Andrew Schell
Department of Pathology & Laboratory Medicine, University of Calgary and Calgary Laboratory Services, Calgary, AB, Canada

Boushab Mohamed Boushab
Department of Internal Medicine and Infectious Diseases, Kiffa Regional Hospital, Assaba, Mauritania

Fatima-Zahra Fall-Malick
National Institute of Hepatitis and Virology, School of Medicine, Nouakchott, Mauritania

Leonardo K. Basco
Aix Marseille Univ, IRD, AP-HM, SSA, VITROME, IHU-Mediterranee Infection, Marseille, France

Saras Mane and Joseph Singer
Medical Research Institute of New Zealand, Wellington, New Zealand

Alex Semprini
Medical Research Institute of New Zealand, Wellington, New Zealand
Victoria University of Wellington, Wellington, New Zealand

Andrew Corin
Clinical Horizons New Zealand, Tauranga, New Zealand

Chelsea Casey and Stephen E. Weis
Department of Internal Medicine, University of North Texas Health Science Center, Texas College of Osteopathic Medicine, Fort Worth, TX, USA

Matthew L. Clark, Angela Sutton and Tricia Ann Missall
Department of Dermatology, Saint Louis University, 1755 S. Grand Blvd., Saint Louis, MO 63104, USA

Courtney A. Tobin
Distinctive Dermatology, 510 Fullerton Rd., Swansea, IL 62226, USA

O. Vanhooteghem
Department of Dermatology, CHU UCL Sainte Elisabeth Hospital, Namur, Belgium

I. Theate
Department of Anatomopathology, IPG, Gosselies, Belgium

Ashley E. Brown
McGovern Medical School, University of Texas Health Science Center at Houston, Houston, TX, USA

Lindsey Schmidtberger, Kathleeen Kroger, Richard R. Jahan-Tigh and Sarah S. Pinney
Department of Dermatology, University of Texas McGovern Medical School at Houston, Houston, TX, USA

Joy Tao
Stritch School of Medicine, Loyola University Chicago, Chicago, IL, USA

Courtney Hentz, Michael L. Mysz, Issra Rashed and Bahman Emami
Department of Radiation Oncology, Stritch School of Medicine, Loyola University Chicago, Chicago, IL, USA

David Eilers
Section of Dermatology, Hines Veterans Affairs Hospital, Hines, IL, USA

James Swan and Rebecca Tung
Division of Dermatology, Department of Medicine, Stritch School of Medicine, Loyola University Chicago, Chicago, IL, USA

Lauren Bonomo and Jacob Levitt
Department of Dermatology, Icahn School of Medicine at Mount Sinai, 5 East 98th Street, 5th Floor, New York, NY 10029, USA

Sara Ghoneim
Saba University School of Medicine, the Bottom, Saba, Netherlands

Birgül Özkesici
Clinic of Dermatology, Adıyaman University Training and Research Hospital, Adıyaman, Turkey

Saliha Koç
Clinic of Dermatology, Kepez State Hospital, Antalya, Turkey

Ayşe Akman-Karakaş, Ertan Yılmaz and Soner Uzun
Department of Dermatology and Venereology, Akdeniz University School of Medicine, Antalya, Turkey

İbrahim Cumhur Başsorgun
Department of Pathology, Akdeniz University School of Medicine, Antalya, Turkey

Bonnie Fergie and Andrew Miller
Canberra Hospital, ACT Health, Canberra, ACT, Australia

Nishant Valecha
Woden Dermatology, Phillip, ACT, Australia

Jeffrey S. Dickman and McKay D. Frandsen
Midwestern University, Arizona College of Osteopathic Medicine, 19555 N 59th Ave, Glendale, AZ 85308, USA

Andrew J. Racette
Omni Dermatology, Inc., KCU-GMEC Phoenix Dermatology Residency Program, 4840 E Indian School Rd, Suite 102, Phoenix, AZ 85018, USA

Bayaki Saka, Waguena Gnassingbe, Garba Mahamadou, Sefako Akakpo, Aurel Abilogun-Chokki and Palokinam Pitché
Service de Dermatologie et IST, CHU Sylvanus Olympio, Universite de Lome, Lome, Togo

Julienne Teclessou and Koussake Kombate
Service de Dermatologie et IST, CHU Campus de Lome, Universite de Lome, Lome, Togo

Abas Mouhari-Toure
Service de Dermatologie et IST, CHU de Kara, Universite de Kara, Kara, Togo

Alexander K. C. Leung
Department of Pediatrics, The University of Calgary, Calgary, AB, Canada T2M 0H5
The Alberta Children's Hospital, Calgary, AB, Canada T2M 0H5

Benjamin Barankin
Toronto Dermatology Centre, Toronto, ON, Canada M3H 5Y8

Dustin Taylor
University of Texas McGovern Medical School, Houston, TX, USA

Natalie Kash and Sirunya Silapunt
Department of Dermatology, University of Texas McGovern Medical School, Houston, TX, USA

Amir Hossein Siadat, Anis Bostakian and Masoom Shahbazi
Skin Diseases and Leishmaniasis Research Center, School of Medicine, Isfahan University of Medical Sciences, Isfahan, Iran

Bahareh Abtahi-Naeini
Cancer Research Center, Semnan University of Medical Sciences, Semnan, Iran
Skin Diseases and Leishmaniasis Research Center, Department of Dermatology, Isfahan University of Medical Sciences, Isfahan, Iran

Dimple Chopra, Aastha Sharma and Shivali Aggarwal
Department of Dermatology, Government Medical College, Patiala, Punjab, India

Vishal Chopra and Deepak Goyal
Department of Pulmonary Medicine, Government Medical College, Patiala, Punjab, India

Siddharth Chopra
Government Medical College, Patiala, Punjab, India

Pinky Jha
Section of Hospital Medicine, Division of General Internal Medicine, Medical College of Wisconsin, Milwaukee, WI, USA

Kurtis Swanson, Jeremiah Stromich and Basia M. Michalski
Medical College of Wisconsin, Milwaukee, WI, USA

Edit Olasz
Department of Dermatology, Medical College of Wisconsin, Milwaukee, WI, USA

Pablo Vargas, Fernando Valenzuela, Viera Kaplan and Montserrat Arceu
Department of Dermatology, Faculty of Medicine, University of Chile, Santiago, Chile

Jacob Yumha
Faculty of Medicine, University of Chile, Santiago, Chile

Claudia Morales
Pathology Service, University of Chile Clinical Hospital, Santiago, Chile

Sharon Chi
Internal Medicine Residency Program, Tripler Army Medical Center, 1 Jarrett White Road, Honolulu, HI 96859, USA

Marcia Leung
John A. Burns School of Medicine, University of Hawaii, Honolulu, HI, USA

Mark Carmichael
Hematology-Oncology Service, Tripler Army Medical Center, Honolulu, HI, USA

Michael Royer
Department of Pathology, Walter Reed National Military Medical Center, Bethesda, MD, USA

Sunghun Cho
Dermatology Service, Tripler Army Medical Center, Honolulu, HI, USA

Daria Marley Kemp, Jun Kang and Young C. Kauh
Department of Dermatology and Cutaneous Biology, Thomas Jefferson University, Philadelphia, PA, USA

Anusha G. Govind and Caroline C. Brugger
Department of Infectious Disease, Thomas Jefferson University, Philadelphia, PA, USA

Zabeer Bhatti, Sharon Brangman, Kerry Whiting and Amit Dhamoon
State University of New York Upstate Medical University, 750 E. Adams Street Syracuse, NY 13210, USA

Rameez Bhatti
Avalon University School of Medicine, 122-124 Santa Rosaweg, Curacao, Netherlands

Astrid-Helene Ravn Jørgensen and Yiqiu Yao
Department of Dermato-Venereology and Wound Healing Centre, Bispebjerg Hospital, Copenhagen, Denmark

Simon Francis Thomsen
Department of Dermato-Venereology and Wound Healing Centre, Bispebjerg Hospital, Copenhagen, Denmark
Department of Biomedical Sciences, University of Copenhagen, Copenhagen, Denmark

Mariam S. Al Harbi
Department of Pediatrics, Tawam Hospital, Al-Ain, UAE

Ayman W. El-Hattab
Division of Clinical Genetic and Metabolic Disorders, Tawam Hospital, Al-Ain, UAE

Priscilla R. Powell
Medical City Weatherford, 713 East Anderson St., Weatherford, TX 76086, USA

Juana Irma Garza-Chapa
Medipiel, Centro Dermatologicoy Clinica Laser, Av. Vasconcelos 405Ote., Col. Residencial San Agustin, 66260 Garza Garcia, NL, Mexico

Joseph S. Susa
Cockerell Dermatopathology, University of Texas Southwestern Medical Center, 2110 Research Row, Suite 100, Dallas, TX 75235, USA

Stephen E. Weis
University of North Texas Health Science Center, 855 Montgomery St., Floor 5, Fort Worth, TX 76107, USA

Caspar Weel Krammer
Department of Plastic Surgery, Hospital South West Jutland, Finsensgade 35, 6700 Esbjerg, Denmark

Rami Mossad Ibrahim
Department of Plastic Surgery, Herlev Hospital, Herlev Ringvej 75, 2730 Herlev, Denmark

Kirsten C. Webb, James Swan and Rebecca Tung
Department of Dermatology, Loyola University Chicago, Chicago, IL, USA

Magdalena Harasimowicz and Monica Janeczek
Stritch School of Medicine, Loyola University Chicago, Chicago, IL, USA

Jodi Speiser
Department of Pathology, Loyola University Chicago, Chicago, IL, USA

N. Almaani
Department of Dermatology, Faculty of Medicine, the University of Jordan, Amman, Jordan
Department of Dermatology, Jordan University Hospital, Amman, Jordan

H. Msallam
Department of Dermatology, Jordan University Hospital, Amman, Jordan

A. H. Al-Tarawneh
Department of Dermatology, Jordan University Hospital, Amman, Jordan
Department of Dermatology, Faculty of Medicine, Mutah University, Karak, Jordan

Yoichi Nishii
Division of Plastic Surgery, Uji-Tokushukai Medical Center, Uji 611-0042, Japan

Keisuke Nishimura
Department of Pathology, Uji-Tokushukai Medical Center, Uji 611-0042, Japan

Ali Haydar Eskiocak and Soner Uzun
Department of Dermatology and Venereology, Akdeniz University School of Medicine Hospital, Antalya, Turkey

Cumhur Ebrahim Bassorgun
Department of Pathology, Akdeniz University School of Medicine Hospital, Antalya, Turkey

Sarah Finch
Department of Pathology, Memorial University, St. Johns, NL, Canada

Paul Dancey
Department of Rheumatology, Memorial University, St. Johns, NL, Canada

Ian Landells
Department of Dermatology, Memorial University, St. Johns, NL, Canada

Axel Egal
Department of Radiotherapy, Montfermeil Hospital, France

Basma M'Barek
Department of Radiotherapy, Montfermeil Hospital, France
Department of Radiotherapy, Saint Louis Hospital, AP-HP, Paris, France

Caroline Ram-Wolf and Martine Bagot
Department of Dermatology, Saint Louis Hospital, AP-HP, Paris, France

Laurent Quero and Christophe Hennequin
Department of Radiotherapy, Saint Louis Hospital, AP-HP, Paris, France

Marie-Dominique Vignon-Pennamen
Department of Pathology, Saint Louis Hospital, AP-HP, Paris, France

Yoichi Nishii
Division of Plastic Surgery, Uji-Tokushukai Medical Center, Uji 611-0042, Japan

Sarp Uzun
Hacettepe University School of Medicine, Ankara, Turkey

Patrick O' Emanuel
University of Auckland, Auckland 1010, New Zealand

Sharad P. Paul
Auckland University of Technology, Auckland 1142, New Zealand
School of Medicine, University of Queensland, Brisbane, QLD 4006, Australia
Department of Surgery, University of Auckland, Auckland 1010, New Zealand

Shinsaku Imashuku
Department of Laboratory Medicine, Uji-Tokushukai Medical Center, Uji 6110042, Japan

Miyako Kobayashi
Department of Internal Medicine, Uji-Tokushukai Medical Center, Uji 6110042, Japan

Ana Laura Rosifini Alves Rezende, Fred Bernardes Filho, Natália Aparecida de Paula and Marco Andrey Cipriani Frade
Dermatology Division, Department of Internal Medicine, Ribeirao Preto Medical School, University of Sao Paulo, Ribeirao Preto, Sao Paulo, Brazil

Loan Towersey
AIDS Division, Carlos Tortelly Municipal Hospital, Ministry of Health, Niteroi, Rio de Janeiro, Brazil

Roderick Hay
International Foundation for Dermatology, London, UK

Index